The Ethics of Psychoanalysis

The Seminar of Jacques Lacan

BOOK VII

'Given all that is implied by the phrase, the ethics of psychoanalysis will allow me, far more than anything else, to test the categories that I believe enable me to give you through my teaching the most suitable instruments for understanding what is new both in Freud's work and in the experience of psychoanalysis that derives from it.'

With these words Jacques Lacan begins his famous seminar on ethics, in which he discusses the problem of sublimation, the paradox of *jouissance*, the essence of tragedy (a reading of Sophocles's *Antigone*), and the tragic dimension of analytical experience. Delving into the psychoanalyst's inevitable involvement with ethical questions and the 'attraction of transgression', Lacan clarifies many of his key concepts, as well as his criticisms of certain trends in psychoanalysis. One of the most influential French intellectuals of this century, Lacan is seen here at the height of his powers.

By Jacques Lacan

TELEVISION
THE SEMINAR OF JACQUES LACAN BOOK I
THE SEMINAR OF JACQUES LACAN BOOK II
ECRITS: A SELECTION
FEMININE SEXUALITY
THE FOUR FUNDAMENTAL CONCEPTS
OF PSYCHO-ANALYSIS

THE ETHICS OF
PSYCHOANALYSIS
1959–1960
The Seminar of Jacques Lacan

Edited by Jacques-Alain Miller

BOOK VII

Translated with notes by
Dennis Porter

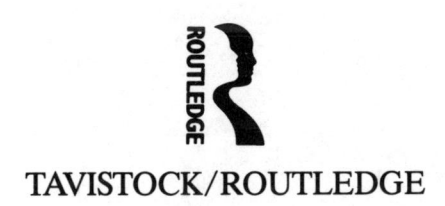

TAVISTOCK/ROUTLEDGE

Originally published in French as *Le Seminaire, Livre VII*
L'ethique de la psychanalyse, 1959–1960
by Les Editions du Seuil, Paris, 1986

First published in English translation in 1992
Published in the US by W.W. Norton & Company, Inc., New York

Published in the UK by Routledge
11 New Fetter Lane, London EC4P 4EE

English translation © W.W. Norton & Company, Inc., 1992

Printed and bound in Great Britain by
Mackays of Chatham PLC, Chatham, Kent

All rights reserved. No part of this book may be reprinted
or reproduced or utilized in any form or by any electronic,
mechanical, or other means, now known or hereafter
invented, including photocopying and recording, or in any
information storage or retrieval system, without permission
in writing from the publishers.

British Library Cataloguing in Publication Data

A catalogue record for this book is available from the British Library.

ISBN 0–415–09054–7 (pbk)

CONTENTS

		page
	Translator's note	vii
I	Outline of the seminar	1

INTRODUCTION TO THE THING

II	Pleasure and reality	19
III	Rereading the *Entwurf*	35
IV	*Das Ding*	43
V	*Das Ding* (II)	57
VI	On the moral law	71

THE PROBLEM OF SUBLIMATION

VII	Drives and lures	87
VIII	The object and the thing	101
IX	On creation *ex nihilo*	115
X	Marginal comments	128
XI	Courtly love as anamorphosis	139
XII	A critique of Bernfeld	155

THE PARADOX OF *JOUISSANCE*

XIII	The death of God	167
XIV	Love of one's neighbor	179
XV	The *jouissance* of transgression	191
XVI	The death drive	205

v

| XVII | The function of the good | 218 |
| XVIII | The function of the beautiful | 231 |

THE ESSENCE OF TRAGEDY
A Commentary on Sophocles's *Antigone*

XIX	The splendor of Antigone	243
XX	The articulations of the play	257
XXI	Antigone between two deaths	270

THE TRAGIC DIMENSION OF ANALYTICAL EXPERIENCE

XXII	The demand for happiness and the promise of analysis	291
XXIII	The moral goals of psychoanalysis	302
XXIV	The paradoxes of ethics *or* Have you acted in conformity with your desire?	311

Acknowledgments	326
Bibliography	327
Index	331

TRANSLATOR'S NOTE

Some of the problems of translating Jacques Lacan's *Seminars* into English have already been pointed out by the translators of *Seminars I* and *II*, John Forester and Sylvana Tomaselli, and there is no point in repeating their helpful comments here. It is, however, important to recall that the *Seminars* now in the process of being translated were delivered from notes to an audience that for the most part had been following the progress of Lacan's thought over many years and was composed to a great extent of psychoanalysts or psychoanalysts in training. These circumstances account in part for his nonacademic mode of exposition and the frequent complexity of the syntax. They also explain the closeness Lacan apparently felt to his audience, the assumptions he was able to make about the knowledge his listeners possessed, the frequent references to previous *Seminars* or to other activities of the *Société Française de Psychanalyse*, and the apparent allusiveness of some of his remarks. The latter in particular seems to derive both from what he felt he could take for granted among those who knew his work well and from a pedagogical style that made great demands on a listener.

Jacques-Alain Miller's French edition of the *Ethique de la Psychanalyse* is without a critical apparatus, like the other Lacan *Seminars* that have so far been published. Miller reproduces Lacan's lectures virtually unmediated, and it seemed proper to model the English edition of the work on the French. As a consequence, footnotes have been kept to a minimum; they are chiefly limited to linguistic difficulties where for one reason or another English is unable to render fully the significance of the French–the most obvious of such cases is Lacan's not infrequent plays on words. However, a bibliography of authors and works cited by Lacan in the course of the *Seminar* is included. I have also followed the French edition in leaving German and Greek words in the original where Lacan did so in the context of analyzing German or Greek texts; in most cases, he gave at the same time a French equivalent or a paraphrase of a concept's meaning. Only in the case of titles have I given the English translation in brackets after the first occurrence.

The task of the translator is, I take it, a critically self-effacing one that insofar as possible avoids the temptation to play editor by reducing ambiguities or by "naturalizing" the strangeness of an original in its passage into the native idiom. Thus, the goals I gave myself were accuracy rather than elegance and a flexibility of tone that matches the different registers of Lacan's expository style. The excitement for those who encounter his *Seminars* in the original French is in the experience of a thought in the making. And it is important to render in the English this liveliness of a distinguished mind at work before an audience, even at the occasional cost of some awkwardnesses. The difficulty was in trying to render in a different linguistic code a captivating spoken word that sometimes meanders, throws out asides, refers backwards or anticipates future problems, moves through passages dense with difficult ideas, narrates an illustrative comic anecdote, draws out the forgotten etymological significance of a word or resorts suddenly to popular speech. The pleasure for the translator is in discovering equivalents for such movements within the very different resources of his own language.

It is for the most part not Lacan's psychoanalytic or philosophical discourse that causes difficulties, but his syntax and, given that the Norton edition of the *Seminars* has as its potential audience the English-speaking world as a whole, his use of familiar language and colloquialisms. As far as the former is concerned, Lacan frequently uses French prepositions and prepositional phrases in startlingly new ways; thus one of the most difficult words to translate turned out to be "de." As for Lacan's colloquialisms, it seemed to me important wherever possible to find equivalents that were not too obviously recognizable as "Americanisms" or as "Britishisms," but have a more general currency. Finally, a few minor errors in the French have been corrected in the translation.

I would like to thank my colleague Edward S. Phinney for help with the Greek and Susan Barrows both for her editorial support and for a careful reading of the manuscript.

DENNIS PORTER
Amherst, Massachusetts, October 1991

I

Outline of the seminar

THE ATTRACTION OF TRANSGRESSION[1]
FROM ARISTOTLE TO FREUD
THE REAL
THE THREE IDEALS

I announced that the title of my seminar this year was *The Ethics of Psychoanalysis*. I do not think that this is a subject whose choice is in any way surprising in itself, although it does leave open for some of you the question of what I might have in mind.

It was certainly not without some hesitation and even trepidation that I decided to tackle it. I, in fact, decided to do so because the subject follows directly from my seminar of last year, if it is true that we can consider that work as completely finished.

In any case, we must move forward. Given all that is implied by the phrase, the ethics of psychoanalysis will allow me, far more than anything else, to test the categories that I believe enable me, through my teaching, to give you the most suitable instruments for understanding what is new both in Freud's work and in the experience of psychoanalysis that derives from it.

New in relation to what? In relation to something that is both very general and very specific. Very general to the extent that the experience of psychoanalysis is highly significant for a certain moment in the history of man, namely, the one we are living in, although this does not imply we are able – far from it – to specify what the collective work we are engaged in means. Very specific, on the other hand, like our daily work, namely, in the way in which we have to respond in experience to what I have taught you to articulate as a demand, a patient's demand, to which our response gives an exact meaning. And in our response itself we must maintain the strictest discipline, so as not to let its deeply unconscious meaning be adulterated by that demand.

---

[1] Lacan's word here, "la faute," is particularly difficult to put into English because of the great range of its potential equivalents – from wrong, error, mistake to blame, misconduct and offense – and because the most obvious choice does not have the moral resonances of the French. "The Attraction of the Fault" not only does not suggest anything, but even manages to sound like pidgin English. And the same is true of "The Universe of the Fault."

In speaking of the ethics of psychoanalysis, I chose a word which to my mind was no accident. I might have said "morality" instead. If I say "ethics," you will soon see why. It is not because I take pleasure in using a term that is less common.

1

Let us begin by noting this – something that, in a word, makes the subject eminently accessible and even tempting. It is my belief that no one who is involved with psychoanalysis has not been drawn to treat the subject of its ethics. I am not the one who created the expression. Moreover, it is impossible not to acknowledge that we are submerged in what are strictly speaking moral problems.

Our experience has led us to explore further than has been attempted before the universe of transgression. That is the expression which, with an extra adjective, my colleague Hesnard uses. He refers to the morbid universe of transgression. And it is doubtless from this morbid point of view that we approach it at its highest point.

In truth, that point of view is impossible to dissociate from the universe of transgression as such. And the link between transgression and morbidity has not failed in our time to mark with its seal all thought about morals. It is even strange sometimes – something I have drawn your attention to before in my asides – to see in religious circles a certain vertigo seize those who are engaged in thinking about moral questions when they come face to face with what our experience has to offer. It is remarkable to see how they, as it were, give in to the temptation of an excessive and even comic optimism, and start to think that a decline of morbidity might lead transgression to vanish.

In fact, what we are dealing with is nothing less than the attraction of transgression.

And what is this transgression? It is certainly not the same as the one the patient commits with the expectation of being punished or punishing himself. When we speak of the need for punishment, we are certainly referring to a transgression which is on the path of this need and which is sought out to obtain this punishment. But that way we are only carried a little further toward some yet more obscure transgression which calls for punishment.

Is it the transgression that Freud's work points to from the beginning, the murder of the father, the great myth that he places at the origin of the development of civilization? Or is it that even more obscure and original transgression for which he finds a name at the end of his work, in a word, the death instinct, to the extent that man finds himself anchored deep within to its formidable dialectic?

It is between these two terms that one finds in Freud a body of thought, a development whose precise significance it will be our task to determine. But it is not, in truth, in the sphere either of practice or of theory that is to be found all that which makes me emphasize the importance of the ethical dimension in my experience and my teaching of Freud. In effect, as has been quite properly pointed out, not everything in ethics is simply related to the sense of obligation.

Moral experience as such, that is to say, the reference to sanctions, puts man in a certain relation to his own action that concerns not only an articulated law but also a direction, a trajectory, in a word, a good that he appeals to, thereby engendering an ideal of conduct. All that, too, properly speaking constitutes the dimension of ethics and is situated beyond the notion of a command, beyond what offers itself with a sense of obligation. That is why I believe it necessary to relate the dimension of our experience to the contribution of those who have attempted in our time to advance moral thought – I am, in fact, alluding to Fritz Rauh, whom we will be concerned with as one of our reference points in this exercise.

But I am certainly not one of those who gladly sets the sense of obligation aside. If there is, in fact, something that psychoanalysis has drawn attention to, it is, beyond the sense of obligation properly speaking, the importance, I would even say the omnipresence, of a sense of guilt. Certain internal tendencies of ethical thought attempt to evade what it must be said is this disagreeable aspect of moral experience. If I am certainly not one of those who attempt to soften, blunt, or attenuate the sense of guilt, it is because in my daily experience I am too insistently brought back to it and reminded of it.

It nevertheless remains true that analysis is the experience which has restored to favor in the strongest possible way the productive function of desire as such. This is so evidently the case that one can, in short, say that the genesis of the moral dimension in Freud's theoretical elaboration is located nowhere else than in desire itself. It is from the energy of desire that that agency is detached which at the end of its development will take the form of the censor.

Thus something is enclosed in a circle that was imposed on us, deduced from what is most characteristic in our experience.

A certain philosophy – it immediately preceded the one which is the nearest relative to the Freudian enterprise, the one which was transmitted to us in the nineteenth century – a certain eighteenth-century philosophy assumed as its task what might be called the naturalist liberation of desire. One might characterize this thought, this particularly practical thought, as that of the man of pleasure. Now the naturalist liberation of desire has failed. The more the theory, the more the work of social criticism, the more the sieve of that experience, which tended to limit obligation to certain precise functions in the social order, have raised in us the hope of relativizing the imperative, the contrary, or, in a word, conflictual character of moral experience, the more we have, in fact, witnessed a growth in the incidence of genuine pathologies. The naturalist liberation of desire has failed historically. We do not find ourselves in the presence of a man less weighed down with laws and duties than before the great critical experience of so-called libertine thought.

If we find ourselves led to consider even in retrospect the experience of that man of pleasure – through reflection on what psychoanalysis has contributed to the knowledge and the circumstances of perverse experience – we will soon see that in truth everything in this moral theory was to destine it to failure.

In effect, although the experience of the man of pleasure presents itself with an ideal of naturalist liberation, one has only to read the major authors – I mean those who in expressing themselves on the subject have adopted the boldest approaches to libertinage, and even to eroticism itself – to realize that this experience contains a note of defiance, a kind of trial by ordeal in relation to that which remains the terminal point of this argument, an undoubtedly diminished but nevertheless fixed term. And that is nothing less than the divine term.

As the creator of nature, God is summoned to account for the extreme anomalies whose existence the Marquis de Sade, Mirabeau, and Diderot, among others, have drawn our attention to. This challenge, this summoning, this trial by ordeal ought not to allow any other way out than the one that was, in effect, realized historically. He who submits himself to the ordeal finds at the end its premises, namely, the Other to whom this ordeal is addressed, in the last analysis its Judge. That is precisely what gives its special tone to this literature, which presents us with the dimension of the erotic in a way that has never been achieved since, never equaled. In the course of our investigation, we definitely must submit to our judgment that which in analysis has retained an affinity with, a relationship to, and a common root with, such an experience.

Here we are touching on a prespective that has been little explored in analysis. It seems that from the moment of those first soundings, from the sudden flash of light that the Freudian experience cast on the paradoxical origins of desire, on the polymorphously perverse character of its infantile forms, a general tendency has led psychoanalysts to reduce the paradoxical origins in order to show their convergence in a harmonious conclusion. This movement has on the whole characterized the progress of analytical thought to the point where it is worth asking if this theoretical progress was not leading in the end to an even more all-embracing moralism than any that has previously existed. Psychoanalysis would seem to have as its sole goal the calming of guilt – although we know well through our practical experience the difficulties and obstacles, indeed the reactions, that such an approach entails. This approach involves the taming of perverse *jouissance,* which is assumed to emerge from the demonstration of its universality, on the one hand, and its function, on the other.

No doubt the term "component," used for designating the perverse drive, is in this situation given its full weight. Last year we explored the expression "component drive"; in a whole section of our remarks we were concerned with the insights that analysis affords concerning the function of desire and with the deep finality of that really remarkable diversity, which explains the value of the catalogue of human instincts that analysis has allowed us to draw up.

Perhaps the question will only be seen in sharp relief, when one compares the position that our point of view of the term desire has led us to, with that which is, for example, articulated in the work of Aristotle in connection with ethics. I will give him an important place in my discussion, including particularly that work which lays out Aristotelian ethics in its most elaborate form, the *Nicomachean Ethics*. There are two points in Aristotle's work in which he shows how a whole register of desire is literally situated by him outside of the field of morality.

Where a certain category of desires is involved, there is, in effect, no ethical problem for Aristotle. Yet these very desires are nothing less than those notions that are situated in the forefront of our experience. A whole large field of what constitutes for us the sphere of sexual desires is simply classed by Aristotle in the realm of monstrous anomalies – he uses the term "bestiality" with reference to them. What occurs at this level has nothing to do with moral evaluation. The ethical questions that Aristotle raises are located altogether elsewhere – I will give you an idea later of their thrust and essence. That is a point of special importance.

On the other hand, if one believes that the whole of Aristotle's morality has lost none of its relevance for moral theory, then one can measure from that fact how subversive our experience is, since it serves to render his theory surprising, primitive, paradoxical and, in truth, incomprehensible.

But all that is just a stop on our journey. What I really want to do this morning is to give you an outline of this seminar.

2

We are faced with the question of what analysis allows us to formulate concerning the origin of morality.

Is its contribution limited to the elaboration of a mythology that is more credible and more secular than that which claims to be revealed? I have in mind the reconstructed mythology of *Totem and Taboo*, which starts out from the experience of the original murder of the father, from the circumstances that give rise to it and its consequences. From this point of view, it is the transformation of the energy of desire which makes possible the idea of the genesis of its repression. As a result, the transgression is not in this instance just something which is imposed on us in a formal way; it is instead something worthy of our praise, *felix culpa*, since it is at the origin of a higher complexity, something to which the realm of civilization owes its development.

In short, is everything limited to the genesis of the superego whose description is formulated, perfected, deepened, and made more complex as Freud's work progresses? We will see that this genesis of the superego is not simply a psychogenesis and a sociogenesis. Indeed, it is impossible to articulate it by limiting oneself merely to the register of collective needs. Something is imposed there whose jurisdiction is to be distinguished from pure and simple social necessity – it is properly speaking something whose unique scope I am trying to make you appreciate here in terms of the relation to the signifier and to the law of discourse. We must maintain the autonomy of this term if we want to be able to locate our experience precisely or simply correctly.

Here no doubt the distinction between culture and society contains something that might appear new or even divergent in comparison with what is found in a certain kind of teaching of the analytical experience. I hope, in fact, to point out to you the references to such a distinction and the scope they occupy in Freud himself, a distinction whose authority I am far from alone in promoting or emphasizing the need for.

And in order to draw your attention immediately to the work in which we will take up the problem, I refer you to *Civilization and Its Discontents*, published in 1922 and written by Freud after the working out of his second topic, that is to say after he had placed in the foreground the highly problematic notion of the death instinct. You will find expressed there in striking phrases the idea that what, in brief, happens in the progress of civilization, those discontents that are to be explored, is situated, as far as man is concerned, far above him – the man involved here being the one who finds himself at that turning point in history where Freud himself and his work are situated. We will come back to the significance of Freud's formula and I will draw your attention to its significance in the text. But I believe it to be important enough for me to point it out to you right away, and already sufficiently illuminated in my teaching, where I show the originality of the Freudian conversion in the relation of man to the logos.

This *Civilization and Its Discontents* that I invite you to get to know or to reread in the context of Freud's work is not just a set of notes. It is not the kind of thing one grants a practitioner or a scientist somewhat indulgently, as his way of making an excursion into philosophical inquiry without our giving it all the technical importance one would accord to such a thought coming from someone who considers himself to belong to the category of philosopher. Such a view of this work of Freud's is widespread among psychoanalysts and is definitely to be rejected. *Civilization and Its Discontents* is an indispensable work, unsurpassed for an understanding of Freud's thought and the summation of his experience. It illuminates, emphasizes, dissipates the ambiguities of wholly distinct points of the analytical experience and of what our view of man should be – given that it is with man, with an immemorial human demand, that we have to deal on a daily basis in our experience.

As I have already said, moral experience is not limited to that acceptance of necessity, to that form in which such experience presents itself in every individual case. Moral experience is not simply linked to that slow recognition of the function that was defined and made autonomous by Freud under the term of superego, nor to that exploration of its paradoxes, to what I have called the obscene and ferocious figure in which the moral agency appears when we seek it at its root.

The moral experience involved in psychoanalysis is the one that is summed up in the original imperative proposed in what might be called the Freudian ascetic experience, namely, that *Wo es war, soll Ich werden* with which Freud concludes the second part of his *Vorlesungen (Introductory Lectures)* on psychoanalysis. The root of this is given in an experience that deserves the term "moral experience," and is found at the very beginning of the entry of the patient into analysis.

That "I" which is supposed to come to be where "it" was, and which analysis has taught us to evaluate, is nothing more than that whose root we already found in the "I" which asks itself what it wants. It is not only questioned, but as it progresses in its experience, it asks itself that question and asks it precisely in the place where strange, paradoxical, and cruel commands are suggested to it by its morbid experience.

Will it or will it not submit itself to the duty that it feels within like a stranger, beyond, at another level? Should it or should it not submit itself to the half-unconscious, paradoxical, and morbid command of the superego, whose jurisdiction is moreover revealed increasingly as the analytical exploration goes forward and the patient sees that he is committed to its path?

If I may put it thus, isn't its true duty to oppose that command? One finds here something which belongs to the givens of our experience as well as to the givens of preanalysis. It is enough to see how the experience of an obsessional is structured at the beginning to know that the enigma concerning the term "duty" as such is always already formulated even before he formulates the demand for help, which is what he goes into analysis for.

In truth, although the response to the problem that we are proposing here is obviously illustrated in the conflict of an obsessional, it nevertheless has a universal validity; that is why there are different ethics and there is ethical thought. It is not simply the philsosopher's thought alone that seeks to justify duty, that duty on which we have shed a variety of light – genetical and originary, for example. The justification of that which presents itself with an immediate feeling of obligation, the justification of duty as such – not simply in one or other of its commands, but in the form imposed – is at the heart of an inquiry that is universal.

Are we analysts simply something that welcomes the suppliant then, something that gives him a place of refuge? Are we simply, but it is already a lot, something that must respond to a demand, to the demand not to suffer, at least without understanding why? – in the hope that through understanding the subject will be freed not only from his ignorance, but also from suffering itself.

Isn't it obvious that analytical ideals are normally to be found here? They are certainly not lacking. They grow in abundance. The evaluation, location, situation, and organization of values, as they say in a certain register of moral thought, that we propose to our patients, and around which we organize the assessments of their progress and the transformation of their way into a path, is supposed to be part of our work. For the moment I will mention three of these ideals.

The first is the ideal of human love.

Do I need to emphasize the role that we attribute to a certain idea of "love fulfilled"? That is an expression you must have learned to recognize and not only here, since, in truth, there is hardly an analyst who writes who has not drawn attention to it. And you know that I have often taken aim at the approximative and vague character, so tainted with an optimistic moralism, which marks the original articulations taking the form of the genitalization of desire. That is the ideal of genital love – a love that is supposed to be itself alone the model of a satisfying object relation: doctor-love, I would say if I wanted to emphasize in a comical way the tone of this ideology; love as hygiene, I would say, to suggest what analytical ambition seems to be limited to here.

It is a problem that I will not expand on indefinitely, since I have not stopped making you think about it since this seminar began. But so as to give it a more marked emphasis, I will point out that analytical thought seems to shirk its task when faced with the convergent character of our experience. This character is certainly not deniable, but the analyst seems to find in it a limit beyond which it is difficult for him to go. To say that the problems of moral experience are entirely resolved as far as monogamous union is concerned would be a formulation that is imprudent, excessive, and inadequate.

Analysis has brought a very important change of perspective on love by placing it at the center of ethical experience; it has also brought an original note, which was certainly different from the way in which love had previously been viewed by the *moralistes* and the philosophers in the economy of interhuman relations. Why then has analysis not gone further in the direction of the investigation of what should properly be called an erotics? That is something that deserves reflection.

In this connection the topic I have placed on the agenda of our forthcoming conference, namely, feminine sexuality, is one of the clearest of signs in the development of analysis of the lack I am referring to with regard to such an investigation. It is hardly necessary to recall what Jones learned from a source that to my mind is not especially qualified, but which, believe it or not, is nevertheless supposed at the very least to have transmitted in his exact words what it heard from Freud's own mouth. Jones tells us that this person told him confidentially that one day Freud said something like "After some thirty years of experience and thought, there is still one question to which I am still unable to find an answer; it is 'Was will das Weib?' " What does woman want? Or more precisely, "What does she desire?" The term "will" in this expression may have that meaning in German.

Have we gone much further on that subject? It will not be a waste of time if I show you the kind of avoidance that the progress of research in analysis has practiced in answering a question that cannot be said to have been invented by it. Let us just say that analysis, and the thought of Freud in particular, is connected to a time that articulated this question with a special emphasis. The Ibsenian context of the end of the nineteenth century in which Freud's thought matured cannot be overlooked here. And it is, in brief, very strange that analytical experience has if anything stifled, silenced, and evaded those areas of the problem of sexuality which relate to the point of view of feminine demand.

The second ideal, which is equally as remarkable in analytical experience, is what I shall call the ideal of authenticity.

I do not think I need to emphasize it particularly. It will not have escaped you that if psychoanalysis is a technique of unmasking, it presupposes such a point of view. But, in fact, it goes further than that.

It is not simply as a path, stage, or measure of progress that authenticity suggests itself to us; it is also quite simply as a certain norm for the finished product, as something desirable and, therefore, as a value. It is an ideal, but one on which we are led to impose clinical norms that are very precise. I will illustrate the point in the very subtle observations of Helene Deutsch concerning a type of character and of personality that one cannot describe as maladjusted or as failing to meet any of the norms demanded by social relations, but whose whole attitude and behavior are visible in the recognition – of whom? – of the other, of others, as if marked by that note that she calls in English "as if," and which in German is "als ob." I am touching here on the point that a certain register – which is not defined and is not simple and cannot be situated other than from a moral perspective – is present, controlling, insisted on in all our experience, and that it is necessary to calculate to what extent we are adequate to it.

That something harmonious, that full presence whose lack we as clinicians can so precisely gauge – doesn't our technique stop half-way toward what is required to achieve it, the technique that I have christened "unmasking"? Wouldn't it be interesting to wonder about the significance of our absence from the field of what might be called a science of virtues, a practical reason, the sphere of common sense? For in truth one cannot say that we ever intervene in the field of any virtue. We clear ways and paths, and we hope that what is called virtue will take root there.

Similarly, we have recently forged a third ideal, which I am not sure belongs to the original space of analytical experience, the ideal of non-dependence or, more precisely, of a kind of prophylaxis of dependence.

Isn't there a limit there, too, a fine boundary, which separates what we indicate to an adult subject as desirable in this register and the means we accord ourselves in our interventions so that he achieves it?

It is enough to remember the fundamental, constitutive reservations of the Freudian position concerning education in the broad sense. There is no doubt that all of us, and child analysts in particular, are led to encroach on this domain, to practice in the space of what I have called elsewhere an orthopedics in its etymological sense. But it is nevertheless striking that both in the means we employ and in the theoretical competence we insist on, the ethics of analysis – for there is one – involves effacement, setting aside, withdrawal, indeed, the absence of a dimension that one only has to mention in order to realize how much separates us from all ethical thought that preceded us. I mean the dimension of habits, good and bad habits.

It is something we refer to very little because psychoanalytic thought defines itself in very different terms, in terms of traumas and their persistence. We have obviously learned to decompose a given trauma, impression, or mark, but the very essence of the unconscious is defined in a different register from the one which Aristotle emphasizes in the *Ethics* in a play on words, ἔθος / ἦθος.[2]

There are extremely subtle distinctions that may be centered on the notion of character. Ethics for Aristotle is a science of character: the building of character, the dynamics of habits and, even more, action with relation to habits, training, education. You must take a look at his exemplary work, if only to understand the difference between our modes of thought and those of one of the most eminent forms of ethical thought.

---

[2] Both ἦθος and ἔθος derive from a Greek verb meaning "to repeat." Their meanings came to be differentiated insofar as ἦθος is active and refers to the capacity of creatures to form habits, whereas ἔθος connotes a condition in a passive sense.

3

So as to emphasize what today's premises are leading us toward, I will simply note that although the topics on which I have attempted to open up different perspectives are varied, I will try next time to start from a radical position. In order to point out the originality of the Freudian position in ethical matters, I must underline a slippage or a change of attitude relative to the question of morality as such.

In Aristotle the problem is that of a good, of a Sovereign Good. We will have to consider why he emphasized the problem of pleasure, its function in the mental economy of ethics from the beginning. It is something that we cannot avoid, not least because it is the reference point of the Freudian theory concerning the two systems φ and ψ, the two psychical agencies that he called the primary and secondary processes.

Is the same pleasure function at work in both of these articulations? It is almost impossible to isolate this difference if we do not realize what took place in the interval. Even if it is not my role and if the place I occupy here doesn't seem to make it obligatory, I will not, in fact, be able to avoid a certain inquiry into historical progress.

It is at this point that I must refer to those guiding terms, those terms of reference which I use, namely, the symbolic, the imaginary, and the real.

More than once at the time when I was discussing the symbolic and the imaginary and their reciprocal interaction, some of you wondered what after all was "the real." Well, as odd as it may seem to that superficial opinion which assumes any inquiry into ethics must concern the field of the ideal, if not of the unreal, I, on the contrary, will proceed instead from the other direction by going more deeply into the notion of the real. Insofar as Freud's position constitutes progress here, the question of ethics is to be articulated from the point of view of the location of man in relation to the real. To appreciate this, one has to look at what occurred in the interval between Aristotle and Freud.

At the beginning of the nineteenth century, there was the utilitarian conversion or reversion. We can define this moment – one that was no doubt fully conditioned historically – in terms of a radical decline of the function of the master, a function that obviously governs all of Aristotle's thought and determines its persistence over the centuries. It is in Hegel that we find expressed an extreme devalorization of the position of the master, since Hegel turns him into the great dupe, the magnificent cuckold of historical development, given that the virtue of progress passes by way of the vanquished, which is to say, of the slave, and his work. Originally, when he existed in his plenitude in Aristotle's time, the master was something very different from the Hegelian fiction, which is nothing more than his obverse, his negation, the sign of his disappearance. It is shortly before that terminal moment that in the wake of a certain revolution affecting interhuman relations, so-called utilitarian thought arose, and it is far from being made up of the pure and simple platitudes one imagines.

It is not just a matter of a thought that asks which goods are available on the market to be distributed and the best way to effect the distribution. One finds there an investigation of something of which Mr. Jakobson, who is here today, first found the key, the little latch, in a hint he gave me concerning the interest of a work of Jeremy Bentham's that is ordinarily neglected in the summary of his contribution traditionally given.

This personage is far from meriting the discredit, indeed the ridicule, which a certain critical philosophy might formulate concerning his role in the history of the development of ethics. We will see that it is in relation to a critical philosophy or, more properly, a linguistic one that his thought is developed. It is impossible to measure so well anywhere else the emphasis given in the course of this revolution to the term real, which in his thought is placed in opposition to the English term "fictitious."[3]

"Fictitious" does not mean illusory or deceptive as such. It is far from being translatable into French by "fictif," although this is something that the man who was the key to his success on the continent, Etienne Dumont, did not fail to do – he was also responsible for popularizing Bentham's thought. "Fictitious" means "fictif" but, as I have already explained to you, in the sense that every truth has the structure of fiction.

Bentham's effort is located in the dialectic of the relationship of language to the real so as to situate the good – pleasure in this case, which, as we will see, he articulates in a manner that is very different from Aristotle – on the side of the real. And it is within this opposition between fiction and reality that is to be found the rocking motion of Freudian experience.

Once the separation between the fictitious and the real has been effected, things are no longer situated where one might expect. In Freud the characteristic of pleasure, as that dimension which binds man, is to be found on the side of the fictitious. The fictitious is not, in effect, in its essence that which deceives, but is precisely what I call the symbolic.

That the unconscious is structured as a function of the symbolic, that it is the return of a sign that the pleasure principle makes man seek out, that the pleasurable element in that which directs man in his behavior without his knowledge (namely, that which gives him pleasure, because it is a form of euphony), that that which one seeks and finds again is the trace rather than the trail – one has to appreciate the great importance of all of this in Freud's

---

[3] In English in the original.

thought, if one is to understand the function of reality.

Certainly Freud leaves no doubt, any more than Aristotle, that what man is seeking, his goal, is happiness. It's odd that in almost all languages happiness offers itself in terms of a meeting – $\tau \nu \chi \eta$. Except in English and even there it's very close. A kind of favorable divinity is involved. *Bonheur* in French suggests to us *augurum*, a good sign and a fortunate encounter. *Glück* is the same as *gelück*. "Happiness" is after all "happen"[4]; it, too, is an encounter, even if one does not feel the need to add the prefix, which strictly speaking indicates the happy character of the thing.

It is nevertheless not clear that all these terms are synonyms – I hardly need to remind you of the story of the individual who emigrated from Germany to America and who was asked, "Are you happy?" "Oh, yes, I am very happy," he answered, "I am really very, very happy, *aber nicht glücklich!*"

It does not escape Freud's attention that happiness as far as we are concerned is what must be offered as the goal of our striving, however ethical it might be. But what stands out clearly – in spite of the fact that it is not given sufficient importance on the grounds that we cease to listen to a man as soon as he steps outside his sphere of expertise – is that I prefer to read in *Civilization and Its Discontents* the idea Freud expresses there concerning happiness, namely, that absolutely nothing is prepared for it, either in the macrocosm or the microcosm.

That is the point which is completely new. Aristotle's thought on the subject of pleasure embodies the idea that pleasure has something irrefutable about it, and that it is situated at the guiding pole of human fulfillment, insofar as if there is something divine in man, it is in his bond to nature.

You should consider how far that notion of nature is different from ours, since it involves the exclusion of all bestial desires from what is properly speaking human fulfillment. Since Aristotle's time we have experienced a complete reversal of point of view. As far as Freud is concerned, everything that moves toward reality requires a certain tempering, a lowering of tone, of what is properly speaking the energy of pleasure.

That has a huge importance, although it may seem to you as men of our time rather banal. I have even heard it said that Lacan doesn't say much more than "The king is naked." Perhaps after all I was the one referred to, but let us assume the best, namely, that it had to do with my teaching. Of course, I do teach in a somewhat more humorous way than my critic thinks – I don't under the circumstances have to reflect on his hidden intentions. If I do say "The king is naked," it is not in the same way as the child who is supposed to have exposed the universal illusion, but more in the manner of Alphonse Allais, who gathered a crowd around him by announcing in a sono-

---

[4] In English in the original.

rous voice, "How shocking! Look at that woman! Beneath her dress she's stark naked!" Yet in truth I don't even say that.

If the king is, in fact, naked, it is only insofar as he is so beneath a certain number of clothes – no doubt fictitious but nevertheless essential to his nudity. And in connection with these clothes, as another good story of Alphonse Allais demonstrates, his very nakedness might never be naked enough. After all, a king can be skinned alive as easily as a female dancer.

In truth, the point of view of this absolutely closed character reminds us of the way in which the fictions of desire are organized. It is in this respect that the formulas I gave you last year on the fantasm are significant and that the notion of desire as desire of the Other assumes its full weight.

I will end today with a note concerning the *Traumdeutung (The Interpretation of Dreams)* taken from the *Introduction to Psychoanalysis*. A second factor that guides us, writes Freud, one that is much more important and is completely overlooked by the layman, is the following. It is certainly true that the satisfaction of a wish does give pleasure but, as is well known, the dreamer – I don't think I am going too far when I find here a Lacanian emphasis in a certain way of posing the problem – does not have a simple and unambiguous relationship to his wish. He rejects it, he censures it, he doesn't want it. Here we encounter the essential dimension of desire – it is always desire in the second degree, desire of desire.

In truth, we can expect Freudian analysis to create a little order in that sphere to which critical thought has turned in recent years, namely, the famous, indeed over-famous, theory of values – the very one that allows one of its proponents to say that the value of a thing is its desirability. Pay attention now – the point is to know if it is worthy of being desired, if it is desirable for one to desire it. The result is a kind of catalogue that in many ways might be compared to a second-hand clothes store in which one finds piled up the different judgments that down through the ages and up to our time have dominated human aspirations in their diversity and even their chaos.

The structure embodied in the imaginary relation as such, by reason of the fact that narcissistic man enters as a double into the dialectic of fiction, will perhaps find its explanation at the end of the inquiry we are conducting this year into the ethics of psychoanalysis. In the end you will see emerge the question posed by the fundamental character of masochism in the economy of the instincts.

No doubt something should remain open relative to the place we currently occupy in the development of erotics and to the treatment to be given, not simply to one individual or other, but to civilization and its discontents. Perhaps we should give up the hope of any genuine innovation in the field of ethics – and to a certain extent one might say that a sign of this is to be found in the fact that, in spite of all our theoretical progress, we haven't even been able to create a single new perversion. But it would be a definite sign that we have really arrived at the heart of the problem of existing perversions, if we managed to deepen our understanding of the economic role of masochism.

Since it is useful to give oneself a goal that is attainable, that will, I hope, in the end be the point with which we will conclude this year.

November 18, 1959

INTRODUCTION TO THE THING

II

Pleasure and reality

THE MORAL AGENCY ACTUALIZES THE REAL
INERTIA AND RECTIFICATION
REALITY IS PRECARIOUS
OPPOSITION AND INTERSECTION OF THE PRINCIPLES

Honey is what I am trying to bring you, the honey of my reflections on something that, my goodness, I have been doing for a number of years and which is beginning to add up, but which, as time goes by, ends up not being that much out of proportion with the time you devote to it yourselves.

If the communication effect here sometimes presents difficulties, reflect on the experience of honey. Honey is either very hard or very fluid. If it's hard, it is difficult to cut, since there are no natural breaks. If it's very liquid, it is suddenly all over the place – I assume that you are all familiar with the experience of eating honey in bed at breakfast time.

Hence the problem of pots. The honey pot is reminiscent of the mustard pot that I have already dealt with. The two have exactly the same meaning now that we no longer imagine that the hexagons in which we tend to store our harvest have a natural relationship to the structure of the world. Consequently, the question we are raising is in the end always the same, i.e., what is the significance of the word?

This year we are more specifically concerned with realizing how the ethical question of our practice is intimately related to one that we have been in a position to glimpse for some time, namely, that the deep dissatisfaction we find in every psychology – including the one we have founded thanks to psychoanalysis – derives from the fact that it is nothing more than a mask, and sometimes even an alibi, of the effort to focus on the problem of our own action – something that is the essence and very foundation of all ethical reflection. In other words, we need to know if we have managed to do anything more than take a small step outside ethics and if, like the other psychologies, our own is simply another development of ethical reflection, of the search for a guide or a way, that in the last analysis may be formulated as follows: "Given our condition as men, what must we do in order to act in the right way?"

This reminder seems to me difficult to disagree with, when every day of our lives our action suggests to us that we are not far removed from that. Of course, things present themselves differently to us. Our way of introducing this action, of presenting and justifying it, is different. Its beginning is characterized by features of demand, appeal and urgency, whose specialized meaning places us closer to earth as far as the idea of the articulation of an ethics is concerned. But that does not change the fact that we may in the end, or at any point whatsoever, discover such an articulation once again in its completeness – the kind of articulation that has always given both meaning and arguments to those who have reflected on morals and have tried to elaborate their different ethics.

1

Last time I sketched an outline of what I wish to cover this year. It extends from the recognition of the omnipresence of the moral imperative, of its infiltration into all our experience, to the other pole, that is to say, the pleasure in a second degree we may paradoxically find there, namely, moral masochism.

In passing, I pointed out the unexpected and original approach I intend to develop with reference to those fundamental categories of the symbolic, the imaginary, and the real, that I use to orient you in your experience. My thesis, as I already indicated – and don't be surprised if it first appears confused, since it is the development of my argument that will give it weight – my thesis is that the moral law, the moral command, the presence of the moral agency in our activity, insofar as it is structured by the symbolic, is that through which the real is actualized – the real as such, the weight of the real.

A thesis that may appear to be both a trivial truth and a paradox. My thesis involves the idea that the moral law affirms itself in opposition to pleasure, and we can sense that to speak of the real in connection with the moral law seems to put into question the value of what we normally include in the notion of the ideal. Thus for the moment I will not attempt to polish further the blade of my argument, since what will likely constitute the thrust of my purpose has precisely to do with the meaning to be given to the term real – within that system of categories that I profess as a function of our practice as analysts.

That meaning isn't immediately accessible, although those among you who have wondered about the final significance I might give the term will nevertheless have already noticed that its meaning must have some relationship to that movement which traverses the whole of Freud's thought. It is a movement which makes him start with a first opposition between reality principle and pleasure principle in order, after a series of vacillations, oscillations and imperceptible changes in his references, to conclude at the end of the theoretic formulations by positing something beyond the pleasure principle that might well leave us wondering how it relates to the first opposition. Beyond the pleasure principle we encounter that opaque surface which to some has seemed so obscure that it is the antimony of all thought – not just biological but scientific in general – the surface that is known as the death instinct.

What is the death instinct? What is this law beyond all law, that can only be posited as a final structure, as a vanishing point of any reality that might be attained? In the coupling of pleasure principle and reality principle, the reality principle might seem to be a prolongation or an application of the pleasure principle. But, on the other hand, this dependent and limited position seems to cause something to emerge, something which controls in the broadest of senses the whole of our relationship to the world. It is this unveiling, this rediscovery, that *Beyond the Pleasure Principle* is about. And in this process, this progress, we see before our eyes the problematic character of that which Freud posits under the term reality.

Is it a question of daily reality, of immediate, social reality? Of conformity to established categories or accepted practices? Of the reality discovered by science or of the one which is yet to be discovered? Is it psychic reality?

It is on the road to the investigation of this reality that we find ourselves as analysts, and it leads us a long way from something that can be expressed under the category of wholeness. It leads us into a special area, that of psychic reality, which presents itself to us with the problematic character of a previously unequaled order.

I will, therefore, begin by attempting to explore the function that the term reality played in the thought of the inventor of psychoanalysis and, at the same time, in our own thought, the thought of those of us who have followed in his path. On the other hand, I will straight away point out to those who might be inclined to forget it, or who might think that I am following in this direction only by referring to the moral imperative in our experience – I will point out that moral action poses problems for us precisely to the extent that if analysis prepares us for it, it also in the end leaves us standing at the door.

Moral action is, in effect, grafted on to the real. It introduces something new into the real and thereby opens a path in which the point of our presence is legitimized. How is it that psychoanalysis prepares us for such action, if it is indeed true that this is the case? How is it that psychoanalysis leaves us ready, so to speak, to get down to work? And why does it lead us in that way? Why, too, does it stop at the threshold? That's where one finds the other pole on which I will focus what I hope to formulate here – it being understood that what I pointed to last time constitutes the limits of the things I have to say – and the extent to which we claim to be able to formulate an ethics. I will say right off that the ethical limits of psychoanalysis coincide with the limits of its practice. Its practice is only a preliminary to moral action as such – the so-called action being the one through which we enter the real.

Among all those who have undertaken the analysis of an ethics before me, Aristotle is to be classed among the most exemplary and certainly the most valid. Reading him is an exciting activity and I cannot recommend too highly that by way of an exercise you find out for yourselves – you will not be bored for a moment. Read the *Nicomachaen Ethics*, which of all his treatises scholars seem to attribute to him with the least hesitation and which is certainly the most readable. There are no doubt a number of difficulties to be found at the level of the text, in its digressions and in the order of his arguments. But skip over the passages that seem too complicated or acquire an edition with good notes that refers you to what it is sometimes essential to know about his logic in order to understand the problems that he raises. Above all, don't overburden yourself by trying to grasp everything paragraph by paragraph. Try instead to read him from beginning to end and you will certainly be rewarded.

One thing at least will emerge, something that to some extent the work has in common with all the other ethics – it tends to refer to an order. This order presents itself first of all as a science, an ἐπιστήμη, the science of what has to be done, the uncontested order which defines the norm of a certain character, ἔθος. Thus the problem is raised of the way in which that order may be established in a subject. How can a form of adequation be achieved in a subject so that he will enter that order and submit himself to it?

The establishment of an ἦθος is posited as differentiating a living being from an inanimate, inert being. As Aristotle points out, no matter how often you throw a stone in the air, it will never acquire the habit of its trajectory; man, on the other hand, acquires habits – that's what is meant by ἦθος. And this ἦθος has to be made to conform to the ἤθος, that is to an order that from the point of view of Aristotle's logic has to be brought together in a Sovereign Good, a point of insertion, attachment or convergence, in which a particular order is unified with a more universal knowledge, in which ethics becomes politics, and beyond that with an imitation of the cosmic order. The notions of macrocosm and microcosm are presupposed from the beginning in Aristotle's thought.

It is then a question of having a subject conform to something which in the real is not contested as presupposing the paths of that order. What is the problem constantly taken up and posed within Aristotelian ethics? Let us start with him who possesses this science. Of course, the one whom Aristotle addresses, that is the pupil or disciple, by the very fact that he listens is supposed to participate in this scientific discourse. The discourse in question, the ὀρθὸς λόγος, the right discourse, the appropriate discourse, is therefore already introduced by the very fact that the ethical question is posed. In that way the problem is clearly returned to the point where Socrates had left it with an excessive optimism that did not fail to strike his immediate successors – if the rule of action is in ὀρθὸς λόγος, if there can be no good action except in conformity with the latter, how is it possible that what Aristotle calls intemperance can survive? How is it possible that a subject's impulses draw him elsewhere? How is that to be explained?

However superficial this demand for an explanation may seem to us, since we believe we know so much more about the matter, it nevertheless constitutes the greater part of the substance of Aristotle's thought in the *Ethics*. I will come back to this later in connection with Freud's reflections on the same topic.

For Aristotle the problem is delimited by the conditions imposed by a certain human ideal that I already briefly referred to in passing as that of the master. It is a question for him of elucidating the relationship that may exist between ἀκολασία, intemperance, and the fault revealed relative to the essential virtue of the master, that is of the man whom Aristotle is addressing.

I think I indicated enough last time that the master in antiquity isn't exactly the heroic brute who is represented in the Hegelian dialectic, and who functions for Hegel as an axis and turning point. I will not elaborate here on what is representative of the type; it is enough to know that it is something that enables us to appreciate properly the contribution of Aristotle's ethics. This comment undoubtedly causes us to set limits on the value of his ethics, to historicize them, but one would be wrong to assume that that is the only conclusion to draw. From an Aristotelian perspective, the master in antiquity is a presence, a human condition joined in a much less narrowly critical way to the slave, than Hegel's perspective affirms. In fact, the problem posed is one that goes unresolved from an Hegelian perspective, that of a society of masters.

Other comments, too, may contribute equally to limit the significance for us of Aristotle's ethics. Note for example that the ideal of this master, like that of god at the center of an Aristotelian world governed by νοῦς, seems to be to avoid work as much as possible. I mean to leave the control of his slaves to his steward in order to concentrate on a contemplative ideal without which the ethics doesn't achieve its proper aim. That tells you how much idealization there is in the point of view of Aristotelian ethics.

Consequently, his ethics is localized, I would almost say limited to a social type, to a privileged representative of leisure – the very term σχολαστικός suggests it. Yet, on the other hand, it is all the more striking to realize how an ethics articulated within such specific conditions still remains full of resonances and lessons. The schemas it proposes are not useless. They may be found in partially unrecognizable forms at the level of our approach to Freud's experience. These schemas may be recomposed or transposed in such a way that we will not be putting our new honey into the same old containers.

One can say right off that the search for a way, for a truth, is not absent from our experience. For what else are we seeking in analysis if not a liberating truth?

But we must be careful. One must not always trust words and labels. This truth that we are seeking in a concrete experience is not that of a superior law. If the truth that we are seeking is a truth that frees, it is a truth that we will look for in a hiding place in our subject. It is a particular truth.

But if the form of its articulation that we find is the same in everyone though always different, it is because it appears to everyone in its intimate specificity with the character of an imperious *Wunsch*. Nothing can be compared to it that allows it to be judged from the outside. The quality that best characterizes it is that of being the true *Wunsch*, which was at the origin of an aberrant or atypical behavior.

We encounter this *Wunsch* with its particular, irreducible character as a modification that presupposes no other form of normalization than that of an experience of pleasure or of pain, but of a final experience from whence it springs and is subsequently preserved in the depths of the subject in an irreducible form. The *Wunsch* does not have the character of a universal law but, on the contrary, of the most particular of laws – even if it is universal that this particularity is to be found in every human being. We find it in a form that we have categorized as a regressive, infantile, unrealistic phase, characterized by a thought abandoned to desire, by desire taken to be reality.

That surely constitutes the text of our experience. But is that the whole of our discovery, is that the whole of our morality? That attenuation, that exposure to the light of day, that discovery of the thought of desire, of the truth of that thought? Do we expect that as a result of its mere disclosure the area will be swept clean for a different thought? In one way, it is indeed so, it is as simple as that. Yet at the same time if we formulate things thus, then everything remains veiled for us.

If the reward or the novelty of the psychoanalytic experience were limited to that, it wouldn't go much further than the dated notion that was born long before psychoanalysis, namely, that the child is father of the man. The phrase comes from Wordsworth, the English romantic poet, and is quoted respectfully by Freud.

It is no accident that we discover it in that period with its fresh, shattering, and even breathtaking quality, bursting forth at the beginning of the nineteenth century with the industrial revolution, in the country that was most advanced in experiencing its effects, in England. English romanticism has its own special features, which include the value given to childhood memories, to the whole world of childhood, to the ideals and wishes of the child. And the poets of the time drew on this not only for the source of their inspiration, but also for the development of their principal themes – in this respect they are radically different from the poets who preceded them and especially from that wonderful poetry of the seventeenth and early eighteenth century, which for a reason that escapes me is called metaphysical.

That reference to childhood, the idea of the child in man, the idea that something demands that a man be something other than a child, but that the demands of the child as such are perpetually felt in him, all of that in the sphere of psychology can be historically situated.

Another man who lived in the first half of the nineteenth century, a Victorian from the early period, the historian Macaulay, noted that at the time, rather than call you a dishonest man or a perfect idiot, one preferred the excellent weapon of affirming that your mind was not fully adult, that you retained characteristics of a juvenile mentality. This attitude, which is historically datable since you find no evidence of it in any previous history, is the sign of an interval, a break in historical development. In Pascal's time, when one speaks of childhood, it is simply to say that a child is not a man. And if one speaks of adult thought, it is in no way in order to discover there traces of infantile thought.

For us, the question is not posed in those terms. If we do nevertheless constantly pose it thus, if it is justified by the contents and the text of our relationship to the neurotic and by the reference in our experience to individual genesis, this also disguises what lies behind it. For in the end, no matter how true it may be, there is a very different tension between the thought that we have to deal with in the unconscious and the thought that we characterize, goodness knows why, as adult. We constantly come upon the fact that this adult thought runs out of steam relative to the famous child's thought that we use to judge our adult. We use it not as a foil, but as a reference point, a vanishing point, where unfulfillments and even degradations come together and reach their end. There is a perpetual contradiction in the reference we make to these things.

Before coming here today I read in Jones a kind of celebration of the sublime virtues of social pressure, without which our contemporaries, our fellow humans, would be vain, egotistical, sordid, sterile, etc. One is tempted to comment in the margin, "What are they but that?" And when we speak of the adult human being, what is our reference? Where is this model of the adult human being?

These considerations incite us to reexamine the true, solid backbone of Freud's thought. No doubt psychoanalysis has ended up ordering all the material of its experience in terms of an ideal development. But at its beginning it finds its terms in a wholly different system of references, to which development and genesis only give intermittent support – this is, I believe, something that I have made you appreciate sufficiently, even if I am obliged on this occasion to refer to it only in passing. The fundamental reference is the tension or, to designate it finally by its name, the opposition between the primary process and the secondary process, between the pleasure principle and the reality principle.

2

Freud in the course of his so-called auto-analysis writes in a short letter, it is number 73: "*Meine Analyse geht weiter,* my analysis continues. It is my principal interest, *meine Hauptinteresse.* Everything remains obscure, even the problems involved, but there is a feeling of comfort. It is as if," he writes, "one had only to reach into a larder and take what one wanted. The unpleasant thing," he says, "are the *Stimmungen,*" in the most general sense we can give to that word, which has a special resonance in German, namely, moods or feelings, which by their very nature cover, hide – what precisely? *Die Wirklichkeit,* reality.

It is in terms of *Wirklichkeit* that Freud questions what presents itself to him as a *Stimmung.* The *Stimmung* is that which reveals to him what he has to look for in his auto-analysis, what he is questioning, the moment when he has the feeling of having, as in a dark room, in a larder or *Vorratskammer,* everything he needs, and that it is waiting there for him, in store for him. But he isn't led toward it by his *Stimmungen.* Such is the meaning of his sentence – the most unpleasant experience, *das Unangenehmste,* is the *Stimmungen.* Freud's experience begins with the search for the reality that is somewhere inside himself. And it is this that constitutes the originality of his point of departure. Moreover, he adds in the same vein that "even sexual excitement is for someone like me unusable in this approach. Even there I do not trust myself to see where are the final realities." And he adds, "I maintain my good humor in this whole business." Before achieving results, we must be patient a little longer.

I bring to your attention in passing a recent little book by Erich Fromm that I won't say I recommend to you, since it is a strangely discordant, almost insidious work, that is close to being defamatory. It is called *Sigmund Freud's Mission* and it makes insinuating points that are not without interest and that concern the special traits of Freud's personality, invariably seen from an obviously belittling point of view. In particular, he selects from the text Freud's sentences on sexual excitation in order to have us draw the conclusion that by the age of forty Freud was already impotent.

We are now in a position to analyze Freud's 1895 manuscript concerning his fundamental conception of the structure of the psyche, a manuscript that chance has placed in our hands. He had thought of calling it *Psychology for the Use of Neurologists.* Since he never published it, the draft remained attached to a packet of letters to Fliess, and it is available to us thanks to the acquisition of these collections.

It is, therefore, not only proper but necessary that we begin at that point our analysis of the meaning in Freud's thought of the thematics of the reality principle in opposition to the pleasure principle. Is there or is there not something distinctive relative to the development of his thought there, and at the same time to the directions taken by our own experience? It is here that we may find that hidden backbone which, I believe, is required on this occasion.

The opposition between the pleasure principle and the reality principle was rearticulated throughout Freud's work – 1895, the *Entwurf (Project for a Scientific Psychology)*; 1900, Chapter VII of the *Traumdeutung*, with the first public rearticulation of the so-called primary and secondary processes, the one governed by the pleasure principle and the other by the reality principle; 1914, return to the article from which I selected the dream that I discussed at length last year, the dream of the dead father, "he didn't know"; the article, "Formulierungen über die Zwei Prinzipen des Psychischen Geschehens," that one might translate as "Of the Structure of the Psyche"; 1930, that *Civilization and Its Discontents* which, I promised you, we will get to by way of conclusion.

Others before Freud spoke of pleasure as a guiding function of ethics. Not only does Aristotle set great store by it, but he finds it impossible not to place it at the center of his ethical teaching. What is happiness if it doesn't contain the bloom of pleasure? A significant part of the discussion of the *Nicomachaen Ethics* is designed to restore the true function of pleasure to its proper place; strangely enough it is introduced in such a way that it is given a value that is not merely passive. Pleasure in Aristotle is an activity that is compared to the bloom given off by youthful activity – it is, if you like, a radiance. In addition, it is also the sign of the blossoming of an action, in the literal sense of ἐνέργεια, a word that expresses the true praxis as that which includes its own end.

Pleasure has no doubt been given other modulations down through the ages as sign, stigmatum, reward, or substance of the psychic life. But let us consider the case of the man who questions us directly, of Freud.

What cannot fail to strike us right away is that his pleasure principle is an inertia principle. Its function is to regulate by a kind of automatism everything that comes together through a process that, in his first formulation, Freud tends to present as dependent on a preformed apparatus that is strictly limited to the neuronic apparatus. The latter regulates the facilitations that it retains after having suffered their effects. It is essentially a matter of everything that results from a fundamental tendency to discharge in which a given quantity is destined to be expended. That is the point of view from which the functioning of the pleasure principle is first articulated.

That attempt at a hypothetical formulation is offered in a way that is unique in Freud's extant writings. And one shouldn't forget that he came to dislike it and didn't want to publish it. No doubt he wrote it in response to certain demands for coherence he made of himself when confronted by himself. But it must be said that this formulation apparently makes no reference to the clinical facts, which doubtless constituted for him the whole force of the demands he had to deal with. He discusses those questions with himself or with Fliess, which under the circumstances comes to the same thing. He presents himself with a probable and coherent representation, a working hypothesis, in order to respond to something whose concrete, experimental dimension is masked and avoided here.

He claims it is a question of explaining a normal functioning of the mind. In order to do this he starts with an apparatus whose basis is wholly antithetical to a result involving adequation and equilibrium. He starts with a system which naturally tends toward deception and error. That whole organism seems designed not to satisfy need, but to hallucinate such satisfaction. It is, therefore, appropriate that another apparatus is opposed to it, an apparatus that operates as an agency of reality; it presents itself essentially as a principle of correction, of a call to order. I am not exaggerating things. Freud himself insists that there must be a distinction between the two apparatuses, although he admits he can find no trace of them in the anatomical structures sustaining them.

The reality principle or that to which the functioning of the neuronic apparatus in the end owes it efficacy appears as an apparatus that goes much further than a mere checking up; it is rather a question of rectification. It operates in the mode of detour, precaution, touching up, restraint. It corrects and compensates for that which seems to be the natural inclination of the psychic apparatus, and it radically opposes it.

The conflict is introduced here at the base, at the origins of an organism which, let us say, seems after all to be destined to live. Nobody before Freud, and no other account of human behavior, had gone so far to emphasize its fundamentally conflictual character. No one else had gone so far in explaining the organism as a form of radical inadequation – to the point where the duality of the systems is designed to overcome the radical inadequation of one of them.

This opposition between the φ system and the ψ system, which is articulated throughout, seems almost like a wager. For what is there to justify it, if it isn't that experience of ungovernable quantities which Freud had to deal with in his experience of neurosis? That is the driving imperative behind the whole system.

We sense directly that the justification for giving such prominence to quantity as such has nothing to do with Freud's desire to bring his theory into conformity with the mechanistic ideas of Helmholtz and Brücke. For him it corresponds rather to the most direct kind of lived experience, namely, that of the inertia which at the level of symptoms presented him with obstacles whose irreversible character he recognized. It is here that one finds his first advance in darkness toward that *Wirklichkeit*, which is the point to which his questioning returns; it is the key, the distinctive feature of his whole system. I ask you to reread this text, without wondering along with the annotators, commentators and connotators who have edited it whether this or that is closer to psychological or physiological thought, whether this or that refers to Herbart, Helmholtz, or anyone else. And you will see that beneath a manner that is cool, abstract, scholastic, complex and arid, one can sense a lived experience, and that this experience is at bottom moral in kind.

People play the historian on this topic, as if to explain an author like Freud in terms of influences had any value, to explain him by means of a greater or lesser similarity between one of his formulas and those which had been used by some previous thinker in a context that was different. But since it is an exercise that people engage in, why shouldn't I do the same, in my own way? Isn't the functioning of the apparatus that supports the reality principle strangely similar to what one finds in Aristotle?

Freud's task is to explain how the activity of review and restraint functions or, in other words, how the apparatus which supports the secondary processes avoids the occurrence of catastrophes that would inevitably follow the lapse of too much or too little time or the abandonment to its own devices of the pleasure principle. If the latter is released too soon, the movement will be triggered simply by a *Wunschgedanke;* it will necessarily be painful and will give rise to unpleasure. If on the other hand the secondary apparatus intervenes too late, if it doesn't give the little discharge required to attempt the beginning of an adequate solution through action, then there will be a regressive discharge, that is to say, an hallucination, which is also a source of displeasure.

Well now, this theory is not unrelated to Aristotle's ideas concerning the question of how it is that someone who knows may be intemperate. Aristotle offers several solutions. I will skip the earlier ones, which introduce syllogistic and dialectical elements that are relatively remote from our concerns here. He also attempts a solution that is not dialectical but physical – he nevertheless advances it in the form of a syllogism of the desirable.

I believe that Chapter V of Book VII on pleasure is worth reading in its entirety. Beside the major premise – one must always taste what is sweet – there is a particular, concrete minor premise, i.e., this is sweet. And the principle of wrong action is to be found in the error of a particular judgment relative to the minor premise. Where is the error found? Precisely in the circumstance that the desire which is subjacent to the major premise causes the wrong judgment to be made concerning the reality of the supposed sweetness toward which the action is directed.

I can't help thinking that Freud, who had attended the lecture series given by Brentano on Aristotle in 1887, is transposing here the properly ethical articulation of the problem on to a hypothetical, mechanistic point of view. And he does so in a way that is purely formal and gives the question a completely different accent.

In truth, it is no more of a psychology than any other of those that were devised at the time. Let us have no illusions; as far as psychology is concerned, nothing has been achieved so far that is superior to Freud's *Entwurf*. Everything that has been devised concerning the functioning of the psyche under the assumption that the mechanisms of the nervous system can account for what is concretely perceived by us as the field of psychological action has a similar air of fanciful hypothesis.

If Freud returns to the logical and syllogistic articulations, which have always been used by ethical philosophers in their field, it is in order to give them a very different meaning. We must remember that in interpreting the true content of his thought, which is to say what I have taught you. The ὀρθὸς λόγος that concerns us here are not simply major premises; they concern rather the way in which I have taught you to articulate what goes on in the unconscious; they concern the discourse that is employed on the level of the pleasure principle.

It is in relation to this ὀρθός, ironically highlighted by inverted commas, that the reality principle has to guide the subject in order for him to complete a possible action.

3

From a Freudian point of view, the reality principle is presented as functioning in a way that is essentially precarious.

No previous philosophy has gone so far in that direction. It is not that reality is called into question; it is certainly not called into question in the way that the idealists did so. Compared to Freud the idealists of the philosophical tradition are small beer indeed, for in the last analysis they don't seriously contest that famous reality, they merely tame it. Idealism consists in affirming that we are the ones who give shape to reality, and that there is no point in looking any further. It is a comfortable position. Freud's position, or that of any sensible man for that matter, is something very different.

Reality is precarious. And it is precisely to the extent that access to it is so precarious that the commandments which trace its path are so tyrannical. As guides to the real, feelings are deceptive. That intuition which animates the whole auto-analysis of Freud expresses itself thus concerning the approach to the real. Its very movement can only begin to occur by means of a primary defense. The profound ambiguity of this approach to the real demanded by man is first inscribed in terms of a defense – a defense that already exists even before the conditions of repression as such are formulated.

In order to emphasize what I am calling the paradox of the relationship to the real in Freud, I will put this on the board – the pleasure principle on the one hand and reality principle on the other. Once you have been gently reassured by these two terms, things seem to go along by themselves. Speaking broadly, one can say that the unconscious is on one side and the conscious on the other. Please bear that in mind in your attempt to follow the points I am trying to bring out.

What are we led to articulate the apparatus of perception onto? Onto reality, of course. Yet, if we follow Freud's hypothesis, on what theoretically is the control of the pleasure principle exercised? Precisely on perception, and it is here that one finds the originality of his contribution. The primary process, as he tells us in the seventh part of the *Traumdeutung*, tends to be exercised toward an identity of perception. It doesn't matter whether it is real or hallucinated, such an identity will always tend to be established. If it isn't lucky enough to coincide with reality, it will be hallucinated. The risk is in the possibility of the primary process winning out.

On the other hand, what does the secondary process tend toward? Once again you should look at Chapter VII, but it is already articulated in the *Entwurf*. It tends toward an identity of thought. What does that mean? It means that the interior functioning of the psychic apparatus – I will discuss next time how it might be represented schematically – occurs as a kind of groping forward, a rectifying test, thanks to which the subject, led on by the discharges that follow along the *Bahnungen* already established, will conduct the series of tests or of detours that will gradually lead him to anastomosis and to moving beyond the testing of the surrounding system of different objects present at that moment of its experience. One might say that the backcloth of experience consists in the construction of a certain system of *Wunsch* or of *Erwartung* of pleasure, defined as anticipated pleasure, and which tends for this reason to realize itself autonomously in its own sphere, theoretically without expecting anything from the outside. It moves directly toward a fulfillment highly antithetical to whatever triggers it.

In this preliminary approach, thought ought to appear to be on the level of the reality principle, in the same column as the reality principle. But it is by no means the case, since as described by Freud, this process is in itself and by nature unconscious. Understand that unlike that which reaches the subject in the perceptual order from the outside world, nothing that takes place at the level of these tests – thanks to which, by means of approximations in the psyche, the facilitations are realized that enable the subject to make his action adequate – is perceptible as such. All thought by its very nature occurs according to unconscious means. It is doubtless not controlled by the pleasure principle, but it occurs in a space that as an unconscious space is to be considered as subject to the pleasure principle.

Of everything that occurs at the level of inner processes, and thought itself is such a process, according to Freud, the only signs of which the subject is consciously aware are signs of pleasure or pain. As with all the other unconscious processes, nothing else reaches the level of consciousness but those signs there.

How then do we have some apprehension of those processes of thought? Here again Freud responds in a fully articulated way – only insofar as words are uttered. An idea that, with the tendency to facility characteristic of all thought that in spite of itself is tainted by a kind of parallelism, is commonly interpreted as follows: "It is, of course, clear that what Freud is telling us there is that words are that which characterizes the transition into the preconscious." But the transition of what precisely?

Of what else but movements that belong to the unconscious? Freud tells us that the thought processes are only known to us through words, what we know of the unconscious reaches us as a function of words. The idea is articulated in the most precise and the most powerful of ways in the *Entwurf*. For example, without the cry that it elicits, we would only have the most confused notion of an unpleasant object, a notion that would indeed fail to detach it from the context of which it would simply be the evil center, the object would instead be stripped of the particularity of its context. Freud tells us that a hostile object is only acknowledged at the level of consciousness when pain causes the subject to utter a cry. The existence of the *feindlicher Objekt* as such is the cry of the subject. This notion is expressed in the *Entwurf*. The cry fulfills the function of a discharge; it plays the role of a bridge where something of what is happening may be seized and identified in the consciousness of the subject. This something would remain obscure and unconscious if the cry did not lend it, as far as the conscious is concerned, the sign that gives it its own weight, presence, structure. It gives it as well a potentiality due to the fact that the important objects for a human subject are speaking objects, which will allow him to see revealed in the discourse of others the processes that, in fact, inhabit his own unconscious.

We only grasp the unconscious finally when it is explicated, in that part of it which is articulated by passing into words. It is for this reason that we have the right – all the more so as the development of Freud's discovery will demonstrate – to recognize that the unconscious itself has in the end no other structure than the structure of language.

It is this that gives value to atomistic theories. The latter do not cover any of those things they claim to cover, namely, a certain number of atoms of the neuronic apparatus, supposedly individualized elements of the nervous system. But, on the other hand, the theories of relations of contiguity and continuity illustrate admirably the signifying structure as such, insofar as it is involved in any linguistic operation.

What do we see offered with this double intersection of the respective effects of the reality and pleasure principles on each other?

The reality principle controls what happens at the level of thought, but it is only insofar as something emerges from thought which can be articulated in words in interhuman experience that it is able as a principle of thought to come to the knowledge of the subject in his consciousness.

Conversely, the unconscious itself is to be situated at the level of elements, of logical components which are of the order of λόγος, articulated in the form of an ὀρθὸς λόγος hidden at the heart of the spot where the transitions, the transferences motivated by attraction and necessity, and the inertia of pleasure occur for the subject, those operations, in short, which cause one sign rather than another to be valorized for him – to the extent that this sign may be substituted for the earlier sign or, on the contrary, have transferred to it the affective charge attached to a first experience.

Thus at these three levels we see three orders emerge as follows.

First, let us say, there is a substance or a subject of psychic experience, which corresponds to the opposition reality principle / pleasure principle.

Next, there is the process of experience, which corresponds to the opposition between thought and perception. And what do we find here? The process is divided according to whether it is a question of perception, and, therefore, linked to the activity of hallucinating, to the pleasure principle, or to a question of thought. This is what Freud calls psychic reality. On one side is the process as fictional process. On the other are the processes of thought through which instinctual activity is effectively realized, that is to say, the appetitive process – a process of search, of recognition and, as Freud explained later, of recovery of the object. That is the other face of psychic reality, its unconscious process, which is also its appetitive process.

Finally, on the level of objectification or of the object, the known and the unknown are in opposition. It is because that which is known can only be known in words that that which is unknown offers itself as having a linguistic structure. This allows us to ask again the question of what is involved at the level of the subject.

Consequently, the oppositions fiction / appetite, knowable / unknowable divide up what takes place at the level of the process and of the object. What is involved at the level of the subject? We need to ask ourselves, what is the division of the two sides between the two principles at this level?

I would propose the following. As far as the pleasure principle is concerned, that which presents itself to the subject as a substance is his good.

Insofar as pleasure controls subjective activity, it is the good, the idea of the good, that sustains it. That is why ethical thinkers have at all times not been able to avoid trying to identify these two terms, which are after all fundamentally antithetical, namely, pleasure and the good.

But over and against that, how does one qualify the substratum of reality of subjective activity?

What is the new figure that Freud gave us in the opposition reality principle / pleasure principle? It is without a doubt a problematic figure. Freud doesn't for a moment consider identifying adequacy to reality with a specific good. In *Civilization and Its Discontents* he tells us that civilization or culture certainly asks too much of the subject. If there is indeed something that can be called his good or his happiness, there is nothing to be expected in that regard from the microcosm, nor moreover from the macrocosm.

It is with this question mark that I will end today.

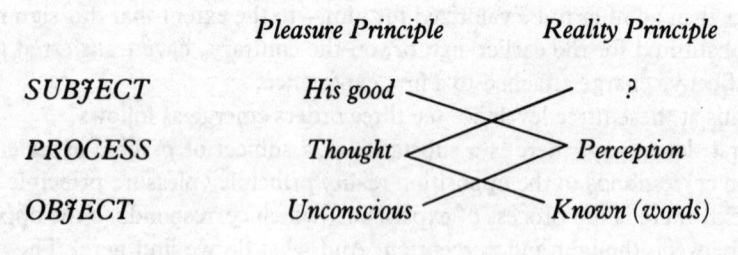

	Pleasure Principle	*Reality Principle*
SUBJECT	His good	?
PROCESS	Thought	Perception
OBJECT	Unconscious	Known (words)

November 25, 1959

III

Rereading the *Entwurf*

AN ETHICS NOT A PSYCHOLOGY
HOW REALITY IS CONSTITUTED
A TOPOLOGY OF SUBJECTIVITY

I have up till now taken account of a number of points in Freud's work. And last time you saw how I was led in particular to refer to that curiously situated work, the *Entwurf*.

You are aware of the reservations that one might have relative to the correspondence with Fliess. It is not a work as such; the text we have isn't complete. But it is certainly extremely valuable, and especially its supplementary material, among which the *Entwurf* has a special place.

1

The *Entwurf* is very revealing of a kind of substructure of Freud's thought. Its obvious relationship to all the formulations of his experience that Freud was led to offer subsequently makes it especially precious.

What I had to say about it last time expressed well enough the way in which it will appear in my commentary this year. Contrary to received opinion, I believe that the opposition between the pleasure principle and the reality principle or between the primary process and the secondary process concerns not so much the sphere of psychology as that of ethics properly speaking.

There was in Freud the perception of the proper dimension in which human action unfolds. And in the appearance of an ideal of mechanistic reduction acknowledged in the *Entwurf*, one should simply see a compensatory movement or the other face of Freud's discovery of the fact of neurosis, which is from the beginning seen in that ethical dimension where it is, in effect, situated. The proof of this is in the fact that conflict is in the foreground, and that from the outset this conflict concerns the moral order in what we might call a massive way.

That's not such a novelty. Every builder of an ethics has had to face the same problem. It is, in fact, in this connection that it is interesting to write a history, or a genealogy, of morals. Not in Nietzsche's sense, but as a series of ethical systems, i.e., of theoretical reflection on moral experience. That way one understands the central significance of problems that have been posed since the beginning and that have been pursued with a notable constancy.

After all, why is it necessary that thinkers in the field of ethics always return to the ethical problem of the relation of pleasure to the final good, whenever the guidance of human action from a moral point of view is concerned? Why do they always return to this same theme of pleasure? How does one explain that internal demand which constrains the ethical philosopher to try to reduce the antimonies associated with this theme? – from the fact that pleasure appears in many cases to be the end which is in opposition to moral effort, but that the latter has nevertheless to locate its ultimate point of reference there, a point of reference to which the good that is supposed to orient human action is finally reduced. That's an example, and by no means the only one, of the kind of knot which one comes upon in solutions to the problem. It is instructive for us to see the constancy with which the problem of conflict is posed within every discussion of morals.

Freud in this respect appears as no more than a descendent. Yet he contributes something unmatched in significance, something that has changed the problems of the ethical perspective for us to a degree that we are not yet aware of. That is why we need reference points, and I have already alluded to some of those that we will need to take account of this year.

One has to choose, since I don't intend to highlight all those writers who have discussed morals. I have discussed Aristotle because I believe that the *Nicomachean Ethics* is properly speaking the first book to be organized around the problem of an ethics. As you know, there are plenty of others around, before, after, and in Aristotle's work itself, who focus primarily on the problemn of pleasure. I will not be referring to Epictetus or Seneca here, but I will be discussing utilitarian theory insofar as it is significant for the new direction which culminated in Freud.

I will indicate today the interest of the analysis I will be giving of certain works in the same terms that Freud used in the *Entwurf*, when he designated something which, to my mind at least, is close to the language that I have taught you over the years to pay attention to in the functioning of the primary process, namely, *Bahnung* or facilitation.

As far as the statement of the problem of ethics is concerned, Freud's discourse facilitates something that allows us to go further than anyone has gone before in a domain that is essential to the problems of morality. That will be the inspiration for our discussion this year; it is around the term reality in the true meaning of the word – a term we always use in such a careless way – that the power of Freud's conception is situated. And it is a power that one can measure through the persistence of Freud's name in the development of our analytical activity.

It is obvious that it is not the poor little contribution to a physiology of fantasy involved, which explains the passionate interest we might take in reading the *Entwurf*.

You will no doubt be told that this text is difficult, but it is also exciting. Not so much in French as in German, for the French translation is extraordinarily awkward. It is wanting in precision, emphasis, and resonance throughout. In brief, I am obliged to evoke or to provoke at this point the sense of regret some of you may have that you don't know German. In German it is a brilliant, pure text; it suggests a virgin source and is altogether remarkable. The outlines of the French translation obliterate that and make it grey. Make the effort to read it and you will realize how true my comment is that one finds there something very different from a work constructed of hypotheses. It is Freud's first skirmish with that hyperbole of reality he had to deal with in his patients. There we have it; around forty years old he discovers the true dimensions, the profoundly meaningful life, of that reality.

It is not out of a vain concern to refer you to a text that I draw your attention to the *Entwurf*. Yet why not, after all? You all know that on occasion I know how to take liberties with Freud's texts and affirm my distance. If for example I have taught you the doctrine of the dominance of a signifier in a subject's unconscious chain, it is so as to emphasize certain characteristics of our experience. By virtue of a distinction that I don't fully agree with, a distinction that does nevertheless express something, the paper we heard last night called the above "the experience of the content." And it affirmed in opposition to it the scaffolding of concepts. Well now, this year I am proposing not simply to be faithful to the text of Freud and to be its exegete, as if it were the source of an unchanging truth that was the model, mold and dress code to be imposed on all our experience.

What are we going to do? We are going to look for the phylum and the development of the concepts in Freud – in the *Entwurf*, in Chapter VII of the *Traumdeutung* – where he publishes for the first time the opposition between the primary and the secondary processes, and his conception of the relationship between the conscious, the preconscious and the unconscious – in the introduction of narcissism into this economy; then in what is called the second topic, with its emphasis on the reciprocal functioning of the ego, the superego and the outside world, which gives a complete expression to things that we may have glimpsed as new shoots in the *Entwurf*; and finally in the later texts that are still centered around the same theme, "How is reality constituted for man?", namely, in the 1925 article on *Verneinung*, which we will look at again together, and in *Civilization and Its Discontents*, the discontents of man's situation in the world. The German term is *Kultur*, and we will perhaps have to try to define its exact meaning in Freud's writings. He never takes over concepts in a neutral, conventional sense; a concept has always for him a fully assumed significance.

It turns out then that if we are following so closely the development of

Freud's metapsychology this year, it is in order to uncover the traces of a theory that reflects an ethical thought. The latter is, in fact, at the center of our work as analysts, however difficult it may be to realize it fully, and it is also the latter which holds together all those who constitute the analytic community – that dispersion, which often gives the impression of being a mere scattering, of a fundamental intuition that is taken up by each one of us from one perspective or another.

If we always return to Freud, it is because he started out with an initial, central intuition, which is ethical in kind. I believe it essential to emphasize that, if we are to understand our experience and animate it, and if we are not to lose our way and allow it to be degraded. That's the reason why I am tackling this subject this year.

2

Last time I was pleased to hear an echo, a kind of response.

Two of you who for other reasons are involved in rereading the *Entwurf* – because they are working on a lexicon and perhaps for personal reasons – came to tell me after my seminar how happy they were with the way in which I had discussed Freud's text; it helped justify the interest of their own rereading.

I, therefore, had no difficulty remembering – it is something of which I am painfully aware – that this seminar is a seminar, and that it would be a good idea if it were not simply the signifier "seminar" alone that maintained its right to such a denomination. That is why I asked one of the two people to come and tell us the thoughts inspired in him by the way in which I related the subject of this seminar to the *Entwurf*. You will hear Jean-Bertrand Lefèvre-Pontalis, but his colleague, Jean Laplanche, and he are currently equally on top of the *Entwurf*, a work that, as Valabrega noted just now, you really have to have fresh in your memory, if you are to say anything valid about it. Is that really true? I don't know, for one ends up realizing that it's not as complicated as all that.

Mr. Lefèvre-Pontalis: "There is a slight misunderstanding that I would like to clear up. I am by no means a specialist of the *Entwurf* and I haven't reread it – I am in the process of reading it. Dr. Lacan asked me to go over a number of points made in his seminar last week, including especially the question of the relation to reality, that he described as particularly problematic, if not downright paradoxical, in this early text of Freud." (Mr. Lefèvre-Pontalis's presentation followed.)

3

I would like to thank you for what you have done today. It will perhaps enable us to introduce this year a way of dividing up the seminar that will allow me to stop now and then, to take a rest, and at the same time have another use.

It seems to me that you presented with remarkable elegance the vital armature of a problem where one risks getting lost in details that are, I must say, extraordinarily tempting. I did occasionally regret that you didn't enter into the detail of the position of the *Bahnung*, on the one hand, and the *Befriedigungserlebnis*, on the other. I also regretted that you didn't remind us of the topology that the system φ, ψ, ω, presupposes. All that might perhaps have illuminated things. But it is clear that one could spend a whole term, indeed a year, simply in the attempt to rectify the distortions of certain of the *Entwurf*'s original intuitions, distortions caused by the English translation.

I notice an example of this more or less at random. *Bahnung* is translated into English by "facilitation." It is obvious that the word has an exactly opposite meaning. *Bahnung* suggests the creation of a continuous way, a chain, and I even have the feeling that it can be related to the signifying chain insofar as Freud says that the development of the ψ apparatus replaces simple quantity by quantity plus *Bahnung*, that is to say its articulation. The English translation, "facilitation," slides over the thing.

The French translation was modeled on the English text. As a result, all its mistakes have been multiplied, and there are even cases where its text is absolutely unintelligible compared to a simple German text.

Nevertheless, I do believe that you emphasized the points that our following discussions will take up, discussions that will lead us back to the relationship between the reality principle and the pleasure principle. You showed the paradox involved by indicating that the pleasure principle cannot be inscribed in a biological system. Yet, my goodness, the mystery isn't so great if we see that this state of affairs is supported in the following way, namely, that the subject's experience of satisfaction is entirely dependent on the other, on the one whom Freud designates in a beautiful expression that you didn't emphasize, I am sorry to say, the *Nebenmensch*. I will have the opportunity to proffer a few quotations so as to show that it is through the intermediary of the *Nebenmensch* as speaking subject that everything that has to do with the thought processes is able to take shape in the subjectivity of the subject.

I ask you to refer to the double column table that I drew for you last time. This diagram will be of use to us until the end of our presentation and will enable us to conceive of the pleasure function and the reality function in a relationship that we will have to bind together more and more closely. If you approach them in another way, you end up with the paradox that you perhaps overemphasized today, namely, that there is no plausible reason why reality should be heard and should end up prevailing. Experience proves it to be overbundant for the human species, which for the time being is not in danger of extinction. The prospect is exactly the opposite. Pleasure in the human economy is only ever articulated in a certain relationship to this point, which is no doubt always left empty, enigmatic, but which presents a certain relationship to what man takes to be reality. And it is through this that we manage to approach ever more closely that intuition, that apperception of reality which animates the whole development of Freud's thought.

Freud posits that the ψ system must always contain a certain level of $Q\dot\eta$ quantity, which will play to the end an essential role. The discharge cannot, in effect, be complete, reach a zero level, after which the psychic apparatus achieves a final state of rest. The latter is certainly not the plausible goal or end of the functioning of the pleasure principle. Freud wonders, therefore – and this is something that the translation misses – how one can justify that it is at such a level that the quantity which regulates everything is maintained.

You perhaps skipped a little quickly over the reference to the ψ system and the φ system. If the one is related to exogenous stimulations, it isn't enough to say that the other is related to endogenous stimulations. An important part of the ψ system is, in fact, constituted of raw Q quantities from the outside which are transformed into quantities that are by no means comparable to those that characterize the ψ system, among which the latter system organizes whatever reaches it from the outside, and does so in a way that is clearly expressed by Freud as apparently being similar to Fechner's theory – it is a matter of the transformation of what is pure and simple quantity into "complication." Freud uses the same Latin term, *complicationes*.

Thus we have the following scheme. On the one hand is the φ system. On the other is the ψ system, which is a highly complex network capable of shrinkage and of *Aufbau*, that is to say of extension. At this point of the theory, there occurs between the two a crossing over, which is indicated in Freud's little diagram. Once a certain limit is passed, that which arrives as quantity is completely transformed as far as its structure is concerned. This notion of structure, of *Aufbau*, is represented by Freud as essential. He distinguishes in the ψ apparatus between its *Aufbau*, to retain quantity, and its function, which is to discharge it, *die Funktion der Abfuhr*. The function isn't simply to circulate and discharge; it appears at this level as split.

One must realize that this apparatus is presented to us as isolated in a living being. It is the nervous system that is being studied and the totality of the organism. The latter is an extremely important point whose significance is to my mind obvious. It affirms and sustains itself in a very different way from the hypotheses that Freud evokes nicely when he says that if one has a taste for them, one should only take them seriously once their arbitrary nature has been attenuated – *die Willkürlichkeit der Constructio ad hoc*. It seems obvious to me that this apparatus is a topology of subjectivity, of subjectivity insofar as it arises and is constructed on the surface of an organism.

There is also in the ψ system an important portion that Freud distinguishes from the part called the nucleus, namely, the *Spinalneuronen*, which are open to endogenous stimulation, a stimulation on the side where there is no apparatus transforming the quantities.

One finds there a wealth of material that, given your wholly legitimate purpose to simplify, you failed to mention. By way of linking up with what I will have to say next time, I will do so.

There is, for example, the notion of *Schlüsselneuronen*, which have a certain function in relation to that part of the ψ system which is turned toward endogeny and which receives its quantities. The *Schlüsselneuronen* are a particular form of discharge that occurs within the ψ system. Yet paradoxically that discharge has as its function to increase the pressure. He also calls these *Schlüsselneuronen, motorische Neuronen* and I don't think it is a mistake. They provoke stimulations that occur within the ψ system, a series of movements which increase the tension still further and which as a result are at the origin of current neuroses. And this is a problem which has been particularly neglected, but that is for us of great interest.

We will not go into that now, however. The important point is that everything that happens here offers the paradox of being in the same place as that in which the principle of articulation by the *Bahnung* reigns, the same place, too, in which the whole hallucinatory phenomenon of perception occurs, of that false reality to which, in brief, the human organism is predestined. It is again in this same place that the processes oriented and dominated by reality are unconsciously formed, insofar at least as it is a question of the subject finding the path to satisfaction. In this instance satisfaction should not be confused with the pleasure principle – this is a topic that emerges, oddly enough, at the end of the third part of the text. You could not, of course, lead us right through such a rich text. When Freud sketches out what the normal functioning of the apparatus might represent, he speaks not of specific reaction but of specific action as corresponding to satisfaction. There is a big system behind that *spezifische Aktion*, for it can only correspond, in fact, to the refound object. We find here the foundation of the principle of repetition in Freud, and it is something we will have to come back to. That specific action will always be missing something. It is not distinguishable from what takes place when a motor reaction occurs, for it is, in effect, a reaction, a pure act, the discharge of an action.

There is a very long passage that I will have occasion to come back to and to distill for you. There is no more vibrant commentary on the gap that is inherent in human experience, on the distance that is manifested in man between the articulation of a wish and what occurs when his desire sets out on the path of its realization. Freud expresses there the reason why there is always something that is far from finding satisfaction and which doesn't include the characteristics sought in a specific action. And he concludes with the words – I seem to remember that they are the last words of his paper –

"monotonous quality." Compared with anything the subject seeks out, that which occurs in the domain of motor discharge always has a diminished character.

We cannot avoid giving that remark the approbation of the most profound moral experience.

By way of concluding these thoughts today, I will draw your attention to the analogy that exists between, on the one hand, that search for an archaic – one might almost say a regressive – quality of indefinable pleasure which animates unconscious instinct as a whole and, on the other, that which is realized and satisfying in the fullest of senses, in the moral sense as such.

That is far more than an analogy; it reaches a level of profundity which has perhaps never previously been articulated as such.

December 2, 1959

IV

Das Ding

SACHE UND WORT
NIEDERSCHRIFTEN
NEBENMENSCH
FREMDE

I am going to try to speak to you about the thing – *das Ding*.

If I introduce this term, it is because there are certain ambiguities, certain insufficiencies, in relation to the true meaning in Freud of the opposition between reality principle and pleasure principle; that is to say in relation to the material which I am trying to explore with you this year, so as to make you understand its importance for our practice as an ethics. And these ambiguities have to do with something that is of the order of the signifier and even of the order of language. What we need here is a concrete, positive and particular signifier. And I don't find anything in the French language – I would be grateful to those who might be sufficiently stimulated by these remarks to suggest a solution – anything that could correspond to the subtle opposition in German, which it is not easy to bring out, between the two terms that mean "thing" – *das Ding* and *die Sache*.

1

We have only one word in French, the word "la chose" (thing), which derives from the Latin word "causa." Its etymological connection to the law suggests to us something that presents itself as the wrapping and designation of the concrete. There is no doubt that in German, too, "thing" in its original sense concerns the notion of a proceeding, deliberation, or legal debate. *Das Ding* may imply not so much a legal proceeding itself as the assembly which makes it possible, the *Volksversammlung*.

Don't imagine that this use of etymology, these insights, these etymological soundings, are what I prefer to guide myself by – although Freud does remind us all the time that in order to follow the track of the accumulated experience of tradition, of past generations, linguistic inquiry is the surest vehicle of the transmission of a development which marks psychic reality. Current practice, taking note of the use of the signifier in its synchrony, is infinitely more precious to us. We attach a far greater weight to the way in which *Ding* and *Sache* are used in current speech. Moreover, if we look up an etymological dictionary, we will find that *Sache,* too, originally had to do with a legal proceeding. *Sache* is the thing that is juridically questioned or, in our vocabulary, the transition to the symbolic order of a conflict between men.

Nevertheless, the two terms are not at all equivalent. For that matter you may have noted last time in Mr. Lefèvre-Pontalis's remarks a quotation of terms whose thrust, as he brought out in his presentation, was to raise this question, it seems to me, in opposition to my doctrine – and it is all the more praiseworthy in his case since he doesn't know German. It had to do with that passage in Freud's article entitled "The Unconscious," in which the representation of things, *Sachvorstellung,* is on every occasion opposed to that of words, *Wortvorstellung.*

I will not enter today into the discussion of the factors that would allow one to respond to that passage, so often invoked at least in the form of a question mark, by those of you who are inspired by my lectures to read Freud. It is a passage which appears to them to constitute an objection to the emphasis I place on signifying articulation as providing the true structure of the unconscious.

The passage in question seems to go against that, since it opposes *Sachvorstellung,* as belonging to the unconscious, to *Wortvorstellung,* as belonging to the preconscious. I would just beg those who stop at that passage – the majority of you presumably do not go and verify in Freud's texts what I affirm here in my commentaries – I would beg them to read together, one after the other, the article called *"Die Verdrängung"* or "Repression," which precedes the article on the unconscious, then that article itself, before arriving at the passage involved. I will just note for the rest of you that it has precisely to do with the question that the schizophrenic's attitude poses for Freud, that is to say, the manifestly extraordinary prevalence of affinities between words in what one might call the schizophrenic world.

Everything that I have just discussed seems to me to lead in only one direction, namely, that *Verdrängung* operates on nothing other than signifiers. The fundamental situation of repression is organized around a relationship of the subject to the signifier. As Freud emphasizes, it is only from that perspective that it is possible to speak in a precise, analytical sense – I would call it operational – of unconscious and conscious. He realizes that the special situation of the schizophrenic, more clearly than that of any other form of neurosis, places us in the presence of the problem of representation.

I will perhaps have the opportunity to come back to this text later. But you will note that by offering the solution he seems to be offering in opposing *Wortvorstellung* to *Sachvorstellung,* there is a problem, an impasse, that Freud himself emphasizes and that can be explained by the state of linguistics in his time. He, nevertheless, understood and formulated admirably the distinction to be made between the operation of language as a function – namely, the moment when it is articulated and, in effect, plays an essential role in the preconscious – and the structure of language, as a result of which those elements put in play in the unconscious are organized. In between, those coordinations are set up, those *Bahnungen*, that concatenation, which dominate its whole economy.

I have digressed too much, since today I only want to restrict myself to the remark that Freud speaks of *Sachvorstellung* and not *Dingvorstellung*. Moreover, it is no accident if the *Sachvorstellungen* are linked to *Wortvorstellungen*, since it tells us that there is a relationship between thing and word. The straw of words only appears to us as straw insofar as we have separated it from the grain of things, and it was first the straw which bore that grain.

I don't want to begin developing a theory of knowledge here, but it is obvious that the things of the human world are things in a universe structured by words, that language, symbolic processes, dominate and govern all. When we seek to explore the frontier between the animal and the human world, it is apparent to what extent the symbolic process as such doesn't function in the animal world – a phenomenon that can only be a matter of astonishment for us. A difference in the intelligence, the flexibility, and the complexity of the apparatuses involved cannot be the only means of explaining that absence. That man is caught up in symbolic processes of a kind to which no animal has access cannot be resolved in psychological terms, since it implies that we first have a complete and precise knowledge of what this symbolic process means.

The *Sache* is clearly the thing, a product of industry and of human action as governed by language. However implicit they may first be in the genesis of that action, things are always on the surface, always within range of an explanation. To the extent that it is subjacent to and implicit in every human action, that activity of which things are the fruit belongs to the preconscious order, that is to say, something that our interest can bring to consciousness, on condition that we pay enough attention to it, that we take notice of it. The word is there in a reciprocal position to the extent that it articulates itself, that it comes to explain itself beside the thing, to the extent also that an action – which is itself dominated by language, indeed by command – will have separated out this object and given it birth.

Sache and *Wort* are, therefore, closely linked; they form a couple. *Das Ding* is found somewhere else.

I would like today to show you this *Ding* in life and in the reality principle that Freud introduces at the beginning of his thought and that persists to the end. I will point out the reference to it in a given passage of the *Entwurf* on the reality principle and in the article entitled "Die Verneinung" or "Denegation" in which it is an essential point.

This *Ding* is not in the relationship – which is to some extent a calculated one insofar as it is explicable – that causes man to question his words as referring to things which they have moreover created. There is something different in *das Ding*.

What one finds in *das Ding* is the true secret. For the reality principle has a secret that, as Lefèvre-Pontalis pointed out last time, is paradoxical. If Freud speaks of the reality principle, it is in order to reveal to us that from a certain point of view it is always defeated; it only manages to affirm itself at the margin. And this is so by reason of a kind of pressure that one might say, if things didn't, in fact, go much further, Freud calls not "the vital needs" – as is often said in order to emphasize the secondary process – but *die Not des Lebens* in the German text. An infinitely stronger phrase. Something that *wishes*. "Need" and not "needs." Pressure, urgency. The state of *Not* is the state of emergency in life.

This *Not des Lebens* intervenes at the level of the secondary process, but in a deeper way than through that corrective activity; it intervenes so as to determine the $Q\dot{\eta}$ level – the quantity of energy conserved by the organism in proportion to the response – which is necessary for the conservation of life. Take note that it is at the level of secondary process that the level of this necessary determination is exercised.

Let us return to the reality principle that is thus invoked from the point of view of its necessity effect. This remark puts us on the track of what I call its secret, namely, the following: As soon as we try to articulate the reality principle so as to make it depend on the physical world to which Freud's purpose seems to require us to relate it, it is clear that it functions, in fact, to isolate the subject from reality.

We find in it nothing more than that which biology, in effect, teaches us, namely, that the structure of a living being is dominated by a process of homeostasis, of isolation from reality. Is that all Freud has to tell us when he speaks of the functioning of the reality principle? Apparently, yes. And he shows us that neither the quantitative element nor the qualitative element in reality enters the realm – the term he uses is *Reich* – of the secondary process.

Exterior quantity enters into contact with the apparatus called the φ system, that is to say, that part of the whole neuronic apparatus which is directly turned to the exterior or, roughly speaking, the nerve ends at the level of the skin, the tendons, and even the muscles and the bones, deep sensitivity. Everything is done so that Q quantity is definitely blocked, stopped in relation to that which is supported by another quantity, the $Q\dot{\eta}$ quantity – the latter determines the level that distinguishes the ψ apparatus within the neuronic whole. For the *Entwurf* is, in fact, the theory of a neuronic apparatus in relation to which the organism remains exterior, just as much as the outside world.

Let us turn to quality. There, too, the outside world doesn't lose all quality. But, as the theory of the sensory organs shows, this quality is inscribed in a discontinuous way, according to a scale cut off at each end and shortened in relation to the different sensory fields in question. A sensory apparatus, Freud tells us, doesn't only play the role of extinguisher or of shock-absorber, like the φ apparatus in general, but also plays the role of sieve.

He doesn't go any further in the direction of potential solutions that properly belong to the domain of the physiologist, of the man who wrote *The Sensations*, Mr. Piéron. The question of whether, in the field likely to provoke visual, auditory or other perceptions, the choice is made in this way or that is not pursued further. Still, we do have there also the notion of a deep subjectivization of the outside world. Something sifts, sieves, in such a way that reality is only perceived by man, in his natural, spontaneous state at least, as radically selected. Man deals with selected bits of reality.

In truth, that only occurs in a function which is localized in relation to the economy of the whole; it doesn't concern quality to the extent that it provides deeper information, that it achieves an essence, but only signs. Freud only sees them playing a role insofar as they are *Qualitätszeichen,* but the function of sign isn't significant in relation to opaque and enigmatic quality. It is a sign to the extent that it alerts us to the presence of something that has, in effect, to do with the outside world; it signals to consciousness that it has to deal with the outside world.

Consciousness has to come to terms with that outside world, and it has had to come to terms with it ever since men have existed and thought and tried out theories of knowledge. Freud doesn't take the problem any further except to note that it is certainly highly complex and that we are still a long way from being able to outline a solution of that which organically determines its particular genesis so precisely.

But given this, is that all that is involved when Freud speaks to us of the reality principle? Isn't this relation no more than that which certain theorists of behaviorism suggest to us? The kind which represents the fortunate encounters of an organism faced with a world where it doubtless finds something to eat and of which it is capable of assimilating certain elements, but which is in principle made up of random events and chance meetings, chaotic. Is that all Freud expresses when he speaks of the reality principle?

That is the question I am raising here today with the notion of *das Ding*.

2

Before going any further, I will once again draw your attention to the contents of the little table with its double column that I introduced two weeks ago (see p. 34).

In one column there is the *Lustprinzip;* in the other, the *Realitätsprinzip.* Unconscious activity is on the side of the pleasure principle. The reality principle dominates that which, whether conscious or preconscious, is in any case present in the order of reasoned discourse, articulatable, accessible and emerging from the preconscious. I pointed out that to the extent that they are dominated by the pleasure principle, the thought processes are unconscious, as Freud emphasizes. They are only available to consciousness to the extent that they can be verbalized, that a reasoned account brings them within range of the reality principle, within range of a consciousness that is perpetually alert, interested through the investment of its attention in discovering something that may happen, so as to allow it to find its bearings in the real world.

It is in his own words that the subject in the most precarious of ways manages to grasp the ruses thanks to which his ideas are made to fit together in his thought, ideas that often emerge in the most enigmatic of ways. The need to speak them, to articulate them, introduces within them an often artificial order. Freud liked to insist on this point when he said that one always finds reasons for finding this attitude or that mood come over one, one after the other, but there is after all nothing to confirm that the true cause of their successive emergence is given us. It is precisely this that analysis adds to our experience.

There is always an abundance of reasons to make us believe in some rational explanation for the sequentiality of our endopsychic forms. However, as we know, in the majority of cases their true connections are to be found somewhere completely different.

Thus the process of thought is to be found in the field of the unconscious – I mean that thought process through which access to reality finds its way, the *Not des Lebens,* which maintains at a certain level the investment of the apparatus. It is only accessible through the artifice of the spoken word. Freud even goes so far as to say that it is only insofar as relations are spoken that we can hear ourselves speak, that there is *Bewegung,* movement of speech – I don't think the use of this word is very common in German, and if Freud uses it, it is to emphasize the strangeness of the notion he insists on. It is only insofar as this *Bewegung* announces itself in the ω system that something may be known concerning whatever is introduced into the circuit to any degree – into the circuit that at the level of the φ apparatus tends above all to discharge itself through movement, so as to maintain tension at the lowest possible level.

The conscious subject is aware of what is involved in the process of *Abfuhr*, and appears under the sign of the pleasure principle only insofar as there is something centripetal in the movement, that there is a sense of movement toward speech, a sense of effort. And that would be limited to a dim perception, capable at the most of opposing in the world the two important qualities that Freud doesn't fail to characterize as monotonous – i.e., immobility and mobility, that which can move and that which it is impossible to move – if certain movements of a different structure didn't exist, that is, the articulated movements of words. That is once again something that is characterized by monotony, pallor, lack of color, but that is also the way everything that has to do with the thought processes reaches consciousness, with those tiny attempts to proceed from *Vorstellung* to *Vorstellung*, from representation to representation, around which the human world is organized. It is only insofar as something in the sensory-motor circuit manages to interest the ψ system at a certain level that something is perceived retroactively, something tangible, in the form of a *Wortvorstellung*.

That is how the conscious system, the ω system, can register something that happens in the psyche. Freud refers to it on a number of occasions, not without caution and sometimes ambiguously, as an endopsychic perception.

Let me emphasize further what is going on in the ψ system. From the *Entwurf* on, Freud isolates an *Ich* system. We will see its metamorphoses and transformations in subsequent developments of the theory, but it appears right away with all the ambiguity that Freud will reaffirm later when he says that the *Ich* is to a great extent unconscious.

The *Ich* is precisely defined in the *Einführung des Ichs* as a system that is uniformly invested with something which has a *Gleichbesetzung* – Freud did not write that term but I am following the drift of what he says relative to an equal, uniform investment. There is in the ψ system something that is constituted as an *Ich* and which is "eine Gruppe von Neuronen . . . . die konstant besetz ist, also dem durch die sekundäre Funktion erforderten Vorratsträger entspricht" – the term *Vorrat* in particular is repeated here. The maintenance of this investment characterizes a regulatory function there. And I am speaking of function here. If there is an unconscious, it is the *Ich* insofar as it is an unconscious function. And we have to deal with it insofar as it is regulated by that *Besetzung*, by that *Gleichbesetzung*. Whence the value of the decussation on which I insist and which we will see maintained in its duality throughout the development of Freud's thought.

Now the system which perceives and registers, and which will later be called the *Wahrnehmungsbewusstsein*, is not on the level of the ego to the extent that it maintains equal and uniform and, as far as possible constant, the *Besetzung* that regulates the functioning of thought. Consciousness is elsewhere; it is an apparatus that Freud has to invent, that he tells us is intermediary between the ψ system and the φ system, yet that at the same time everything in the text informs us we should not put at the boundary between them. The fact is that the ψ system enters directly, doubtless through an apparatus, and spreads itself directly throughout the φ system, where it only gives up a part of the quantity that it brings with it.

The ω system functions elsewhere in a more isolated position, one that is less easily situated than any other apparatus. In fact, it isn't from exterior quantity that the ω neurons extract their energy, Freud tells us; one can assume at most that they "sich die Periode aneignen," they appropriate the period. That is what I was alluding to just now when I was referring to the choice of sensory apparatus. It plays a guiding role there in relation to the contributions coming from the *Qualitätszeichen*, in order to allow with the least movement all those departures that are individualized as attention paid to this or that chosen point on the circuit, and that will permit a better approximation to the process than the pleasure principle would tend to make automatically.

As soon as Freud tries to articulate the function of this system, something strikes us about this coupling, this union, which seems a fusion, between *Wahrnenhmung*, perception, and *Bewusstsein*, consciousness, expressed in the symbol W-Bw. I enjoin you to refer to letter 52 that, as Lefèvre-Pontalis noted last time, I have remarked on a number of times.[1] It is a letter in which Freud begins to explain to Fliess in confidence his conception of how the unconscious must work. His whole theory of memory has to do with the sequence of *Niederschriften*, of inscriptions. The fundamental demand to which the whole system responds is that of ordering, in a coherent conception of the psychic apparatus, the different fields of that which he finds effectively functioning in the memory traces.

In letter 52 *Wahrnehmung*, that is to say the impression of the external world as raw, original, primitive, is outside the field which corresponds to a notable experience, namely, one that is effectively inscribed in something that, it is quite striking to note, Freud expresses right at the beginning of his thought as a *Niederschrift*, something that presents itself not simply in terms of *Prägung* or of impression, but in the sense of something which makes a sign and which is of the order of writing. And I wasn't the one who made him choose that term.

The first *Niederschrift* occurs at a certain age that his first estimate has him situate before four years old, but that's not important. Later, up to the age

---

[1] *The Complete Letters of Sigmund Freud to Wilhelm Fliess*, pp. 158–162.

of eight, another, more organized *Niederschrift,* one that is organized in terms of memories, seems to me to constitute more precisely an unconscious. It's not important if Freud is right or wrong; we have seen since how we can trace the unconscious and its organization of thought much further back. What is important is that next we have the level of the *Vorbewusstsein* and then that of the *Bewusstsein* insofar as it is not the sign of a time but of a terminus. In other words, that discussion which takes us forward from a meaning of the world to speech that can be formulated, the chain that extends from the most archaic unconscious to the articulate form of speech in a subject, all that takes place between *Wahrnehmung* and *Bewusstsein,* between glove and hand, so to speak. The progress that interests Freud is then situated somewhere that, from the point of view of the topology of the subject, is not easily identified with a neuronic apparatus. Yet what goes on between *Wahrnehmung* and *Bewusstsein* must after all have to do with the unconscious, since that's how Freud represents it to us – this time not simply in the form of a function, but of an *Aufbau,* of a structure, as he puts it himself in making the opposition.

In other words, it is to the extent that the signifying structure interposes itself between perception and consciousness that the unconscious intervenes, that the pleasure principle intervenes. Yet it is no longer in the form of a *Gleichbesetzung* or the function of the maintenance of a certain investment, but insofar as it concerns the *Bahnungen.* The structure of accumulated experience resides there and remains inscribed there.

At the level of the *Ich,* of the functioning unconscious, something regulates itself that tends to exclude the outside world. On the other hand, what is expressed at the level of *Übung* is discharge. And one finds the same intersection as in the whole economy of the apparatus. The structure regulates discharge; the function restrains it. Freud also calls that *Vorrat,* provisions; this is the word he uses for the larder of his own unconscious, *Vorratskammer. Vorratsträger* is the *Ich* as the basis of quantity and of energy that constitutes the core of the psychic apparatus.

On that basis there enters into play what we will see function as the first apprehension of reality by the subject. And it is at this point that that reality intervenes, which has the most intimate relationship to the subject, the *Nebenmensch.* The formula is striking to the extent that it expresses powerfully the idea of beside yet alike, separation and identity.

I ought really to read you the whole passage but I will limit myself to the climactic sentence: "Thus the complex of the *Nebenmensch* is separated into two parts, one of which affirms itself through an unchanging apparatus, which remains together as a thing, *als Ding.*"

That's what the awful French translation you have at your disposal misses when it says "something remains as a coherent whole." It has nothing to do with an allusion to a coherent whole that would occur in the passage from the verb to the noun, quite the contrary. The *Ding* is the element that is initially isolated by the subject in his experience of the *Nebenmensch* as being by its very nature alien, *Fremde*. The complex of the object is in two parts; there is a division, a difference in the approach to judgment. Everything in the object that is quality can be formulated as an attribute; it belongs to the investment of the ψ system and constitutes the earliest *Vorstellungen* around which the destiny of all that is controlled according to the laws of *Lust* and *Unlust*, of pleasure and unpleasure, will be played out in what might be called the primary emergences of the subject. *Das Ding* is something entirely different.

We have here an original division of the experience of reality. We find it as well in *Verneinung*. Look it up in the text. You will find the same function with the same significance of that which, from within the subject, finds itself in the beginning led toward a first outside – an outside which, Freud tells us, has nothing to do with that reality in which the subject will subsequently have to locate the *Qualitätszeichen*, signs that tell him that he is on the right track in his search for satisfaction.

That is something which, even prior to the test of this search, sets up its end, goal and aim. That's what Freud indicates when he says that "the first and most immediate goal of the test of reality is not to find in a real perception an object which corresponds to the one which the subject represents to himself at that moment, but to find it again, to confirm that it is still present in reality."

The whole progress of the subject is then oriented around the *Ding* as *Fremde*, strange and even hostile on occasion, or in any case the first outside. It is clearly a probing form of progress that seeks points of reference, but with relation to what? – with the world of desires. It demonstrates that something is there after all, and that to a certain extent it may be useful. Yet useful for what? – for nothing other than to serve as points of reference in relation to the world of wishes and expectations; it is turned toward that which helps on certain occasions to reach *das Ding*. That object will be there when in the end all conditions have been fulfilled – it is, of course, clear that what is supposed to be found cannot be found again. It is in its nature that the object as such is lost. It will never be found again. Something is there while one waits for something better, or worse, but which one wants.

The world of our experience, the Freudian world, assumes that it is this object, *das Ding*, as the absolute Other of the subject, that one is supposed to find again. It is to be found at the most as something missed. One doesn't find it, but only its pleasurable associations. It is in this state of wishing for it and waiting for it that, in the name of the pleasure principle, the optimum tension will be sought; below that there is neither perception nor effort.

In the end, in the absence of something which hallucinates it in the form of a system of references, a world of perception cannot be organized in a valid way, cannot be constituted in a human way. The world of perception is represented by Freud as dependent on that fundamental hallucination without which there would be no attention available.

3

Here we come to the notion of the *spezifische Aktion* of which Freud speaks on a number of occasions, and that I would like to shed some light on here. There is, in fact, an ambiguity in the *Befriedigungserlebnis*. What is sought is the object in relation to which the pleasure principle functions. This functioning is in the material, the web, the medium to which all practical experience makes a reference. How then does Freud conceive of this experience, this specific action?

In this connection one has to read his correspondence with Fliess to appreciate the significance of it, and in particular that letter referred to above, which still has a lot to tell us. He says that an attack of hysteria is not a discharge. It is a warning to those who always feel the need to place the emphasis on the role of quantity in the functioning of affect. There is no field more favorable than that of hysteria to suggest to what extent in the concatenation of psychic events a fact is a question of relative contingency. It is by no means a discharge, *sondern eine Aktion* – an action, moreover, which is *Mittel von Reproduktion von Lust*.

We will see how what Freud calls an action is made clear. The essential characteristic of any action is to be a *Mittel*, a means of reproduction. In its root at least it is this: "Das ist er [der hysterische Anfall] wenigstens in der Wurzel." And elsewhere "sonst motiviert er sich von dem Vorbewusstsein allerlei Gründen" – an action may be motivated on all kinds of grounds which are located at the level of the preconscious.

Immediately afterwards Freud explains what its essence consists of. And he illustrates at the same time what an action as *Mittel zur Reproduktion* means. In the case of hysteria, of a crisis of tears, everything is calculated, regulated, and, as it were, focused on *den Anderen*, on the Other, the prehistoric, unforgettable Other, that later no one will ever reach.

The thoughts we find expressed here allow us to make a first approach to the problem of neurosis and to understand its correlative or regulatory term. If one goal of the specific action which aims for the experience of satisfaction is to reproduce the initial state, to find *das Ding*, the object, again, we will be able to understand a great many forms of neurotic behavior.

The behavior of the hysteric, for example, has as its aim to recreate a state centered on the object, insofar as this object, *das Ding*, is, as Freud wrote somewhere, the support of an aversion. It is because the primary object is an object which failed to give satisfaction that the specific *Erlebnis* of the hysteric is organized.

On the other hand – this is Freud's distinction and we don't need to give it up – in obsessional neurosis, the object with relation to which the fundamental experience, the experience of pleasure, is organized, is an object which literally gives too much pleasure. Freud perceived this clearly; it was his first apperception of obsessional neurosis.

What in its various advances and many byways the behavior of the obsessional reveals and signifies is that he regulates his behavior so as to avoid what the subject often sees quite clearly as the goal and end of his desire. The motivation of this avoidance is often extraordinarily radical, since the pleasure principle is presented to us as possessing a mode of operation which is precisely to avoid excess, too much pleasure.

So as to move fast – as fast as Freud in his first apperceptions of ethical reality, insofar as it functions in the subject whom he is dealing with – I will outline the positing of the subject in the third of the major categories that Freud distinguishes at the beginning – hysteria, obsessional neurosis, and paranoia. As far as paranoia is concerned, Freud gives us a term that I invite you to reflect on as it first emerged, namely, *Versagen des Glaubens*. The paranoid doesn't believe in that first stranger in relation to whom the subject is obliged to take his bearings.

The use of the term belief seems to me to be emphasized in a less psychological sense than first seems to be the case. The radical attitude of the paranoid, as designated by Freud, concerns the deepest level of the relationship of man to reality, namely, that which is articulated as faith. Here you can see easily how the connection with a different perspective is created that comes to meet it – I already referred to it when I said that the moving force of paranoia is essentially the rejection of a certain support in the symbolic order, of that specific support around which the division between the two sides of the relationship to *das Ding* operates – as we will see in subsequent discussions.

Das Ding is that which I will call the beyond-of-the-signified. It is as a function of this beyond-of-the-signified and of an emotional relationship to it that the subject keeps its distance and is constituted in a kind of relationship characterized by primary affect, prior to any repression. The whole initial articulation of the *Entwurf* takes place around it. Let us not forget that repression still posed a problem for Freud. And everything that he will subsequently say about repression, in its extraordinary sophistication, can only be understood as responding to the need to understand the specificity of repression compared to all the other forms of defense.

It is then in relation to the original *Ding* that the first orientation, the first choice, the first seat of subjective orientation takes place, and that I will sometimes call *Neuronenwahl*, the choice of neurosis. That first grinding will henceforth regulate the function of the pleasure principle.

It remains for us to see that it is in the same place that something which is the opposite, the reverse and the same combined, is also organized, and which in the end substitutes itself for that dumb reality which is *das Ding* – that is to say, the reality that commands and regulates. That is something which emerges in the philosophy of someone who, better than anyone else, glimpsed the function of *das Ding*, although he only approached it by the path of the philosophy of science, namely, Kant. In the end, it is conceivable that it is as a pure signifying system, as a universal maxim, as that which is the most lacking in a relationship to the individual, that the features of *das Ding* must be presented. It is here that, along with Kant, we must see the focal point, aim and convergence, according to which an action that we will qualify as moral will present itself. And which, moreover, we will see present itself paradoxically as the rule of a certain *Gut* or good.

Today I will simply emphasize this: the Thing only presents itself to the extent that it becomes word, hits the bull's eye,[2] as they say. In Freud's text the way in which the stranger, the hostile figure, appears in the first experience of reality for the human subject is the cry. I suggest we do not need this cry. Here I would like to make a reference to something that is more inscribed in the French than in the German language – each language has its advantages. The German *das Wort*, word, is both *le mot* and *la parole* in French. The word *le mot* has a particular weight and meaning. "Mot" refers essentially to "no response." "Mot," La Fontaine says somewhere, is what remains silent; it is precisely that in response to which no word is spoken. The things in question are things insofar as they are dumb – some people might object that these things are placed by Freud at a higher level than the world of signifiers that I have described as the true moving force of the functioning in man of that process designated as primary. And dumb things are not exactly the same as things which have no relationship to words.

It is enough to evoke a face which is familiar to everyone of you, that of the terrible dumb brother of the four Marx brothers, Harpo. Is there anything that poses a question which is more present, more pressing, more absorbing, more disruptive, more nauseating, more calculated to thrust everything that takes place before us into the abyss or void than that face of Harpo Marx, that face with its smile which leaves us unclear as to whether it signifies the most extreme perversity or complete simplicity? This dumb man alone is sufficient to sustain the atmosphere of doubt and of radical annihilation which is the stuff of the Marx brothers' extraordinary farce and the uninterrupted play of "jokes"[3] that makes their activity so valuable.

[2] The French here contains a pun: "faire mouche" means to hit the bull's-eye and by analogy with that Lacan creates the phrase "faire mot," to become word.
[3] In English in the original.

Just one more thing. I have spoken today of the Other as a *Ding*. I would like to conclude with something that is much more accessible to our experience. And that is the isolated use that French reserves for certain forms of the pronoun of interpellation. What does the emission, the articulation, the sudden emergence from out of our voice of that "You!" (*Toi!*) mean? A "You" that may appear on our lips at a moment of utter helplessness, distress or surprise in the presence of something that I will not right off call death, but that is certainly for us an especially privileged other – one around which our principle concerns gravitate, and which for all that still manages to embarrass us.

I do not think that this "You" is simple – this you of devotion that other manifestations of the need to cherish occasionally comes up against. I believe that one finds in that word the temptation to tame the Other, that prehistoric, that unforgettable Other, which suddenly threatens to surprise us and to cast us down from the height of its appearance. "You" contains a form of defense, and I would say that at the moment when it is spoken, it is entirely in this "You," and nowhere else, that one finds what I have evoked today concerning *das Ding*.

So as not to end with something that might seem to you to be so optimistic, I will focus on the weight of the identity of the thing and the word that we can find in another isolated use of the word.

To the "You" which, according to me, tames, but which tames nothing, a "You" of vain incantation and fruitless connection, there corresponds what may happen to us when some order comes from beyond the apparatus where there lurks that which, along with ourselves, has to do with *das Ding*. I am thinking of what we answer when we are made responsible or accountable for something. "Me!" (Moi!).[4] What is this "Me!", this "Me!" all by itself, if it is not a "Me!" of apology, a "Me!" of refusal, a "Me!" that's simply not for me?

Thus from its beginning the "I" as thrust forth in an antagonistic movement, the "I" as defense, the "I" as primarily and above all an "I" that refuses and denounces rather than announces, the "I" in the isolated experience of its sudden emergence – which is also perhaps to be considered as its original decline – this "I" is articulated here.

I will speak about this "I" again next time in order to explore further the way in which moral action presents itself as an experience of satisfaction.

December 9, 1959

[4] It should be noted that the emphatic first pronoun "moi" is also used in French to mean both "self" and "ego."

V

Das Ding (II)

THE *COMBINATOIRE* OF THE *VORSTELLUNGEN*
THE LIMIT OF PAIN
BETWEEN PERCEPTION AND CONSCIOUSNESS
THE INTERSAID OF *VERNEINUNG*
MOTHER AS *DAS DING*

Freud comments somewhere that if psychology succeeded in making some people anxious, by insisting excessively on the reign of the instincts, it nevertheless also promoted the importance of the moral agency.

This is an obvious truth, one that is confirmed every day in our practice.

Furthermore, we still do not rate highly enough in the world outside the exorbitant character of the power of the sense of guilt, which is exercised without the subject's knowledge. Thus it is that which presents itself in the massive guise of the sense of guilt that I believe is important to focus on more narrowly this year. Moreover, it is important to articulate it so as to bring out the originality, the revolution in thought, that was the effect of the Freudian experience in the field of ethics.

1

Last time I tried to show you the meaning in Freudian psychology of the *Entwurf* in connection with which Freud organized his first intuition concerning what takes place in the experience of the neurotic. I tried, in particular, to show you the pivotal function that we must accord something which is to be found in a detour taken by the text. And it is one that it is important not to miss, especially since Freud picks up on it again in a variety of forms right to the end. I mean *das Ding*.

Right at the beginning of the organization of the world in the psyche, both logically and chronologically, *das Ding* is something that presents and isolates itself as the strange feature around which the whole movement of the *Vorstellung* turns – a *Vorstellung* that Freud shows us is governed by a regulatory principle, the so-called pleasure principle, which is tied to the functioning of the neuronic apparatus. And it is around *das Ding* that the whole adaptive development revolves, a development that is so specific to man insofar as the symbolic process reveals itself to be inextricably woven into it.

We find *das Ding* again in the *Verneinung* article of 1925, an article that is full of ideas and also of questions. It occurs in a formula which we must assume to be essential since it is placed at the center of the article and is, so to speak, the crucial enigma. *Das Ding* has, in effect, to be identified with the *Wieder zu finden,* the impulse to find again that for Freud establishes the orientation of the human subject to the object. Yet you should note that this object is not even stated. And here we might give its due to a certain textual criticism, whose attachment to the signifier sometimes seems to take a talmudic turn. It is remarkable that the object in question is nowhere articulated by Freud.

Moreover, since it is a matter of finding it again, we might just as well characterize this object as a lost object. But although it is essentially a question of finding it again, the object indeed has never been lost. In this orientation to the object, the regulation of the thread, the *Vorstellungen* relate to each other in accordance with the laws of a memory organization, a memory complex, a *Bahnung* (that is to say, a facilitator, but also, I would say more decidedly, a concatenation) whose neuronic apparatus perhaps allows us to glimpse those operations in a material form, and whose functioning is governed by the law of the pleasure principle.

The pleasure principle governs the search for the object and imposes the detours which maintain the distance in relation to its end. Even in French the etymology of the word – which replaced the archaic "quérir ("to search")" – refers to *circa*, detour. The transference of the quantity from *Vorstellung* to *Vorstellung* always maintains the search at a certain distance from that which it gravitates around. The object to be found confers on the search its invisible law; but it is not that, on the other hand, which controls its movements. The element that fixes these movements, that models the return – and this return itself is maintained at a distance – is the pleasure principle. It is the pleasure principle which, when all is said and done, subjects the search to encounter nothing but the satisfaction of the *Not des Lebens*.

Thus the search encounters in its path a series of satisfactions that are tied to the relation to the object and are polarized by it. And at every point they model, guide and support its movements according to the particular law of the pleasure principle. This law fixes the level of a certain quantity of excitation which cannot be exceeded without going beyond the limit of the *Lust/ Unlust* polarity – pleasure and unpleasure are the only two forms through which that same and single mode of regulation we call the pleasure principle expresses itself.

The admission of quantity is regulated by the width of the channels that do the conducting, by the individual diameters that a given organism can support – the thing is expressed metaphorically by Freud, but it is almost as if we were to take it literally. What happens once the limit is exceeded? The psychic impulse is not as such capable of advancing any further toward what is supposed to be its goal. Instead it is scattered and diffused within the psychic organism; the quantity is transformed into complexity. In a kind of expansion of the lighted zone of the neuronic organism, here and there in the distance, it lights up according to the laws of associative facilitation, or constellations of *Vorstellungen* which regulate the association of ideas, unconscious *Gedanken*, according to the pleasure principle.

The limit has a name. It is something more than the *Lust/Unlust* polarity Freud speaks of.

I would have you note that it is avoidance, flight, movement, which in the beginning, even before the system starts to function, normally intervenes in order to regulate the invasion of quantity in accordance with the pleasure principle. And it is to the motor system that the function of regulating the bearable or homeostatic level of tension for the organism is handed over in the end. But the homeostatis of the nervous system, which is the site of autonomous regulatory mechanism, is distinct from the general homeostasis (with all the potential for conflict that that implies), the homeostasis which activates the balance of moods. The balancing of moods occurs, but as an order of stimulation arising from within. That is how Freud expresses it. Certain stimulations come from within the nervous system, and he compares them to external stimulations.

I would like us to stop for a moment at this limit of pain.

Those commentators who collected the letters to Fliess consider that Freud slipped up by using the term *motorisch*, motor, instead of *secretorisch*, cell, nucleus, organ. I once said that it did not seem to be clear that it was such a slip. Freud tells us, in effect, that in the majority of cases, the reaction of pain derives from the fact that the motor reaction, the flight reaction, is impossible. And the reason for this is that the stimulation, the excitation, comes from within. Consequently, it seems to me that this so-called slip is only present in order to point to the fundamental homology between the relationship of pain and the motor reaction. Besides – this idea occurred to me a long time ago, and I hope you will not find it absurd – in the organization of the spinal marrow, the neurons and axons of pain coexist at the same level and at the same spot as certain neurons and axons of the tonic motor system.

Thus, even pain must not be simply attributed to the register of sensory reactions. I would say, and this is something that the surgery of pain reveals, that it is not a question of something simple, which can be considered a simple quality of sensory reaction. The complex character of pain, the character that, so to speak, makes it an intermediary between afferent and efferent, is suggested by the surprising results of certain operations, which in the case of some internal illnesses, including some cancers, allow the notation of pain to be preserved, when the suppression or removal of a certain subjective quality has been effected, which accounts for the fact that it is unbearable.

All this belongs to the sphere of modern physiological research, and it does not yet allow us to explain the problem fully. I will, therefore, limit myself to suggesting that we should perhaps conceive of pain as a field which, in the realm of existence, opens precisely onto that limit where a living being has no possibility of escape.

Isn't something of this suggested to us by the insight of the poets in that myth of Daphne transformed into a tree under the pressure of a pain from which she cannot flee? Isn't it true that the living being who has no possibility of escape suggests in its very form the presence of what one might call petrified pain? Doesn't what we do in the realm of stone suggest this? To the extent that we don't let it roll,[1] but erect it, and make of it something fixed, isn't there in architecture itself a kind of actualization of pain?

What happened during the period of the Baroque, under the influence of an historical movement that we will come back to later, would support this idea. Something was attempted then to make architecture itself aim at pleasure, to give it a form of liberation, which, in effect, made it blaze up so as to constitute a paradox in the history of masonry and of building. And that goal of pleasure gave us forms which, in a metaphorical language that in itself takes us a long way, we call "tortured."

I hope you will pardon my digression, since it does, in fact, point in the direction of the themes we will take up again later, in connection with the man of pleasure and the eighteenth century, and the very style it introduced into the investigation of eroticism.

Let us return to our *Vorstellungen,* and try to understand them now, to surprise them in their operations, so as to understand what is involved in Freudian psychology.

The character of imaginary composition, of the imaginary element of the object, makes of it what one might call the substance of appearance, the material of a living lure – an apparition open to the deception of an *Erscheinung,* I would say, if I took the liberty of speaking German; that is to say, that by means of which the appearance is sustained, but which is also at the same time an unremarkable apparition – something that creates that *Vor,* that third element, something that is produced starting from the Thing. *Vorstellung* is something that is essentially fragmented. It is that around which Western philosophy since Aristotle and φαντασία has always revolved.

Vorstellung is understood by Freud in a radical sense, in the form in which it appears in a philosophy that is essentially marked by the theory of knowl-

---

[1] The pun here involves a reference to the French proverb "Pierre qui roule n'amasse pas mousse." – "A rolling stone gathers no moss."

edge. And that is the remarkable thing about it. He assigned to it in an extreme form the character philosophers themselves have been unable to reduce it to, namely, that of an empty body, a ghost, a pale incubus of the relation to the world, an enfeebled *jouissance*, which through the age-old interrogations of the philosophers makes it the essential feature. And by isolating it in this function, Freud removes it from its tradition.

And the sphere, order, and gravitation of the *Vorstellungen*, where does he locate them? I told you last time that if one reads Freud carefully, one has to locate them between perception and consciousness, between the glove and the hand.

It is between perception and consciousness that is inserted that which functions at the level of the pleasure principle. Which is what precisely? – The thought processes insofar as they regulate by means of the pleasure principle the investment of the *Vorstellungen*, and the structure in which the unconscious is organized, the structure in which the underlying unconscious mechanisms are flocculated. And it is this which makes the small curds of representation, that is to say, something which has the same structure as the signifier – a point on which I insist. That is not just *Vorstellung*, but as Freud writes later in the same article on the unconscious, *Vorstellungsrepräsentanz*; and he thus turns *Vorstellung* into an associative and combinatory element. In that way the world of *Vorstellung* is already organized according to the possibilities of the signifier as such. Already at the level of the unconscious there exists an organization that, as Freud says, is not necessarily that of contradiction or of grammar, but the laws of condensation and displacement, those that I call the laws of metaphor and metonymy.

Why should it be a surprise, therefore, if Freud tells us that these thought processes that take place between perception and consciousness would not mean anything to consciousness, if they were not transmitted there by the mediation of a discourse, of that which can be clarified in the *Vorbewusstsein*, in preconsciousness? But what does that mean? Freud leaves us with little doubt; it is a question of words. And we must, of course, situate the *Wortvorstellungen* that are involved in relation to our argument here.

Freud tells us this is not the same thing as the *Vorstellungen* whose thought processes of superposition, metaphor and metonymy we follow through the unconscious mechanism. It is something entirely different. The *Wortvorstellungen* inaugurate a discourse that is articulated on the thought processes. In other words, we know nothing about our thought processes, unless we engage in psychology – allow me to say that to make my point more forcefully. We only know them because we are speaking of something which goes on inside us, because we are speaking of them in terms that are unavoidable – terms whose indignity, emptiness and vanity we are also aware of. It is from that moment when we speak of our will and our understanding as distinct faculties that we have a preconscious, and that we are able, in effect, to articulate in a discourse something of that chattering by means of which we articulate ourselves inside ourselves, we justify ourselves, or we rationalize for ourselves, with reference to this or that, the progress of our desire.

It is definitely a discourse that is involved. And Freud emphasizes that, after all, we know nothing else except this discourse. That which emerges in the *Bewusstsein* is *Wahrnehmung*, the perception of this discourse, and nothing else. That is exactly what he thinks.

That is why he tends to reject utterly superficial representations or, to use Silberer's term, the functional phenomena. There are no doubt in a given phase of a dream things that represent the functioning of the psyche to us imagistically – a notable example represents the layers of psychic activity in the form of the game of Chutes and Ladders. What does Freud say? Involved here is the production of dreams by a mind given to metaphysics or, in other words, to psychology, which tends to expand on what the discourse necessarily imposes on us when we should be trying to distinguish a certain rhythm in our inner experience. But this representation, Freud tells us, overlooks that structure, that most profound gravitation, which is established at the level of the *Vorstellungen*. And he affirms that these *Vorstellungen* gravitate, operate exchanges and are modulated according to laws that you will recognize, if you have followed my teaching, as the fundamental laws of the signifying chain.

Have I managed to make myself understood? It seems to me difficult to be any clearer as far as this essential point is concerned.

2

We have now reached the point where we must distinguish the effective articulation of a discourse, of the gravitation of the *Vorstellungen*, in the form of *Vorstellungsrepräsentanzen* of these unconscious articulations. We must examine what in such circumstances we mean by *Sachvorstellungen*. The latter are to be set in polar opposition to word play, to *Wortvorstellungen*, but at this level they go together. As far as *das Ding* is concerned, that is something else. *Das Ding* is a primordial function which is located at the level of the initial establishment of the gravitation of the unconscious *Vorstellungen*.

I did not have time last week to make you appreciate how in ordinary German usage there is a linguistic difference between *Ding* and *Sache*.

It is clear that in every case they cannot be used interchangeably. And that even if there are cases where one can use either one, to choose one or the other in German gives a particular emphasis to the discourse. I ask those who know German to refer to the examples in the dictionary. One does not use *Sache* for religious matters, but one nevertheless says that faith is not *jeder-*

man Ding – it is not for everybody. Master Eckhart uses *Ding* to refer to the soul, and heaven knows that for Master Eckhart the soul was a *Grossding*, the biggest of things. He certainly would not use the term *Sache*. If I wanted to make you sense the differences by giving you a general measure of the way in which the use of the signifier breaks down differently in German relative to French, I would cite this sentence that I was on the point of citing last time, but that I held back because I am not after all a Germanist, and I wanted to make use of the interval to test it on the ears of some people whose mother tongue is German. One could say that "Die Sache ist das Wort des Dinges." Or, in French, "L'affaire est le mot de la chose ("The affair is the word of the thing.")."

It is precisely as we shift into discourse that *das Ding*, the Thing, is resolved into a series of effects – in the sense that one can say *meine Sache*. That suggests all my kit and caboodle, and is something very different from *das Ding* – that thing to which we must now return.

You will not be surprised if I tell you that at the level of the *Vorstellungen*, the Thing is not nothing, but literally is not. It is characterized by its absence, its strangeness.

Everything about it that is articulated as good or bad divides the subject in connection with it, and it does so irrepressibly, irremediably, and no doubt with relation to the same Thing. There is not a good and a bad object; there is good and bad, and then there is the Thing. The good and the bad already belong to the order of the *Vorstellung;* they exist there as clues to that which orients the position of the subject, according to the pleasure principle, in connection with that which will never be more than representation, search for a privileged state, for a desired state, for the expectation of what? Of something that is always a certain distance from the Thing, even if it is regulated by the Thing, which is there in a beyond.

We see it at the level of what the other day we noted were the stages of the φ system. Here there are *Wahrnehmungszeichen*, here there is *Vorbewusstsein*, here there are the *Wortvorstellungen*, insofar as they reflect in a discourse what goes on at the level of the thought processes. And the latter are themselves governed by the laws of the *Unbewusst*, that is to say, by the pleasure principle. The *Wortvorstellungen*, as a reflection of discourse, stand in opposition to that which is ordered in the *Vorstellungsrepräsentanzen* according to an economy of words. And in the *Entwurf* Freud calls these *Vorstellungsrepräsentanzen* conceptual memories, which is no more than a first approximation of the same notion.

At the level of the φ system, that is to say, at the level of what takes place before the entry into the ψ system, and the crossover into the space of the *Bahnung* and the organization of the *Vorstellungen*, the typical reaction of the organism as regulated by the neuronic system is avoidance. Things are *ver-*

meidet, avoided. The level of the *Vorstellungsrepräsentanzen* is the special site of *Verdrängung*. The level of *Wortvorstellungen* is the site of *Verneinung*.

I will stop there for a moment to explain the meaning of a point which is still a problem for some of you in connection with *Verneinung*. As Freud notes, it is the privileged means of connotation at the level of discourse for whatever is *verdrängt* or repressed in the unconscious. *Verneinen* is the paradoxical way in which what is hidden, *verborgen*, in the unconscious is located in spoken, enunciated discourse, in the discourse of *Bewusstwerden; verneinen* is the manner in which what is simultaneously actualized and denied comes to be avowed.

One should continue this study of *Verneinung* that I have just begun with a study of the negative particle. Following Pichon's example, I have already pointed out here the subtly differentiated use in French of this pleonastic "ne," which, as I showed, makes it seem paradoxical when, for example, the subject enunciates his own fear.

We do not say "Je crains qu'il vienne" ("I am afraid he may come"), as logic would seem to demand, but "Je crains qu'il ne vienne" ("I am afraid he may [not] come").[2] This "ne" has a floating place between the two levels of the graph that I showed you how to use, so as to distinguish between the level of enunciation and the level of the enunciated. By enunciating "I am afraid that . . .," I make it appear both in its reality, and in its reality as a wish –" . . . he may come." And it is here that in French the little "ne" is interposed, which points to the discordance between the levels of enunciation and of the enunciated.

The negative particle "ne" only emerges at the moment when I really speak, and not at the moment when I am spoken, if I am on the level of the unconscious. And I think it is a good idea to interpret Freud in a similar way when he says that there is no negation at the level of the unconscious. Given that immediately afterwards, he shows us that there is indeed negation. That is to say, in the unconscious there are all kinds of ways of representing negation metaphorically. There are all kinds of ways of representing it in a dream, except, of course, for the little negative particle "ne," because the particle only belongs to discourse.

The concrete examples show us the distinction that exists between the function of discourse and the function of speech.

Thus the *Verneinung*, far from being the pure and simple paradox of that which presents itself in the form of a "no," isn't just any old "no." There is a whole world of no-saying *(non-dit)*, of interdiction *(interdit)*, since it is in that very form that the *Verdrängt*, which is the unconscious, essentially pre-

---

[2] As Lacan's example suggests, the pleonastic "ne" in French grammar is a kind of submerged negation used after verbs of fearing and certain conjunctions. My bracketed "not" is designed to suggest the effect, since it has no equivalent in English.

sents itself. But the *Verneinung* is the most solid beachhead of that which I would call the "intersaid" *(entre dit)* in the same way that we say "interview." One might just as easily explore a little common usage in the sphere of the language of love, in all that is said when, for example, one says, "I do not say that . . ." or quite simply in the way people express themselves in Corneille: "No, I do not hate you."

You can see that in this game of Chutes and Ladders, from a certain point of view *Verneinung* represents the inverse of *Verdrängung*, and that there is a difference of organization between them with relation to the function of avowal. Let me point out to those for whom this still constitutes a problem that there is a correspondence between that which is fully articulated at the level of the unconscious, *Verurteilung*, and that which takes place at the level pointed to by Freud in letter 52, in the first signifying signification of *Verneinung*, that of *Verwerfung*.

One of you who shall remain nameless, Laplanche, in a dissertation on Hölderlin that we will, I hope, have the opportunity to discuss here some time, asked himself and asked me, what *Verwerfung* might be. He wanted to know if it was the paternal No / Name (Nom-*de*-père), as is the case in paranoia, or the No / Name of the Father (Nom-*du*-père).[3] If that's what it is, there are few pathological examples that put us in the presence of its absence, of its effective refusal. If it is the No / Name of the Father, are we not entering into a series of difficulties concerning the fact that something is always signified for the subject who is attached to experience, whether present or absent, something which for one reason or another and to a variety of degrees has come to occupy that place for him?

Of course, the notion of signifying substance cannot fail to create a problem for an alert mind. But don't forget that we are dealing with the system of the *Wahrnehmnungszeichen*, signs of perception, or, in other words, the first system of signifers, the original synchrony of the signifying system. Everything begins when several signifers can present themselves to the subject at the same time, in a *Gleichzeitigkeit*. It is at this level that *Fort* is the correlative of *Da*. *Fort* can only be expressed as an alternative derived from a basic synchrony. It is on the basis of this synchrony that something comes to be organized, something that the mere play of *Fort* and *Da* could not produce by itself.

I have already asked the question here as to what the critical conceivable minimum is for a signifying scale, if the register of the signifier is to begin to organize itself. There cannot be a two without a three, and that, I think, must certainly include a four, the quadripartite, the *Geviert*, to which Hei-

---

[3] In the context of this discussion of forms of denial, it seems appropriate to remind the English-speaking reader of the pun contained in the spoken French of the *Nom-du-Père*.

degger refers somewhere. As we will see, the whole psychology of the psychotic develops insofar as a term may be refused, a term that maintains the basic system of words at a certain distance or relational dimension. Something is missing and his real effort at substitution and "significization" is directed in desperation at that. Let us hope that we will have the opportunity to return to the problem, along with the remarkable analysis that Laplanche has given of a poetic experience which displays and which unveils it, and makes it apparent in a way that is especially revealing, namely, the case of Hölderlin.

The function of this place is to contain words, in the sense in which contain means to keep – as a result of which an original distance and articulation are possible, through which synchrony is introduced, and it is on the foundation of synchrony that the essential dialect is then erected, that in which the Other may discover itself as the Other of the Other.

The Other of the Other only exists as a place. It finds its place even if we cannot find it anywhere in the real, even if all we can find to occupy this place in the real is simply valid insofar as it occupies this place, but cannot give it any other guarantee than that it is in its place.

It is in this way that another typology is established, the typology which institutes the relation to the real. And now we can define this relation to the real, and realize what the reality principle means.

3

The whole function of that which Freud articulates in the term superego, *Uberich*, is tied to the reality principle. And this would be no more than a banal play of words, if it were merely an alternative way of designating what has been called the moral conscience or something similar.

Freud gives us a completely new theory by showing us the root or psychological operation of something that in the human constitution weighs so heavily on all those forms of which there is no reason why we should misunderstand any, including the simplest, namely, that of the commandments and, I would even say, the ten commandments.

I will not avoid discussing these ten commandments that we might assume we know all about. It is clear that we see them functioning, if not in ourselves, at least in things in a singularly lively way. It will, therefore, perhaps be appropriate to look again at what Freud articulates here.

What that is, I will put in the following terms, terms that all the commentaries seem designed merely to make us forget. As far as the formation of morality is concerned, Freud contributes what some call the discovery and others the affirmation, and I believe is the affirmation of the discovery, that the fundamental or primordial law, the one where culture begins in opposition to nature, is the law of the prohibition of incest – nature and culture being precisely distinguished in Freud in a modern sense, that is to say, in the way in which Lévi-Strauss might articulate them today.

The whole development of psychoanalysis confirms it in an increasingly weighty manner, while at the same time it emphasizes it less and less. I mean that the whole development at the level of the mother/child interpsychology – and that is badly expressed in the so-called categories of frustration, satisfaction, and dependence – is nothing more than an immense development of the essential character of the maternal thing, of the mother, insofar as she occupies the place of that thing, of *das Ding*.

Everyone knows that its correlative is the desire for incest, which is Freud's discovery. There is no point in affirming that it is to be found somewhere in Plato, or that Diderot spoke of it in *Rameau's Nephew* or *The Supplement to Bougainville's Voyage*. That is of no interest to me. What is important is that there was a man who at a given historical moment stood up to affirm: "That's the fundamental desire."

And we must grasp this thought firmly in our hand. Freud designates the prohibition of incest as the underlying principle of the primordial law, the law of which all other cultural developments are no more than the consequences and ramifications. And at the same time he identifies incest as the fundamental desire.

Claude Lévi-Strauss in his magisterial work no doubt confirms the primordial character of the Law as such, namely, the introduction of the signifer and its *combinatoire* into human nature through the intermediary of the marriage laws, which are regulated by a system of exchanges that he defines as elementary structures – this is the case to the extent that guidance is given concerning the choice of a proper partner or, in other words, order is introduced into marriage, which produces a new dimension alongside that of heredity. But even when Lévi-Strauss explains all that, and spends a lot of time discussing incest in order to show what makes its prohibition necessary, he does not go beyond suggesting why the father does not marry a daughter – because the daughters must be exchanged. But why doesn't a son sleep with his mother? There is something mysterious there.

He, of course, dismisses justifications based on the supposedly dangerous biological effects of inbreeding. He proves that, far from producing results involving the resurgence of a recessive gene that risks introducing degenerative effects, a form of endogamy is commonly used in all fields of breeding of domestic animals, so as to improve a strain, whether animal or vegetable. The law only operates in the realm of culture. And the result of the law is always to exclude incest in its fundamental form, son / mother incest, which is the kind Freud emphasizes.

If everything else around it may find a justification, this central point nevertheless remains. If one reads Lévi-Strauss's text closely, one can see that it is the most enigmatic and the most stubborn point separating nature from culture.

And I want to make you stop there. What we find in the incest law is located as such at the level of the unconscious in relation to *das Ding*, the Thing. The desire for the mother cannot be satisfied because it is the end, the terminal point, the abolition of the whole world of demand, which is the one that at its deepest level structures man's unconscious. It is to the extent that the function of the pleasure principle is to make man always search for what he has to find again, but which he never will attain, that one reaches the essence, namely, that sphere or relationship which is known as the law of the prohibition of incest.

This metaphysical analysis is not worthy of our interest, however, if it cannot be confirmed at the level of the effective discourse which manages to put itself at the disposition of man's knowledge, that preconscious or unconscious discourse or, in other words, the effective law, or, in other words again, the famous ten commandments I was speaking about just now.

But are there ten commandments? My goodness, perhaps there are. I tried to add them up by going back to the source. I took down my copy of Silvestre de Sacy's Bible. It is the closest thing we have in French to those versions of the Bible that have exercised such a decisive influence on the thought and history of other peoples – in one case, inaugurating Slav culture with Saint Cyril and, in another, that of the authorized version of the English; one can say that, if one does not know it by heart, one finds oneself an outsider among them. We do not have the equivalent of that. But I nevertheless advise you to take a look at the seventeenth-century version, in spite of its inaccuracies and mistakes, since it was the version people read, and on the basis of which generations of clergymen have written and fought over the interpretation of a given prohibition, both past and present, that is inscribed in its pages.

I thus took down the text of that Decalogue that God dictated before Moses on the third day of the third month after the flight from Egypt, in the dark cloud on Mount Sinai, accompanied by flashes of lightning and the command to the people not to come near. I must say I would like one day to have someone more qualified than I to analyze for us the diverse forms that the interpretation of these ten commandments have undergone – from the Hebrew texts to the one in which it appears as the quiet droning of the rhythmic lines of the catechism.

However negative the ten commandments may seem, I will not linger long over their character as prohibitions – we are always being told that morality doesn't only have a negative side, it also has a positive side – but I will note, as I have before in this place, that they are perhaps only the commandments of speech. By that I mean they clarify that without which no speech is possible – notice that I did not say discourse.

I just gave you an indication there, since I could hardly go any further, and I pick up the trail again here. This is what I want to point out. In the ten commandments, which constitute almost everything that, against all odds, is accepted as commandments by the whole of the civilized community – civilized or not, or almost civilized, but since we only know the other, uncivilized part by means of a number of cryptograms, let us limit ourselves to the so-called civilized portions – in the ten commandments, it is nowhere specified that one must not sleep with one's mother. I do not think that the command "to honor" her should be considered as the least suggestive of this, either negatively or positively – in spite of what in the Provençal tales of Marius and Olive is known as "performing honorable service."[4]

Couldn't we next time try to interpret the ten commandments as something very close to that which effectively goes on in repression in the unconscious? The ten commandments may be interpreted as intended to prevent the subject from engaging in any form of incest on one condition, and on one condition only, namely, that we recognize that the prohibition of incest is nothing other than the condition sine qua non of speech.

This brings us back to questioning the meaning of the ten commandments insofar as they are tied in the deepest of ways to that which regulates the distance between the subject and *das Ding* – insofar as that distance is precisely the condition of speech, insofar as the ten commandments are the condition of the existence of speech as such.

I am simply on the point of broaching this topic, but I beg you right away not to stop at the idea that the ten commandments are, so to speak, the condition of all social life. For from another point of view, how can one not in truth see, when one merely recites them, that they are in a way the chapter and verse of our transactions at every moment of our lives? They display the range of what are properly speaking our human actions. In other words, we spend our time breaking the ten commandments, and that is why society is possible.

I do not for all that have to push the paradox to its extreme, like Bernard de Mandeville in *The Fable of the Bees*, when he demonstrates that private vices constitute public wealth. It is not a question of that, but of seeing what kind of preconscious immanence the ten commandments correspond to. I will take up the question there next time – not, however, without making a detour through that fundamental reference I evoked when I spoke to you for the first time of what might be called the real.

---

[4] The reference here is to the Provençal material of Marcel Pagnol's trilogy of plays on Marseilles life, *Marius, Fanny*, and *César*.

The real, I have told you, is that which is always in the same place. You will see this in the history of science and thought. This detour is indispensable if we are to reach the great revolutionary crisis of morality, namely, the systematic questioning of principles there where they need to be questioned, that is, at the level of the imperative. That is the culminating point for both Kant and Sade with relation to the Thing; it is there that morality becomes, on the one hand, a pure and simple application of the universal maxim and, on the other, a pure and simple object.

This point is essential if one is to understand the step taken by Freud. By way of conclusion today I would just like to bring to your attention something that a poet, who happens to be a friend of mine, once wrote: "The problem of evil is only worth raising as long as one has not fixed on the idea of transcendence by some good that is able to dictate to man what his duties are. Till that moment the exalted representation of evil will continue to have the greatest revolutionary value."

Well now, the step taken by Freud at the level of the pleasure principle is to show us that there is no Sovereign Good – that the Sovereign Good, which is *das Ding*, which is the mother, is also the object of incest, is a forbidden good, and that there is no other good. Such is the foundation of the moral law as turned on its head by Freud.

Now we have to consider where the positive moral law comes from that has remained quite intact, and that we are literally capable of "banging our heads against the wall for," to borrow an expression made famous by a film, rather than see it overturned.[5]

What does this mean? It means, and this is where I am leading you, that what you were looking for in the place of the object that cannot be found again is the object that one always finds again in reality. In the place of the object impossible to find again at the level of the pleasure principle, something has happened that is nothing more than the following: something which is always found again, but which presents itself in a form that is completely sealed, blind and enigmatic, the world of modern physics.

You will see that it is in relation to this that the crisis of morality was played out at the end of the eighteenth century at the time of the French revolution. And it is to this that Freud's doctrine constitutes an answer. It sheds a light on the subject that, I hope to be able to show you, has not yet yielded up all its implications.

December 16, 1959

[5] The reference is to Georges Franju's *La Tête contre les Murs*.

VI

On the moral law

THE CRITIQUE OF PRACTICAL REASON
PHILOSOPHY IN THE BOUDOIR
THE TEN COMMANDMENTS
THE EPISTLE TO THE ROMANS

What if we brought a simple soul into this lecture hall, set him down in the front row, and asked him what Lacan means.

The simple soul will get up, go to the board and will give the following explanation: "Since the beginning of the academic year Lacan has been talking to us about *das Ding* in the following terms. He situates it at the heart of a subjective world which is the one whose economy he has been describing to us from a Freudian perspective for years. This subjective world is defined by the fact that the signifier in man is already installed at the level of the unconscious, and that it combines its points of reference with the means of orientation that his functioning as a natural organism of a living being also gives him."

Simply by writing it on the board and putting *das Ding* at the center, with the subjective world of the unconscious organized in a series of signifying relations around it, you can see the difficulty of topographical representation. The reason is that *das Ding* is at the center only in the sense that it is excluded. That is to say, in reality *das Ding* has to be posited as exterior, as the prehistoric Other that it is impossible to forget – the Other whose primacy of position Freud affirms in the form of something *entfremdet*, something strange to me, although it is at the heart of me, something that on the level of the unconscious only a representation can represent.

1

I said "something that only a representation can represent." Do not look upon that as a simple pleonasm, for "represent" and "representation" here are two different things, as the term *Vorstellungsrepräsentanz* indicates. It is a matter of that which in the unconscious represents, in the form of a sign, representation as a function of apprehending – of the way in which every representation is represented insofar as it evokes the good that *das Ding* brings with it.

But to speak of "the good" is already a metaphor, an attribute. Everything that qualifies representations in the order of the good is caught up in refraction, in the atomized system that the structure of the unconscious facilitations imposes, in the complex mechanism of a signifying system of elements. It is only in that way that the subject relates to that which presents itself on the horizon as his good. His good is already pointed out to him as the significant result of a signifying composition that is called up at the unconscious level or, in other words, at a level where he has no mastery over the system of directions and investments that regulate his behavior in depth.

I will use a term here that only those who have present in their minds the Kantian formulas of *The Critique of Practical Reason* will be able to appreciate. I invite those who do not have them present in their minds or who have not yet encountered what is, from more than one point of view, an extraordinary book to make good their memories or their general knowledge.

It is impossible for us to make any progress in this seminar relative to the questions posed by the ethics of psychoanalysis if you do not have this book as a reference point.

So as to motivate you to look at it, let me emphasize that it is certainly extraordinary from the point of view of its humor. To remain poised at the limit of the most extreme conceptual necessity produces an effect of plenitude and content as well as of vertigo, as a result of which you will not fail to sense at some point in the text the abyss of the comic suddenly open up before you. Thus I do not see why it is a door that you would refuse to open. We will in any case see in a minute how we can open it here.

It is then, to be explicit, the Kantian term *Wohl* that I propose in order to designate the good in question. It has to do with the comfort of the subject insofar as, whenever he refers to *das Ding* as his horizon, it is the pleasure principle that functions for him. And it does so in order to impose the law in which a resolution of the tension occurs that is linked to something that, using Freud's phrase, we will call the successful lures – or, better yet, the signs that reality may or may not honor. The sign here is very close to a representative currency, and it suggests an expression that I incorporated into one of my first lectures, that on physical causality, in a phrase that begins one of its paragraphs, i.e., "more inaccessible to our eyes that are made for the signs of the money changer."

Let me carry the image further. "The signs of the money changer" are already present at the base of the structure which is regulated according to the law of *Lust* and *Unlust,* according to the rule of the indestructible *Wunsch* that pursues repetition, the repetition of signs. It is in that way that the subject regulates his initial distance to *das Ding,* the source of all *Wohl* at the level of the pleasure principle, and which at its heart already gives rise to what we may call *das Gut des Objekts*, the good object – following the Kantian example, as the practitioners of psychoanalysis have not failed to do.

On the horizon, beyond the pleasure principle, there rises up the *Gut, das Ding*, thus introducing at the level of the unconscious something that ought to oblige us to ask once again the Kantian question of the *causa noumenon*. *Das Ding* presents itself at the level of unconscious experience as that which already makes the law. Although it is necessary to give this verbal phrase, "makes the law," the emphasis it receives in one of the most brutal games of elementary society and that is evoked in a recent book by Roger Vailland. It is a capricious and arbitrary law, the law of the oracle, the law of signs in which the subject receives no guarantee from anywhere, the law in relation to which he has no *Sicherung*, to use another Kantian term. That is also at bottom the bad object that Kleinian theory is concerned with.

Although it must be said that at this level *das Ding* is not distinguished as bad. The subject makes no approach at all to the bad object, since he is already maintaining his distance in relation to the good object. He cannot stand the extreme good that *das Ding* may bring him, which is all the more reason why he cannot locate himself in relation to the bad. However much he groans, explodes, curses, he still does not understand; nothing is articulated here even in the form of a metaphor. He produces symptoms, so to speak, and these symptoms are at the origin of the symptoms of defense.

And how should we conceive of defense at this level? There is organic defense. Here the ego defends itself by hurting itself as the crab gives up its claw, revealing thereby the connection I developed between the motor system and pain. Yet in what way does man defend himself that is different from an animal practising self-mutilation? The difference is introduced here by means of the signifying structuralization in the human unconscious. But the defense or the mutilation that is proper to man does not occur only at the level of substitution, displacement or metaphor – everything that structures its gravitation with relation to the good object. Human defense takes place by means of something that has a name, and which is, to be precise, lying about evil.

At the level of the unconscious, the subject lies. And this lying is his way of telling the truth of the matter. The ὀρθὸς λόγος of the unconscious at this level – as Freud indicates clearly in the *Entwurf* in relation to hysteria – is expressed as πρῶτον ψεῦδος, the first lie.

Given the amount of time I have been discussing the *Entwurf* with you, do I need to remind you of the example that he gives of a female patient called Emma, whom he doesn't mention elsewhere and who is not the Emma of the *Studies on Hysteria?* It is the case of a woman who has a phobia about going into stores by herself because she is afraid people will make fun of her on account of her clothes.

Everything is related to an early memory. At the age of twelve she went into a store and the shop assistants apparently laughed at her clothes. One of them attracted her and even stirred her in some strange way in her emerging puberty. Behind that we find a causal memory, that of an act of aggression she suffered in a shop at the hands of a *Greis*. The French translation, modeled on the English, which was itself particularly careless, says "shopkeeper" – but an old fogey is involved, an elderly man, who pinched her somewhere under her dress in a very direct manner. This memory thus echoes the idea of a sexual attraction experienced in the other.

All that remains in the symptom is attached to clothes, to the mockery of her clothes. But the path of truth is suggested in a masked form, in the deceiving *Vorstellung* of her clothes. In an opaque way, there is an allusion to something that did not happen on the occasion of the first memory, but on the second. Something that wasn't apprehended in the beginning is apprehended retroactively, by means of the deceitful transformation – *proton pseudos*. Thus in that way we have confirmation of the fact that the relationship of the subject to *das Ding* is marked as bad – but the subject can only formulate this fact through the symptom.

That is what the experience of the unconscious has forced us to add to our premises when we take up again the question of ethics as it has been posed over the centuries, and as it has been bequeathed us in Kantian ethics, insofar as the latter remains, in our thought if not in our experience, the point to which these questions have been brought.

The way in which ethical principles are formulated when they impose themselves on consciousness or when about to emerge from preconsciousness, as commandments, has the closest relationship to the second principle introduced by Freud, namely, the reality principle.

The reality principle is the dialectical correlative of the pleasure principle. One is not simply, as one at first imagines, the application of the consequence of the other; each one is really the correlative of the other. Without this neither one would make any sense. Once again we are led to deepen the reality principle in a way I suggested in connection with the experience of paranoia.

As I have already told you, the reality principle isn't simply the same as it appears in the *Entwurf*, the testing that sometimes takes place at the level of the ω system or the *Wahrnehmungsbewusstsein* system. It doesn't function only on the level of that system in which the subject, probing in reality that which communicates the sign of a present reality, is able to adjust correctly the deceptive emergence of the *Vorstellung* as it is provoked by repetition at the level of the pleasure principle. It is something more. Reality faces man – and that is what interests him in it – both as having already been structured and as being that which presents itself in his experience as something that always returns to the same place.

I pointed it out when I was discussing the case of President Schreber. The function of the stars in the delirious system of that exemplary subject shows us, just like a compass, the polar star of the relation of man to the real. The history of science makes something similar seem plausible. Isn't it strange, paradoxical even, that it was the observations of shepherds and Mediterranean sailors of the return to the same place of an object which might seem to interest human experience least, namely, a star, that revealed to the farmer when he should sow his seeds? Think of the important role that the Pleiades played for Mediterranean navigators. Isn't it remarkable that it was the observation of the return of the stars to the very same places that, repeated over the centuries, led to the structuralization of reality by physics, which is what we mean by science? The fruitful laws involved came down to earth from the sky, to Galileo from the physics of the peripatetic philosophers. However, from that earth, where the laws of the heavens had been rediscovered, Galilean physics returned to the sky by demonstrating that the stars are by no means what we had believed them to be, that they are not incorruptible, that they are subject to the same laws as the terrestrial globe.

Furthermore, if a decisive step in the history of science was already taken by Nicolas of Cuse, who was one of the first to formulate the idea that the stars were not incorruptible, we know something else, we know that they might not be in the same place.

Thus that first demand that made us explore the structuralization of the real down through history in order to produce a supremely efficient and supremely deceptive science, that first demand is the demand of *das Ding* – it seeks whatever is repeated, whatever returns, and guarantees that it will always return, to the same place – and it has driven us to the extreme position in which we find ourselves, a position where we can cast doubt on all places, and where nothing in that reality which we have learned to disrupt so admirably responds to that call for the security of a return.

Yet it is to this search for something that always returns to the same place that what is known as ethics has attached itself over the centuries. Ethics is not simply concerned with the fact that there are obligations, that there is a bond that binds, orders, and makes the social law. There is also something that we have frequently referred to here by the term "the elementary structures of kinship" – the elementary structures of property and of the exchange of goods as well. And it is as a result of these structures that man transforms himself into a sign, unit, or object of a regulated exchange in a way that Claude Lévi-Strauss has shown to be fixed in its relative unconsciousness. That which over generations has presided over this new supernatural order of the structures is exactly that which has brought about the submission of man to the law of the unconscious. But ethics begins beyond that point.

It begins at the moment when the subject poses the question of that good he had unconsciously sought in the social structures. And it is at that moment, too, that he is led to discover the deep relationship as a result of which that which presents itself as a law is closely tied to the very structure of desire. If he doesn't discover right away the final desire that Freudian inquiry has discovered as the desire of incest, he discovers that which articulates his conduct so that the object of his desire is always maintained at a certain distance. But this distance is not complete; it is a distance that is called proximity, which is not identical to the subject, which is literally close to it, in the way that one can say that the *Nebenmensch* that Freud speaks of as the foundation of the thing is his neighbor.

If at the summit of the ethical imperative something ends up being articulated in a way that is as strange or even scandalous for some people as "Thou shalt love thy neighbor as thyself," this is because it is the law of the relation of the subject to himself that he make himself his own neighbor, as far as his relationship to his desire is concerned.

My thesis is that the moral law is articulated with relation to the real as such, to the real insofar as it can be the guarantee of the Thing. That is why I invite you to take an interest in what I have called the high point of the crisis in ethics, and that I have designated from the beginning as linked to the moment when *The Critique of Practical Reason* appeared.

2

Kantian ethics appears at the moment when the disorienting effect of Newtonian physics is felt, a physics that has reached a point of independence relative to *das Ding*, to the human *Ding*.

It was Newtonian physics that forced Kant to revise radically the function of reason in its pure form. And it is also in connection with the questions raised by science that a form of morality has come to engage us; it is a morality whose precise structure could not have been perceived until then – one that detaches itself purposefully from all reference to any object of affection, from all reference to what Kant called the *pathologisches Objekt*, a pathological object, which simply means the object of any passion whatsoever.

No *Wohl*, whether it be our own or that of our neighbor, must enter into the finality of moral action. The only definition of moral action possible is that which was expressed in Kant's well-known formula: "Act in such a way that the maxim of your action may be accepted as a universal maxim." Thus action is moral only when it is dictated by the motive that is articulated in the maxim alone. To translate *allgemeine* as "universal" is not quite right, since it is closer to "common." Kant contrasts "general" with "universal," which he takes up in its Latin form. All of which proves that something here is left in an undetermined state. *Handle so, dass die Maxime deines Willens jederzeit zugleich als Prinzip einer allgemeinen Gesetzgebung gelten könne.* "Act so that the maxim of your will may always be taken as the principle of laws that are valid for all."

That formula, which is, as you know, the central formula of Kant's ethics, is pursued by him to the limit of its consequences. His radicalism even leads to the paradox that in the last analysis the *gute Wille,* good will, is posited as distinct from any beneficial action. In truth, I believe that the achievement of a form of subjectivity that deserves the name of contemporary, that belongs to a man of our time, who is lucky enough to be born now, cannot ignore this text. I simply emphasize it as we continue on our merry way, for one can, in fact, get by with very little – the person to our right and the person to our left are nowadays, if not neighbors, then at the very least people who, from the point of view of volume, are close enough to prevent us from falling down. But one must have submitted oneself to the test of reading this text in order to measure the extreme, almost insane character of the corner that we have been backed into by something that is after all present in history, namely, the existence, indeed the insistence, of science.

If, of course, no one has ever been able to put such a moral axiom into practice – even Kant himself did not believe it possible – it is nevertheless useful to see how far things have gone. In truth, we have built another bridge in our relation to reality. For some time transcendental aesthetics itself – I am referring to that which is designated as such in *The Critique of Pure Reason* – is open to challenge, at the very least on the level of that play of writing where theoretical physics is currently registering a hit. Henceforth, given the point we have reached in the light of our science, a renewal or updating of the Kantian imperative might be expressed in the following way, with the help of the language of electronics and automation: "Never act except in such a way that your action may be programmed." All of which takes us a step further in the direction of an even greater, if not the greatest, detachment from what is known as a Sovereign Good.

Let us be clear about this: when we reflect on the maxim that guides our action, Kant is inviting us to consider it for an instant as the law of a nature in which we are called upon to live. That is where one finds the apparatus that would have us reject in horror some maxim or other that our instincts would gladly lead us to. In this connection he gives us examples that are worth taking note of in a concrete sense, for however obvious they may seem, they perhaps suggest, at least to the analyst, a line of reflection. But note that he affirms the laws of *nature,* not of *society.* It is only too clear that not only do societies live very well by reference to laws that are far from promoting their universal application, but even more remarkably, as I suggested last time, these societies prosper as a result of the transgression of these maxims.

It is a matter then of a mental reference to a nature that is organized according to the laws of an object constructed at the moment when we raise the question of our rule of conduct.

So as to produce the kind of shock or eye-opening effect that seems to me necessary if we are to make progress, I simply want to draw your attention to this: if *The Critique of Practical Reason* appeared in 1788, seven years after the first edition of *The Critique of Pure Reason*, there is another work which came out six years after *The Critique of Practical Reason*, a little after Thermidor in 1795, and which is called *Philosophy in the Boudoir*.

As, I suppose, you all know, *Philosophy in the Boudoir* is the work of a certain Marquis de Sade, who is famous for more than one reason. His notoriety was accompanied from the beginning by great misfortunes, and one might add by the abuse of power concerning him – he did after all remain a prisoner for twenty-five years, which is a long time for someone who, my goodness, as far as we know, never committed a serious crime, and who in certain of our modern ideologies has been promoted to a point where one can also say that there is at the very least some confusion, if not excess.

Although in the eyes of some the work of the Marquis de Sade seems to promise a variety of entertainments, it is not strictly speaking much fun. Moreover, the parts that seem to give the most pleasure can also be regarded as the most boring. But one cannot claim that his work lacks coherence. And, in a word, it is precisely the Kantian criteria he advances to justify his positions that constitute what can be called a kind of anti-morality.

The paradox of this is argued with the greatest coherence in the work that is entitled *Philosophy in the Boudoir*. A short passage is included in it that, given the number of attentive ears here, is the only one that I expressly recommend you read – "Frenchmen, one more effort to become republicans."

As a result of this appeal, which supposedly came from a number of cells that were active at that time in revolutionary Paris, the Marquis de Sade proposes that, given the ruin of those authorities on which (according to the work's premises) the creation of a true republic depends, we should adopt the opposite of what was considered up to that point as the essential minimum of a viable and coherent morality.

And, in truth, he does quite a good job in defending that proposal. It is no accident if we first find in *Philosophy in the Boudoir* the praise of calumny. Calumny, he writes, can in no sense be injurious; if it imputes to our neighbor worse things than one can justifiably impute to him, it nevertheless has the merit that it puts us on guard against his activities. And the author proceeds in like manner to justify point by point the reversal of the fundamental imperatives of the moral law, extolling incest, adultery, theft, and everything else you can think of. If you adopt the opposite of all the laws of the Decalogue, you will end up with the coherent exposition of something which in the last instance may be articulated as follows: "Let us take as the universal maxim of our conduct the right to enjoy any other person whatsoever as the instrument of our pleasure."

Sade demonstrates with great consistency that, once universalized, this law, although it gives libertines complete power over all women indifferently, whether they like it or not, conversely also liberates those same women from all the duties that civilized society imposes on them in their conjugal, matrimonial and other relations. This conception opens wide the flood gates that in imagination he proposes as the horizon of our desire; everyone is invited to pursue to the limit the demands of his lust, and to realize them.

If the same opening is given to all, one will be able to see what a natural society is like. Our repugnance may be legitimately related to that which Kant himself claims to eliminate from the criteria of the moral law, namely, to the realm of sentiment.

If one eliminates from morality every element of sentiment, if one removes or invalidates all guidance to be found in sentiments, then in the final analysis the Sadian world is conceivable – even if it is its inversion, its caricature – as one of the possible forms of the world governed by a radical ethics, by the Kantian ethics as elaborated in 1788.

Believe me, there is no lack of Kantian echoes in the attempts to articulate moral systems that one finds in a vast literature that might be called libertine, the literature of the man of pleasure, which is an equally caricatural form of the problem that for a long time preoccupied the *ancién regime,* and from Fénelon on, the education of girls. You can see that pushed to its comically paradoxical limit in *The Raised Curtain* by Mirabeau.

Well now, we are coming to that on account of which, in its search for justification, for a base and support, in the sense of reference to the reality principle, ethics encounters its own stumbling block, its failure – I mean there where an aporia opens up in that mental articulation we call ethics. In the same way that Kantian ethics has no other consequence than that gymnastic exercise whose formative function for anyone who thinks I have called to your attention, so Sadian ethics has had no social consequences at all. Understand that I don't know if the French have really tried to become republicans, but it is certain that just like all the other nations of the world, including those who had their revolutions after them – bolder, more ambitious, and more radical revolutions, too – they have left what I will call the religious bases of the ten commandments completely intact, even pushing them to a point where their puritan character is increasingly marked. We've reached a situation where the leader of a great socialist state on a visit to other contemporary cultures is scandalized to see dancers on the Pacific coast of the noble country of America raising their legs a little too high.

We are thus faced here with a question, that is to say, the question of the relationship to das Ding.

This relationship seems to me to be sufficiently emphasized in the third chapter of *The Critique of Practical Reason* concerning the motives of practical pure reason. In effect, Kant acknowledges after all the existence of *one* sentient correlative of the moral law in its purity, and strangely enough, I ask you to note, it is nothing other than pain itself. I will read you the passage concerned, the second paragraph of the third part: "Consequently, we can see *a priori* that the moral law as the determining principle of will, by reason of the fact that it sets itself against our inclinations, must produce a feeling that one could call pain. And this is the first and perhaps only case, where we are allowed to determine, by means of *a priori* concepts, the relationship between a knowledge, which comes from practical pure reason, and a feeling of pleasure or pain."

In brief, Kant is of the same opinion as Sade. For in order to reach *das Ding* absolutely, to open the flood gates of desire, what does Sade show us on the horizon? In essence, pain. The other's pain as well as the pain of the subject himself, for on occasions they are simply one and the same thing. To the degree that it involves forcing an access to the Thing, the outer extremity of pleasure is unbearable to us. It is this that explains the absurd or, to use a popular expression, maniacal side of Sade that strikes us in his fictional constructions. We are aware at every moment of the discomfort in living constructions, the kind of discomfort that makes it so difficult for our neurotic patients to confess certain of their fantasms.

In fact, to a certain degree, at a certain level, fantasms cannot bear the revelation of speech.

3

We are then brought back again to the moral law insofar as it is incarnated in a certain number of commandments. I mean the ten commandments, which in the beginning, at a period that is not so remote in the past, were collected by a people that sets itself apart as a chosen people.

As I said, it is appropriate to reconsider these commandments. I noted last time that there is a study to be done for which I would gladly call upon one of you as the representative of a tradition of moral theology. A great many questions deserve our attention. I spoke of the number of commandments. There is also the matter of their form and the way in which they are transmitted to us in the future tense. I would be glad to call upon the help of someone who knows enough Hebrew to answer my questions. In the Hebrew version is it a future tense or a form of the volitive that is used in *Deuteronomy* and *Numbers*, where we see the first formulations of the Decalogue?

The issue I want to raise today concerns their privileged structure in relation to the structure of the law. I want today to consider two of them.

I must leave to one side the huge questions posed by the promulgation of these commandments by something that announces itself in the following form: "I am what I am." It is, in effect, necessary not to draw the text in the direction of Greek metaphysics by translating as "he who is," or "he who am." The English translation, "I am that I am," is, according to Hebrew scholars, the closest to what is meant by the formulation of the verse. Perhaps I am mistaken, but since I do not know Hebrew and while I wait on further information on the subject, I rely on the best authorities, and they are of one mind on the question.

That "I am what I am" is announced first of all to a small people in the form of that which saved it from the misfortunes of Egypt, and it begins by affirming, "You will adore no God but me, before my countenance." I leave open the question of what "before my countenance" means. Does it mean that beyond the countenance of God, i.e., outside Canaan, the adoration of other gods is not inconceivable for a believing Jew? A passage from the second Book of Samuel, spoken by David, seems to confirm this.

It is nevertheless the case that the second commandment, the one that formally excludes not only every cult, but also every image, every representation of what is in heaven, on earth, or in the void, seems to me to show that what is involved is in a very special relationship to human feeling as a whole. In a nutshell, the elimination of the function of the imaginary presents itself to my mind, and, I think, to yours, as the principle of the relation to the symbolic, in the meaning we give that term here; that is to say, to speech. Its principal condition is there.

I leave aside the question of rest on the sabbath day. But I believe that that extraordinary commandment, according to which, in a land of masters, we observe one day out of seven without work – such that according to humorous proverbs, the common man is left no happy medium between the labor of love and the most stultifying boredom – that suspension, that emptiness, clearly introduces into human life the sign of a gap, a beyond relative to every law of utility. It seems to me, therefore, that it has the most intimate relationship to something that we are on the track of here.

I leave aside the prohibition on murder, for we will have to come back to that in connection with the respective significance of the act and its retribution. I want to take up the prohibition on lying insofar as it is related to what presented itself to us as that essential relationship of man to the Thing, insofar as it is commanded by the pleasure principle, namely, the lie that we have to deal with every day in our unconscious.

"Thou shalt not lie" is the commandment in which the intimate link between desire, in its structuring function, with the law is felt most tangibly. In truth, this commandment exists to make us feel the true function of the law. And I can do no better than to place it beside the sophism in which is manifested most strikingly the type of ingenuity that is furthest from the Jewish or talmudic tradition, namely, the paradox of Epimenides, he who affirmed that all men are liars. What am I saying, in proposing the articulation of the unconscious that I gave you; what am I saying, responds the sophism? – except that I, too, lie, and, consequently, I can affirm nothing valid concerning not simply the function of truth, but even the significance of lying.

"Thou shalt not lie" as a negative precept has as its function to withdraw the subject of enunciation from that which is enunciated. Remember the graph. It is there that I can say "Thou shalt not lie" – there where I lie, where I repress, where I, the liar, speak. In "Thou shalt not lie" as law is included the possibility of the lie as the most fundamental desire.

I am going to give you a proof that is to my mind nevertheless valid. It concerns Proudhon's famous phrase: "Property is theft." Another proof is that of the cries of anguish lawyers emit whenever it is a question, in some more or less grotesque and mythical form, of using a lie detector. Must we conclude from this that the respect of the human person involves the right to lie? Surely, it is a question and not an answer to reply "yes, certainly." One might say, it's not so simple.

What is the source of that rebellion against the fact that something exists which may reduce the question of the subject's speech to a universally objectified application? The point is that speech doesn't itself know what it is saying when it lies, and that, on the other hand, in lying it also speaks some truth. Moreover, it is in this antinomic function between the law and desire, as conditioned by speech, that resides the primordial authority which makes this commandment among all ten one of the cornerstones of that which we call the human condition, to the extent that that condition merits our respect.

Since time is getting on, I will skip quickly forward to the issue that is the object of our discussion today relative to the relationship between desire and the law. It is the famous commandment that affirms the following – it makes one smile, but when one thinks about it, one doesn't smile for long: "Thou shalt not covet thy neighbor's house, thou shalt not covet thy neighbor's wife, neither his man servant, nor his maid servant, neither his ox, nor his ass, nor anything that belongs to thy neighbor."

Putting the wife between the house and the donkey has given rise to more than one idea that one can recognize there the exigences of a primitive society—a society of Bedouins, "wogs," and "niggers." Well, I don't agree.

The law affirmed there, the part concerning one's neighbor's wife at least, is still alive in the hearts of men who violate it every day, and it doubtless has a relationship to that which is the object of our discussion today, namely, *das Ding*.

It is not after all a question of just any good here. It is not a question of that which creates the law of exchange and covers with a kind of amusing legality, a kind of social *Sicherung*, the movements, the *impetus*, of human instincts. It is a question of something whose value resides in the fact that none of these objects exists without having the closest possible relationship to that in which the human being can rest as if it were *die Trude, das Ding* – not insofar as it is his good, but insofar as it is the good in which he may find rest. Let me add *das Ding* insofar as it is the very correlative of the law of speech in its most primitive point of origin, and in the sense that this *Ding* was there from the beginning, that it was the first thing that separated itself from everything the subject began to name and articulate, that the covetousness that is in question is not addressed to anything that I might desire but to a thing that is my neighbor's Thing.

It is to the extent that the commandment in question preserves the distance from the Thing as founded by speech itself that it assumes its value.

But where does this take us?

Is the Law the Thing? Certainly not. Yet I can only know of the Thing by means of the Law. In effect, I would not have had the idea to covet it if the Law hadn't said: "Thou shalt not covet it." But the Thing finds a way by producing in me all kinds of covetousness thanks to the commandment, for without the Law the Thing is dead. But even without the Law, I was once alive. But when the commandment appeared, the Thing flared up, returned once again, I met my death. And for me, the commandment that was supposed to lead to life turned out to lead to death, for the Thing found a way and thanks to the commandment seduced me; through it I came to desire death.

I believe that for a little while now some of you at least have begun to suspect that it is no longer I who have been speaking. In fact, with one small change, namely, "Thing" for "sin," this is the speech of Saint Paul on the subject of the relations between the law and sin in the Epistle to the Romans, Chapter 7, paragraph 7.

Whatever some may think in certain milieux, you would be wrong to think that the religious authors aren't a good read. I have always been rewarded whenever I have immersed myself in their works. And Saint Paul's Epistle is a work that I recommend to you for your vacation reading; you will find it very good company.

The relationship between the Thing and the Law could not be better defined than in these terms. And we will come back to it now. The dialectical relationship between desire and the Law causes our desire to flare up only in relation to the Law, through which it becomes the desire for death. It is only because of the Law that sin, ἁμαρτία – which in Greek means lack and nonparticipation in the Thing – takes on an excessive, hyperbolic character. Freud's discovery – the ethics of psychoanalysis – does it leave us clinging to that dialectic? We will have to explore that which, over the centuries, human beings have succeeded in elaborating that transgresses the Law, puts them in a relationship to desire that transgresses interdiction, and introduces an erotics that is above morality.

I don't think that you should be surprised by such a question. It is after all precisely something that all religions engage in, all mysticisms, all that Kant disdainfully calls the *Religionsschwärmereien*, religious enthusiasms – it's not an easy term to translate. What is all this except a way of rediscovering the relationship to *das Ding* somewhere beyond the law? There are no doubt other ways. No doubt, in talking about erotics, we will have to talk about the kind of rules of love that have been elaborated over the centuries. Freud said somewhere that he could have described his doctrine as an erotics, but, he went on, "I didn't do it, because that would have involved giving ground relative to words, and he who gives ground relative to words also gives ground relative to things. I thus spoke of the theory of sexuality."

It's true: Freud placed in the forefront of ethical inquiry the simple relationship between man and woman. Strangely enough, things haven't been able to move beyond that point. The question of *das Ding* is still attached to whatever is open, lacking, or gaping at the center of our desire. I would say – you will forgive the play on words – that we need to know what we can do to transform this dam-age into our "dame" in the archaic French sense, our lady.

Don't laugh at this sleight of hand; it was in the language before I used it. If you look up the etymology of the word "danger," you will see that exactly the same ambiguity exists from the beginning in French: "danger" was originally "domniarium," domination. The word "dame" gradually came to contaminate that word. And, in effect, when we are in another's power, we are in great danger.

Therefore, next year we will try to advance still further into these incontestably perilous waters.

December 23, 1959

THE PROBLEM OF SUBLIMATION

VII

Drives and lures

THE DOMAIN OF THE PASTORAL
THE PARADOX OF THE MORAL CONSCIENCE
WORLD AND BODY
LUTHER
THE PROBLEM OF THE OBJECT RELATION

During the retreat of the vacation, I felt the need to make a little excursion into a certain domain within the treasure house of English and French literature. "Quaerens," not "quem devorem," but rather "quod doceam vobis" – seeking what to teach you and how, on the subject that we are navigating towards under the title of the ethics of psychoanalysis. You can certainly sense that it must be leading us toward a problematic point, not only of Freud's doctrine, but also of what one might call our responsibility as analysts.

It is a point that you haven't yet seen rise up on the horizon. And, my goodness, there is no reason why you should, since up till now this year I have avoided using the term. It is something that is so problematic for the theorists of analysis, as you will see from the testimony of the quotations I will cite; yet it is so essential. It is what Freud called *Sublimierung*, sublimation.

1

Sublimation is, in effect, the other side of the research that Freud pioneered into the roots of ethical feeling, insofar as it imposes itself in the form of prohibitions, of the moral conscience. It is the side that is referred to in the world in a manner that is so improper and so comical to a sensitive ear – I mean in the world outside the field of psychoanalysis – as the philosophy of values.

We who find ourselves, along with Freud, in a position to give a radically new critique of the sources and the incidence of ethical thought, are we in the same fortunate situation concerning its positive side, that of moral and spiritual elevation, that of the scale of values? The problem seems much more uncertain and more delicate there, but one cannot for all that say we may neglect it for the sake of the more immediate concerns of straightforward therapeutic action.

In *Three Essays on the Theory of Sexuality,* Freud uses two correlative terms concerning the effects of the individual libidinal adventure: *Fixierarbeit* is the fixation that is for us the register of explanation of that which is, in fact, inexplicable, and *Haftbarkeit,* which is perhaps best translated by "perseverance" but has a curious resonance in German, since it means also "responsibility," "commitment." And that is what is involved here; it concerns our collective history as analysts.

We are caught up in an adventure that has taken a certain direction, a certain contingency, certain stages. Freud didn't finish at a stroke the trail he blazed for us. And it may be that, on account of Freud's detours, we are attached to a certain moment in the development of his thought, without fully realizing its contingent character, like that of every effect of our human history.

In accordance with a method you are familiar with – for if it isn't mine, it is at least known to me – let us try to take a few steps backwards, two, for example, before taking three steps forward. That way we may hope to gain one.

A step backward then: let us remember that psychoanalysis might seem at first to be of an ethical order. It might seem to be the search for a natural ethics – and, my goodness, a certain siren song might well promote a misunderstanding of that kind. And indeed, through a whole side of its action and its doctrine, psychoanalysis effectively presents itself as such, as tending to simplify some difficulty that is external in origin, that is of the order of a misrecognition or indeed of a misunderstanding, as tending to restore a normative balance with the world – something that the maturation of the instincts would naturally lead to. One sometimes sees such a gospel preached in the form of the genital relation that I have more than once referred to here with a great deal of reservation and even with a pronounced skepticism.

A great many things immediately present themselves in opposition. It is in any case in just such a simple way that analysis leads us in the direction of what, for reasons that I do not believe are merely picturesque, one might call the domain of the pastoral.

The domain of the pastoral is never absent from civilization; it never fails to offer itself as a solution to the latter's discontents. If I use that name, it is because over the centuries that is how it has happened to present itself openly. Nowadays, it is often masked; it appears for example in the more severe and more pedantic form of the infallibility of proletarian consciousness – something that has preoccupied us for so long, although in recent years it has receded a little. It appears also in the form of the somewhat mythical notion I referred to just now concerning the hopes, however vague, that were raised by the Freudian revolution. But it's the same old idea of the pastoral. And, as you will see, it concerns a very serious debate.

Perhaps we need to rediscover it, to rediscover its meaning. There is perhaps a good reason why we should reexamine the archaic form of the pastoral, reexamine a certain return to nature or the hope invested in a nature that you shouldn't imagine our ancestors thought of in simpler terms than we do. We will see whether the inventions that the *ingenium* of our ancestors attempted in this direction teach us something that needs to be elucidated for us, too.

Obviously, as soon as one takes a look at Freud's thought as a whole, one sees immediately that there is something that from the beginning resists being absorbed into this domain. And it is that through which I began to attack the problem of the ethics of psychoanalysis with you this year. Freud allows us, in effect, to measure the paradoxical character or practical aporia of something that is not at all of the order of difficulties that an improved nature or a natural amelioration can present. It is rather something that introduces itself immediately as possessed of a very special quality of malice, of bad influence – that is the meaning of the French word *méchant*. Freud isolates it increasingly in the course of his work up to *Civilization and Its Discontents*, where he gives it its fullest articulation, or in his studies of mechanisms such as the phenomenon of melancholia.

What is this paradox? It is that the moral conscience, as he says, shows itself to be the more demanding the more refined it becomes, crueller and crueller even as we offend it less and less, more and more fastidious as we force it, by abstaining from acts, to go and seek us out at the most intimate levels of our impulses or desires. In short, the insatiable character of this moral conscience, its paradoxical cruelty, transforms it within the individual into a parasite that is fed by the satisfactions accorded it. Ethics punishes the individual relatively much less for his faults than for his misfortunes.

This is the paradox of the moral conscience in what I hesitate to call its spontaneous form. Rather than speak of the investigation of the moral conscience functioning in a natural state – we would never find our way through that – let us choose the other dimension covered by the meaning of the term "natural"; and let's call it the critique, by means of psychoanalysis, of wild, uncultivated ethics, such as we find it functioning all alone, especially in those whom we deal with as we explore the level of affect or pathos, and of pathology.

It is here that analysis sheds some light, and it does so, in the end, on that which in the depths of man might be called self-hate. It is something that is suggested by the classical comedy whose title is *He Who Punishes Himself*.[1]

It is a little comedy which belongs to the New Comedy taken over from

[1] A play by Terence usually translated in Englsh as *The Self-Tormentor*.

Greece by Latin literature. I don't especially recommend that you read it, for after that fine title you would only be disappointed by the text. You would only find, like everything else, a concrete satire of character traits, precise notations of forms of the ridiculous. But don't forget that the function of comedy is only apparently without profundity. Through the very fact of the play of the signifier, through the simple force of signifying articulation, we find ourselves going beyond something that is simply depiction or contingent description, to the revelation of what lies below. Comedy makes us rediscover what Freud showed was present in the practice of nonsense.

We see the depths emerge, we see something that detaches itself beyond the exercise of the unconscious, there where Freudian research invites us to recognize the point where the *Trieb* is unmasked – the *Trieb* and not the *Instinkt*. For the *Instinkt* is not far from the field of *das Ding* in relation to which I invite you to recenter this year the way in which the problems around us are posed.

The *Triebe* were discovered and explored by Freud within an experience founded on the confidence he had in the play of signifiers, in the play of substitutions; the result is that we can in no way confuse the domain of the *Triebe* with a reclassification of human beings' associations with their natural milieu, however new that reclassification may seem. The *Trieb* must be translated insofar as possible with some ambiguity, and I like sometimes to say *dérive* in French, "drift." It is in any case "drive" that is used in English to translate the German word. That drift, where the whole action of the pleasure principle is motivated, directs us toward the mythic point that has been articulated in terms of an object relation. We have to be precise about the meaning of this and to criticize the confusions introduced by ambiguities of signification that are much more serious than the signifying kind.

We are now getting close to the most profound things Freud had to say about the nature of the *Triebe*, and especially insofar as they may give satisfaction to the subject in more than one way, notably, in leaving open a door, a way or a career, of sublimation. Within psychoanalytic thought, this domain has remained until now almost undisturbed; only the boldest spirits have dared to approach it, and even then not without expressing the dissatisfaction or unassuaged thirst Freud's formulations left them with. I will be referring here to a few texts found at more than one point in his work, from the *Three Essays on the Theory of Sexuality* to *Moses and Monotheism*, and including *Five Lectures on Psychoanalysis*, the *Introductory Lectures on Psychoanalysis*, and *Civilization and Its Discontents*.

Freud invites us to reflect on sublimation or, more exactly, he proposes – in a way that enables him to define the field – all kinds of difficulties that merit our attention today.

2

Since the problem of sublimation is situated for us in the field of the *Triebe*, I would like first to look for a moment at a passage taken from the *Introductory Lectures*, that is to say a work that has been translated as *Introductory Lectures on Psychoanalysis*. It is on page 358, Volume XI, of the *Gesammelte Werke*[2]:

> Therefore, we have to take into consideration the fact that the drives *[Triebe]*, the pulsating sexual excitements, are extraordinarily plastic. They may appear in each others' places. One of them may accumulate the intensity of the others. When the satisfaction of one is denied by reality, the satisfaction of another may offer total compensation. They behave in relation to each other like a network, like communicating channels that are filled with water.

We can see there the metaphor that is no doubt at the origin of that surrealist work which is called *Communicating Vases*.

Freud goes on, and I paraphrase, "They behave, therefore, in that way; and this is true in spite of the fact that they may have fallen under the domination or the supremacy of the *Genitalprimat*. Thus the latter must not be thought to be so easy to gather into a single *Vorstellung*, representation."

Freud warns us in this passage – and there are plenty of others – that even when the whole *Netz der Triebe* has fallen beneath the *Genitalprimat*, it is not so easy to conceive of the latter structurally as a unitary *Vorststellung*, a resolution of contradictions.

We know only too well that that in no way eliminates the communicating or fleeting, plastic character, as Freud himself puts it, of the economy of the *Triebregungen*. In short, as I have been teaching you for years, that structure commits the human libido to the subject, commits it to slipping into the play of words, to being subjugated by the structure of the world of signs, which is the single universal and dominant *Primat*. And the sign, as Peirce put it, is that which is in the place of something else for someone.

The articulation as such of the possibilities of *Verschiebbarkeit*, or the displacement of the natural attitude, is elaborated at length and ends up in this passage with the elucidation of the *Partiallust* in the genital libido itself. In short, an approach to the problem of *Sublimierung* must begin with a recognition of the plasticity of the instincts, even if one acknowledges subsequently, for reasons to be explained, that complete sublimation is not possible for the individual. With the individual – and as long as it is a question of the individual with all that that implies concerning internal dispositions and external actions – we find ourselves faced with limits. There is something that cannot

---

[2] S.E., *XV*, p. 345.

be sublimated; libidinal demand exists, the demand for a certain dose, of a certain level of direct satisfaction, without which harm results, serious disturbances occur.

But our point of departure is the relationship of the libido to that *Netz*, that *Flüssigkeit*, that *Verschiebbarkeit* of the signs as such. It is to this in any case that we are always brought back whenever we read Freud with an attentive eye.

Let me posit another essential point of articulation, necessary if we are to move forward once more.

It is obvious that the libido, with its paradoxical, archaic, so-called pregenital characteristics, with its eternal polymorphism, with its world of images that are linked to the different sets of drives associated with the different stages from the oral to the anal and the genital – all of which no doubt constitutes the originality of Freud's contribution – that whole microcosm has absolutely nothing to do with the macrocosm; only in fantasy does it engender world. That's Freud's doctrine, contrary to the direction in which one of his disciples, namely Jung, wanted to take it – this schism within Freud's entourage occurring around 1910.

This is important particularly at a moment when it is obvious that, even if one once located them there, there is no point now in seeking the phallus or the anal ring in the starry sky; they have been definitely expelled. For a long time even in scientific thinking, men seemed to inhabit cosmological projections. For a long time a world soul existed, and thought could comfort itself with the idea that there was a deep connection between our images and the world that surrounds us. This is a point whose importance does not seem to have been noticed, namely, that the Freudian project has caused the whole world to reenter us, has definitely put it back in its place, that is to say, in our body, and nowhere else. Let me remind you in this connection to what extent, in the period which immediately preceded the liberation of modern man, both scientific and theological thought were preoccupied by something that Freud did not hesitate to mention and to call by its name, but about which we never speak anymore, namely, the figure who was for a long time known as the prince of this world, *Diabolus* himself. The symbolic here is united with the diabolic, with all those forms that theological preaching has so powerfully articulated.

Read a little Luther; not just the *Table Talk*, but the *Sermons* as well, if you want to see to what extent the power of images may be affirmed, images that are very familiar to us because they have been invested with the quality of scientific authentification on a daily basis through our psychoanalytic experience. It is to those images that the thought of a prophet refers whose influence was such a powerful one, and who renewed the very basis of Christian teaching when he sought to express our dereliction, our fall in a world where we let ourselves go. His choice of words is in the end far more analytic than all that modern phenomenology has been able to articulate in the relatively gentle terms of the abandonment of the mother's breast; what kind of negligence is that which causes her milk to dry up? Luther says literally, "You are that waste matter which falls into the world from the devil's anus."

That is the essentially digestive and excremental schema forged by a thought that draws the ultimate consequences from the form of exile in which man finds himself relative to any good in the world whatsoever.

That's where Luther leads us. Don't imagine that these things didn't have an effect on the thought and the way of life of people of the time. One finds articulated here precisely the essential turning point of a crisis from which emerged our whole modern immersion in the world. It is to this that Freud came to give his approval, his official stamp, when he made that image of the world, those fallacious archetypes, return once and for all there where they belong, that is in our body.

Henceforth we are to deal with the world where it is. Do these erogenous zones, these fundamental points of fixation, open onto rosy possibilities and pastoral optimism? Does one find here a path that leads to freedom? Or to the strictest servitude? These erogenous zones that, until one has achieved a fuller elucidation of Freud's thought, one can consider to be generic, and that are limited to a number of special points, to points that are openings, to a limited number of mouths at the body's surface, are the points where Eros will have to find his source.

In order to realize what is essential and original in Freud's thought here, it is sufficient to refer to those openings that the exercise of poetic lyricism gives. According to a given poet, to Walt Whitman for example, imagine what as a man one might desire of one's own body. One might dream of a total, complete, epidermic contact between one's body and a world that was itself open and quivering; dream of a contact and, in the distance, of a way of life that the poet points out to us; hope for a revelation of harmony following the disappearance of the perpetual, insinuating presence of the oppressive feeling of some original curse.

Well now, Freud, on the contrary, emphasizes a point of insertion, a limit point, an irreducible point, at the level of what we might call the source of the *Triebe*. And it is precisely that that our experience then encounters in the irreducible character – once again the ambiguity is clear – of these residues of archaic forms of the libido.

These forms, we are told on the one hand, are not susceptible to *Befriedigung*. The most archaic aspirations of the child are both a point of departure and a nucleus that is never completely resolved under some primacy of genitality or a pure and simple *Vorstellung* of man in human form by androgynous fusion, however total one may imagine it. There always remain dreams of these primary, archaic forms of the libido. That is a first point that experience insists on and Freudian discourse articulates.

On the other hand, Freud reveals the opening, which at first sight seems limitless, of the substitutions that may occur at the other end, at the level of the goal.

I have avoided the word *Objekt,* which never fails to appear at the point of one's pen as soon as one begins to differentiate what is involved in sublimation. One cannot characterize the sublimated form of the instinct without reference to the object, whatever one does. In a minute I will read you some passages which will show you the scope of the difficulty.

It is a question of the object. But what does the object mean at that level? When Freud at the beginning of his more emphatic formulations of his doctrine begins his first topic by articulating that which concerns sublimation, notably in the *Three Essays on the Theory of Sexuality,* sublimation is characterized by a change of objects, or in the libido, a change that doesn't occur through the intermediary of a return of the repressed nor symptomatically, indirectly, but directly, in a way that satisfies directly. The sexual libido finds satisfaction in objects; how does it distinguish them? Quite simply and massively, and in truth not without opening a field of infinite complexity, as objects that are socially valorized, objects of which the group approves, insofar as they are objects of public utility. That is how the possibility of sublimation is defined.

Thus we find ourselves here in a position to hold firmly in our hands the two ends of a chain.

On the one hand, there is the possibility of satisfaction, even if it is substitutive, and through the intermediary of what the text calls a *Surrogate.* On the other hand, it is a question of objects that are going to acquire collective social value. We find ourselves here faced with a trap into which thought, with its penchant for facility, would love to leap, merely by constructing a simple opposition and a simple reconciliation between the individual and the collectivity.

It doesn't seem to be a problem that the collectivity might find satisfaction there where the individual happens to need to change his batteries or his rifle from one shoulder to the other; where, moreover, it would be a matter of an individual satisfaction that is taken for granted, all by itself. Yet we were told at the beginning how problematic the satisfaction of the libido is. Everything that has to do with the *Triebe* raises the question of plasticity and of limits. Thus the formulation suggested above is far from being one that Freud could adhere to.

Far from adhering to it, he establishes a relation in the *Three Essays* between sublimation in its most obvious social effects and what he calls *Reaktionsbildung.* That means that right away, at a moment when things cannot yet be articulated powerfully, for want of that component of his topic he will produce later, he introduces the notion of reaction formation. In other words, he illustrates a given character trait, a trait acquired through social regulation, as something which, far from occurring as a direct consequence or as in line with a specific instinctual satisfaction, necessitates the construction of a system of defenses that is, for example, antagonistic to the anal drive. He, therefore, introduces the idea of an opposition, an antinomy, as fundamental in the construction of the sublimation of an instinct. He thus introduces the problem of a contradiction in his own formulation.

Thus, that which is presented as a construction in opposition to an instinctual tendency can in no way be reduced to a direct satisfaction in which the drive itself would be saturated in a way that would have no other characteristic than that it succeeds in receiving the seal of collective approval.

In truth, the problem Freud raises relative to sublimation only comes fully to light at the time of his second topic. We will have to approach that from *Zur Einführung des Narzissmus* ("On Narcissism: An Introduction"), a work that is not only the introduction to narcissism, but also the introduction to the second topic.

3

In this text that our friend Jean Laplanche has translated for the *Society* and that you should look up in the *Gesammelte Werke,* Volume X, pages 161–162[3], you will find the following comment: "What we have to seek is that which now presents itself to us concerning the relations of this formulation of the ideal to sublimation. Sublimation is a process that concerns object libido."

I would just point out that the opposition *Ichlibido / Objektlibido* only begins to be articulated as such on an analytical level with the *Einführung*. This text complements the articulation first given by Freud of the fundamentally conflictual position of man relative to his satisfaction as such. That is why it is essential to introduce *das Ding* at the beginning.

That is *Das Ding* insofar as, if he is to follow the path of his pleasure, man must go around it. One must take one's time to recognize, to find out for oneself, to take one's time to see that Freud is telling us the same thing as Saint Paul, namely, that what governs us on the path of our pleasure is no Sovereign Good, and that moreover, beyond a certain limit, we are in a thoroughly enigmatic position relative to that which lies within *das Ding,* because there is no ethical rule which acts as a mediator between our pleasure and its real rule.

[3] S.E., *XIV*, p. 94.

And behind Saint Paul, you find the teaching of Christ when he is questioned just before the final Easter [la dernière Pâques]. There are two versions, that of the Gospel according to Saint Mathew and that of the Gospels of Mark and Luke. In Saint Mathew's Gospel, where it is clearest, he is asked, "What good must we do to achieve life eternal?" In the Greek version, he answers, "Why do you speak to me of good? Who knows what is good? Only He, He who is beyond, our Father, knows what is good. And He told you, Do this, Do that, Don't go any further." One just has to follow his commandments. Then after that there is the statement, "Thou shalt love thy neighbor as thyself." That's the commandment that appropriately enough, given its obvious relevance, is the terminal point of *Civilization and Its Discontents;* it is the ideal end to which his investigation by necessity leads him – Freud never held back from anything that offered itself to his examination.

I cannot urge you too strongly to appreciate, if you are able, what in Christ's answer has for so long been closed to aural apprehension, apart from that of knowing ears – "They have ears but they hear not," the Gospel tells us. Try to read the words of the man who, it is claimed, never laughed; read them for what they are. From time to time, you will be struck by a form of humor that surpasses all others.

The parable of the unfaithful steward, for example. No matter how seldom one has been to church, one is nevertheless used to having that parable trotted out. And it occurs to no one to be surprised by the fact that the Son of Man, the purest of the pure, tells us that the best way to achieve salvation for one's soul is to embezzle the funds one is in charge of, since that, too, may lead the children of light to grant you, if not a reward, then at least a certain gratitude. From the point of view of a homogeneous, uniform, and stable morality, there is some contradiction there, but perhaps one could confirm it with other insights of a similar kind – such as, for example, the terrific "joke,"[4] "Render unto Caesar that which is Caesar's" – and after that get on with it! It is a form of paradox that may lead to all kinds of evasions or ruptures, to all the gaps opened up by nonsense – those insidious dialogues, for example, in which the interlocutor always manages to slip out of the traps that are set for him.

To come back to our subject for the moment, the good as such – something that has been the eternal object of the philosophical quest in the sphere of ethics, the philosopher's stone of all the moralists – the good is radically denied by Freud. It is rejected at the beginning of his thought in the very notion of the pleasure principle as the rule of the deepest instinct, of the realm of the drives. This is confirmed in a thousand different ways, and is for example consistent with Freud's central question, which concerns, as you know, the Father.

[4] In English in the original.

To understand Freud's position relative to the Father, you have to go and look up the form it is given in Luther's thought, when he had his nostrils tickled by Erasmus. Reluctantly, after a great many years, Erasmus had finally published his *De Libero Arbitrio*, so as to remind the excitable mad man from Wittenberg that the authoritative Christian tradition, from the words of Christ to Saint Paul, Saint Augustine and the Church Fathers, led one to believe that works, good works, were not nothing, and that to be sure the tradition of the philosophers on the subject of the Sovereign Good was not to be just thrown out.

Luther, who up to that point had remained reserved in his relations with the figure of Erasmus – although he did privately indulge in a little irony on the subject – then published his *De Servo Arbitrio* in order to emphasize both the fundamentally bad character of the relations between men and the fact that at the heart of man's destiny is the *Ding*, the *causa*, which I described the other day as analogous to that which is designated by Kant as at the horizon of his *Practical Reason* – except that it is a pendant to it. To coin a phrase whose approximate Greekness I will ask you to forgive, it is the *causa pathomenon*, the *cause* of the most fundamental human passion.

Luther writes of the following – God's eternal hatred of men, not simply of their failures and the works of their free will, but a hatred that existed even before the world was created. You see that there are reasons why I advise you to read religious authors from time to time; I mean good ones, of course, not those who are all sweetness and light, although even they are sometimes rewarding. Saint François de Sales on marriage is, I assure you, better than Van de Velde on ideal marriage. But in my opinion Luther is much more interesting. That hatred which existed even before the world was created is the correlative of the relationship that exists between a certain influence of the law as such and a certain conception of *das Ding* as the fundamental problem and, in a word, as the problem of evil. I assume that it hasn't escaped your attention that it is exactly what Freud deals with when the question he asks concerning the Father leads him to point out that the latter is the tyrant of the primitive horde, the one against whom the original crime was committed, and who for that very reason introduced the order, essence, and foundation of the domain of law.

Not to recognize the filiation or cultural paternity that exists between Freud and a new direction of thought – one that is apparent at the break which occurred toward the beginning of the sixteenth century, but whose repercussions are felt up to the end of the seventeenth century – constitutes a fundamental misunderstanding of the kind of problems Freud's intellectual project addresses.

I have just finished a digression of some twenty-five minutes. And it was designed to tell you that, just after 1914 with the *Einführung*, Freud introduces us to something that dodges the issue again by articulating things that are, of course, essential, but of which one must know the context, namely, the problem of the object relation.

This problem of the object relation has to be read "Freudianly." You can, in fact, see it emerge in a narcissistic relation, an imaginary relation. At this level the object introduces itself only insofar as it is perpetually interchangeable with the love that the subject has for its own image. *Ichlibido* and *Objektlibido* are introduced by Freud in relation to the difference between *Ich-ideal* and *Ideal-ich*, between the mirage of the ego and the formation of an ideal. This ideal makes room for itself alone; within the subject it gives form to something which is preferred and to which it will henceforth submit. The problem of identification is linked to this psychological splitting, which places the subject in a state of dependence relative to an idealized, forced image of itself – something that Freud will emphasize subsequently.

It is through this mirage relation that the notion of an object is introduced. But this object is not the same as that which is aimed at on the horizon of the instinct. Between the object as it is structured by the narcissistic relation and *das Ding*, there is a difference, and it is precisely on the slope of that difference that the problem of sublimation is situated for us.

In a short note in the *Three Essays*, Freud gives us a kind of brief summary in the style of an essay on the difference that strikes us between the love life of antiquity, of pre-Christians, and our own. It resides, he says, in the fact that in antiquity the emphasis was on the instinct itself, whereas we place it on the object. The Ancients feted the instinct, and, through the intermediary of the instinct, were also ready to honor an object of lesser, common value, whereas we reduce the value of the manifestation of the instinct, and we demand the support of the object on account of the prevailing characteristics of the object.

Moreover, Freud wrote a great many other pages where he discussed disparaging commentaries on love life – commentaries made in the name of what? In the name of an incontestable ideal. You can read the following in *Civilization and Its Discontents:* "Among the works of that sensitive English author, Galsworthy, whose worth is universally acknowledged nowadays, I once really enjoyed one story. It was called *The Apple Tree*, and it shows how there is no room anymore in contemporary civilized life for the simple, natural love of two human beings of the pastoral tradition."[5]

The whole passage flows forth spontaneously in a way that I call excessive. How does Freud know that we emphasize the object, whereas the Ancients put the accent on the instinct? You will respond that there is no example of ideal exaltation in any Greek tragedy, unlike our own classical tragedies. Yet Freud hardly explains the question.

[5] S.E., *XXI*, p. 105, Note 2.

Next time we will have to compare our ideal of love with that of the Ancients by referring to some works of history and to a given historical moment that will also have to be defined. It is no more or less than a structuralization, a historical modification of Eros. It is, of course, of great importance that courtly love, the exaltation of woman, a certain Christian style of love that Freud himself discusses, mark a historical change. And I will be leading you into that territory.

It is nevertheless true, as I will show you, that in certain authors of antiquity – and interestingly enough in Latin rather than Greek literature – one finds some and perhaps all the elements that characterize the cult of an idealized object, something which was determinative for what can only be called the sublimated elaboration of a certain relationship. Thus what Freud expresses over-hastily and probably inversely, concerns a kind of degradation which, when one examines it closely, is directed less at love life than at a certain lost cord, a crisis, in relation to the object.

To set out to find the instinct again is the result of a certain loss, a cultural loss, of the object. That such a problem exists at the center of that mental crisis from which Freudianism emerged is a question that we will have to ask ourselves. The nostalgia expressed in the idea that the Ancients were closer than we are to the instinct perhaps means no more, like every dream of a Golden Age or El Dorado, than that we are engaged in posing questions at the level of the instinct because we do not yet know what to do as far as the object is concerned.

At the level of sublimation the object is inseparable from imaginary and especially cultural elaborations. It is not just that the collectivity recognizes in them useful objects; it finds rather a space of relaxation where it may in a way delude itself on the subject of *das Ding*, colonize the field of *das Ding* with imaginary schemes. That is how collective, socially accepted sublimations operate.

Society takes some comfort from the mirages that moralists, artists, artisans, designers of dresses and hats, and the creators of imaginary forms in general supply it with. But it is not simply in the approval that society gladly accords it that we must seek the power of sublimation. It is rather in an imaginary function, and, in particular, that for which we will use the symbolization of the fantasm ($\$ \lozenge a$), which is the form on which depends the subject's desire.

In forms that are historically and socially specific, the *a* elements, the imaginary elements of the fantasm come to overlay the subject, to delude it, at the very point of *das Ding*. The question of sublimation will be brought to bear here. That is why I shall talk to you next time of courtly love in the Middle Ages, and, in particular, of *Minnesang*.

In an anniversary way, since last year I talked to you about *Hamlet*, I shall speak about the Elizabethan theater, which is the turning point in European eroticism, and civilized as well. It is at that moment, in effect, that the celebration of the idealized object occurs that Freud talks about in his note.

Freud left us with the problem of a gap once again at the level of *das Ding*, which is that of religious men and mystics, at a time when we could no longer rely on the Father's guarantee.

January 13, 1960

VIII

The object and the thing

THE PSYCHOLOGY OF AFFECTS
THE KLEINIAN MYTH OF THE MOTHER
KANTIAN FABLES
SUBLIMATION AND PERVERSION
THE FABLE OF JACQUES PRÉVERT, COLLECTOR

We are progressing this year around an axis that I take to be essential, namely, that *Ding*, which is not without causing problems, indeed, not without causing some doubts to emerge as to its Freudian legitimacy, at least among those who reflect and who retain their critical intelligence, as they should, in the presence of what I formulate here before you.

I take full responsibility for *das Ding*, whose exact importance you can imagine to the extent that it has proved to be necessary if we are to make any progress. You will be able to appreciate its merits in the use made of it. But I will also be talking about it specifically again.

1

Some might say or think that I have only taken up a small detail of Freud's text in the *Entwurf*.

But experience tells us precisely that in texts like those of Freud nothing is outdated, in the sense that it is simply borrowed from somewhere, the product of scholarly parroting; nothing goes unmarked by that powerful articulatory necessity that distinguishes his discourse. That's what makes it so significant when one notices places where his discourse remains open, gaping, but nevertheless implying a necessity that I think I have made you sense on a number of occasions.

And that's not all. This *Ding*, whose place and significance I have tried to make you feel, is absolutely essential as far as Freud's thought is concerned; and as we go forward, you will see why.

What is involved is that excluded interior which, in the terminology of the *Entwurf*, is thus excluded in the interior. In the interior of what then? Of something that is precisely articulated at that moment as the *Real-Ich*, which means then the final real of the psychic organization, a real conceived of as hypothetical, to the extent that it necessarily presupposes the *Lust-Ich*. It is in the latter that one finds the first sketches of the psychic organization, that is to say, of the organism whose development shows us that it is dominated by the function of *Vorstellungsrepräsentanzen*. And these are not only representations but the representatives of representation – something that corresponds very precisely to the path taken by so-called psychological knowledge before Freud, insofar as it first took its form from atomism. That ideational elementarity is in brief the truth of the atomism involved.

Through a kind of essential need, the whole effort of psychology has been to try to free itself from that. But it can only free itself or rebel against atomism by failing to recognize that flocculation which submits its material – and the material here is psychic – to the texture on which thought is founded, in other words, the texture of discourse as signifying chain. It is the very web on which logic rises up, with both the surplus and the essential it brings with it, which is the negation, the "splitting," the *Spaltung*, the division, the rending, that the inmixing of the subject introduces there. Psychology is subjected to the atomic condition of having to use *Vorstellungsrepräsentanzen* because it is in them that psychic material if flocculated. Doubtless psychology attempts to free itself from this necessity, but its efforts to achieve it have thus far been crude.

I don't need to do more than remind you of the confused nature of the recourse to affectivity; it reaches a point where, even when the reference is made within analysis, it always leads us toward an impasse, toward something that we feel is not the direction in which our research can really make progress.

Of course, it is not a matter of denying the importance of affects. But it is important not to confuse them with the substance of that which we are seeking in the *Real-Ich*, beyond signifying articulation of the kind we artists of analytical speech are capable of handling.

As far as the psychology of affects is concerned, Freud always manages to give in passing significant and suggestive hints. He always insists on their conventional and artificial character, on their character not as signifiers but as signals, to which in the last analysis they may be reduced. This character also explains their displaceable significance, and, from the economic point of view, presents a certain number of necessities, such as irreducibility. But affects do not throw light on the economic or even dynamic essence which is sought at the horizon or limit from an analytical perspective. That is something more opaque, more obscure, namely, analytical metaphysics's notions concerning energy.

It is true that this metapsychology has come nowadays to be organized in strangely qualitative categories. One only has to remember the function recently advanced of the term desexualized libido. That reference to a qualitative notion is increasingly difficult to maintain on the basis of any experience, and even less on the basis of an experience that could be called affective.

We will perhaps look into the psychology of affects together someday. In order to impress upon you the inadequacy of what has so far been done on the subject, especially in psychoanalysis, I should simply like to propose to you a few incidental subjects to reflect on – an affect such as anger, for example. I am giving you there a few practical little exercises in passing. The use of precise categories that I invite you to refer to might perhaps explain why there has been so much interest in anger in the history of psychology and of ethics, and why we have been so little interested in it in psychoanalysis.

Does, for example, what Descartes says about anger satisfy you fully? The working hypothesis that I am suggesting, and we will have to see whether it does the trick or not, is that anger is no doubt a passion which is manifested by means of an organic or physiological correlative, by a given more or less hypertonic or even elated feeling, but that it requires perhaps something like the reaction of a subject to a disappointment, to the failure of an expected correlation between a symbolic order and the response of the real. In other words, anger is essentially linked to something expressed in a formulation of Charles Péguy's, who was speaking in a humorous context – it's when the little pegs refuse to go into the little holes.

Think about that and see if you find it useful. It has all kinds of possible applications, up to and including offering a clue as to the possible outline of a symbolic organization of the world among the rare animal species where one can, in fact, observe something that resembles anger. It is, after all, surprising that anger is remarkably absent throughout the animal realm as a whole.

The direction taken by Freudian thought has involved locating affect under the heading of a signal. A sufficient indication of this is that, by the end, Freud came to evaluate anxiety itself as a signal. What we are looking for, however, is beyond the organization of the *Lust-Ich* insofar as it is entirely linked in a phenomenal way to the greater or lesser investment of the system of the *Vorstellungsrepräsentanzen*, or, in other words, of the signifying elements in the psyche. This is something that is calculated to allow us to define the field of *das Ding* at least operationally, as we attempt to advance on the terrain of ethics. And since Freud's thought progressed from a therapeutic starting point, we can try to define the field of the subject insofar as it is not simply the field of the intersubjective subject, the subject subjected to the mediation of the signifier, but what is behind this subject.

With this field that I call the field of *das Ding*, we are projected into something that is far beyond the domain of affectivity, something moving, obscure and without reference points owing to the lack of a sufficient organization of its register, something much more primitive that I have already tried to describe to you in our previous discussion this year. It isn't just the register of the

Wille in Schopenhauer's sense of the word, insofar as, in opposition to representation, it is the essence of life whose support it is. It is a register where there is both good and bad will, that *volens nolens*, which is the true meaning of the ambivalence one fails to grasp, when one approaches it on the level of love and hate.

It is on the level of good and bad will, indeed of the preference for the bad at the level of negative therapeutic reaction, that Freud at the end of his thinking discovers once again the field of *das Ding*, and points out to us the space beyond the pleasure principle. It is an ethical paradox that the field of *das Ding* is rediscovered at the end, and that Freud suggests there that which in life might prefer death. And it is along this path that he comes closer than anyone else to the problem of evil or, more precisely, to the project of evil as such.

This is pointed to in everything that we have seen at the beginning of this year's seminar. Is it to be found in a corner of Freud's work where one might overlook it, might consider it as merely contingent or even outmoded? I believe that everything in Freud's thought proves that that is by no means the case. And in the end Freud refers to this field as that around which the field of the pleasure principle gravitates, in the sense that the field of the pleasure principle is beyond the pleasure principle. Neither pleasure nor the organizing, unifying, erotic instincts of life suffice in any way to make of the living organism, of the necessities and needs of life, the center of psychic development.

Clearly, the term "operational" has its value on this occasion as it does in all thought processes. This *Ding* is not fully elucidated, even if we make use of it. The label "operational" may leave you with a certain comic dissatisfaction, since what we are trying to point to there is precisely that which each and every one of us has to deal with in the least operational of ways.

I don't want to indulge in overdramatization. All ages have thought they had reached the most extreme point of vision in a confrontation with something terminal, some extra-worldly force that threatened the world. But our world and society now bring news of the shadow of a certain incredible, absolute weapon that is waved in our faces in a way that is indeed worthy of the muses. Don't imagine that the end will occur tomorrow; even in Leibnitz's time, people believed in less specific terms that the end of the world was at hand. Nevertheless, that weapon suspended over our heads which is one hundred thousand times more destructive than that which was already hundreds of thousands of times more destructive than those which came before – just imagine that rushing toward us on a rocket from outer space. It's not something I invented, since we are bombarded everyday with the news of a weapon that threatens the planet itself as a habitat for mankind.

Put yourself in that spot, which has perhaps been made more present for us by the progress of knowledge than it was before in men's imagination – although that faculty never ceased to toy with the idea; confront that moment when a man or a group of men can act in such a way that the question of existence is posed for the whole of the human species, and you will then see inside yourself that *das Ding* is next to the subject.

You will see that you will beg the subject of knowledge who has given birth to the thing in question – the other thing, the absolute weapon – to take stock, and you will also wish either that the true Thing be at that moment within him (in other words that he not let the other go or, in common parlance, "let it all blow up") or that we know why.

Well now, after that short digression that was suggested to me by the word "operational," and from a less dramatic point of view – one no longer dares say eschathological, given the very precise materialization of things – I will take up our discussion again where we are in effect concerned with the essence of *das Ding*. Or, more exactly, in what way are we concerned with it in the domain of ethics?

2

It is not just a matter of drawing close to *das Ding,* but also to its effects, to its presence at the core of human activity, namely, in that precarious existence in the midst of the forest of desires and compromises that these very desires achieve with a certain reality, which is certainly not as confused as one might imagine.

The demands of reality, in effect, present themselves readily in the form of social demands. Freud cannot not consider them seriously, but one has to indicate immediately the special approach he adopts; it permits him to transcend the simple opposition between individual and society, in which the individual is straightway posited as the eventual site of disorder.

Note right off that it is quite unthinkable nowadays to speak abstractly of society. It is unthinkable historically, and it is unthinkable philosophically, too, for the reason that a certain Hegel revealed to us the modern function of the state, and the link between a whole phenomenology of mind and the necessity which renders a legal system perfectly coherent. A whole philosophy of law, derived from the state, encloses human existence, up to and including the monogamous couple that is its point of departure.

I am concerned with the ethics of psychoanalysis, and I can't at the same time discuss Hegelian ethics. But I do want to point out that they are not the same. At the end of a certain phenomenology, the opposition between the individual and the city, between the individual and the state, is obvious. In Plato, too, the disorders of the soul are also referred to the same dimension – it's a matter of the reproduction of the disorders of the city at the level of the psyche. All of that is related to a problematic that is not at all Freudian. The sick individual whom Freud is concerned with reveals another dimension than that of the disorders of the state and of hierarchical disturbances. Freud addresses the sick individual as such, the neurotic, the psychotic; he addresses directly the powers of life insofar as they open onto the powers of death; he addresses directly the powers that derive from the knowledge of good and evil.

Here we are then in the company of *das Ding*, trying to get along with it.

What I am saying should in no way surprise, for I am only trying to point out to you what is going on in the psychoanalytical community. The analysts are so preoccupied with the field of *das Ding*, which responds so well to the internal necessity of their experience, that the development of analytic theory is dominated by the existence of the so-called Kleinian school. And it is striking to note that whatever reservations or even scorn another branch of the analytic community may express for that school, it is the latter that polarizes and orients the whole development of analytic thought, including the contribution of our group.

Let me suggest then that you reconsider the whole of Kleinian theory with the following key, namely, Kleinian theory depends on its having situated the mythic body of the mother at the central place of *das Ding*.

To begin with, it is in relation to that mythic body that the aggressive, transgressive, and most primordial of instincts is manifested, the primal aggressions and inverted aggressions. Also in that register which currently interests us, namely, the notion of sublimation in the Freudian economy, the Kleinian school is full of interesting ideas – not only Melanie Klein herself but also Ella Sharpe, insofar as on this point she follows Klein completely. Recently, an American author, who isn't at all Kleinian, has written on sublimation as the principle of creation in the fine arts. In an article that I shall come back to later, entitled "A Theory Concerning Creation in the Free Arts," after a more or less exhaustive critical examination of Freudian formulations on sublimation and of Kleinian attempts to explain its full meaning, the author, M. Lee, ends up attributing to it a restitutive function. In other words, she finds there more or less of an attempt at symbolic repair of the imaginary lesions that have occurred to the fundamental image of the maternal body.

I will bring the texts involved, if you don't know them. But I can tell you right away that the reduction of the notion of sublimation to a restitutive effort of the subject relative to the injured body of the mother is certainly not the best solution to the problem of sublimation, nor to the topological, metapsychological problem itself. There is nevertheless there an attempt to approach the relations of the subject to something primordial, its attachment to the fundamental, most archaic of objects, for which my field of *das Ding*, defined operationally, establishes the framework. It allows us to conceive of the conditions that opened onto the blossoming of what one might call the Kleinian myth, allows us also to situate it, and, as far as sublimation is concerned, to reestablish a broader function than that which one necessarily arrives at if one accepts Kleinian categories.

The clinicians who do on the whole accept them end up – I will tell you so now and explain why later – with a rather limited and puerile notion of what might be called an atherapy. All of that which is included under the heading fine arts, namely, a number of gymnastic, dance and other exercises, is supposed to give the subject satisfactions, a measure of solution to his problems, a state of equilibrium. That is noted in a number of observations that are still rewarding. I am thinking especially of Ella Sharpe's articles, which I am far from depreciating – "Certain Aspects of Sublimation and Delirium" or "Similar and Divergent Unconscious Determinants, which Subtend the Sublimations of Pure Art and Pure Science."

To read these papers is to realize how such an orientation reduces the problem of sublimation and yields somewhat puerile results. The approach involves valorizing activities that seem to be located in the register of a more or less transitory explosion of supposedly artistic gifts, gifts which appear in the cases described to be highly doubtful. Completely left out is something that must always be emphasized in artistic production and something that Freud paradoxically insisted on, to the surprise of many writers, namely, social recognition. These objects play an essential role in a question that Freud doesn't perhaps take as far as one would like, but which is clearly linked to the championship of a certain progress – and God knows that such a notion is far from being unilinear in Freud – to the celebration of something that achieves social recognition. I won't go any further for the moment. It is enough to note that Freud articulates it in a way that may seem completely foreign to the metapsychological register.

Note that no correct evaluation of sublimation in art is possible if we overlook the fact that all artistic production, including especially that of the fine arts, is historically situated. You don't paint in Picasso's time as you painted in Velazquez's; you don't write a novel in 1930 as you did in Stendhal's time. This is an absolutely essential fact that does not for the time being need to be located under the rubric of the collectivity or the individual – let's place it under the rubric of culture. What does society find there that is so satisfying? That's the question we need to answer.

The problem of sublimation is there, of sublimation insofar as it creates a certain number of forms, among which art is not alone – and we will concentrate on one art in particular, literary art, which is so close to the domain of ethics. It is after all as a function of the problem of ethics that we have to judge sublimation; it creates socially recognized values.

In order to refocus our discussion onto the level of ethics, one could hardly do better than to refer to that which, however paradoxical it may seem, has proved to be pivotal, namely, the Kantian perspective on the field.

Alongside *das Ding*, however much we may hope that its weight will be felt on the good side, we find in opposition the Kantian formula of duty. That is another way of making one's weight felt. Kant invokes the universally applicable rule of conduct or, in other words, the weight of reason. Of course, one still has to prove how reason may make its weight felt.

There is always an advantage to reading authors in the original. The other day I brought to your attention the passage on the theme of *Schmerz*, of pain, as a correlative of the ethical act. I observed then that even some of you to whom these texts were once familiar didn't pick up on the reference. Well now, if you open up *The Critique of Pure Reason*, you will see that in order to impress upon us the influence of the weight of reason, Kant invents for his didactic purposes an example which is magnificent in its freshness. A double fable is involved that is designed to make us feel the weight of the ethical principle pure and simple, the potential dominance of duty as such against all, against all that is conceived as vitally desirable.

The key to the proof lies in a comparison between two situations. Suppose, says Kant, that in order to control the excesses of a sensualist, one produces the following situation. There is in a bedroom the woman he currently lusts after. He is granted the freedom to enter that room to satisfy his desire or his need, but next to the door through which he will leave there stands the gallows on which he will be hanged. But that's nothing, and is certainly not the basis of Kant's moral; you will see in a moment where the key to the proof is. As far as Kant is concerned, it goes without saying that the gallows will be a sufficient deterrent; there's no question of an individual going to screw a woman when he knows he's to be hanged on the way out. Next comes a situation that is similar as far as the tragic outcome is concerned, but here it is a question of a tyrant who offers someone the choice between the gallows and his favor, on the condition that he bear false witness against his friend. Kant quite rightly emphasizes here that one can conceive of someone weighing his own life against that of bearing false witness, especially if in this case the false witness is without fatal consequences for the person bearing it.

The striking point is that the power of proof is here left to reality – to the real behavior of the individual, I mean. It is in the real that Kant asks us to examine the impact of the weight of reality, which he identifies here with the weight of duty.

To follow him onto this ground is to discover that he misses something. It is after all not impossible that under certain conditions the subject of the first scenario will not so much offer himself up to be executed – at no point is the fable taken to this point – but will at least consider doing so.

Our philosopher from Königsberg was a nice person, and I don't intend to imply that he was someone of limited stature or feeble passions, but he doesn't seem to have considered that under certain conditions of what Freud would call *Überschätzung* or overevaluation of the object – and that I will henceforth call object sublimation – under conditions in which the object of a loving passion takes on a certain significance (and, as you will see, it is in this direction that I intend to introduce the dialectic through which I propose to teach you how to identify what sublimation really is), under certain conditions of sublimation of the feminine object or, in other words, the exaltation we call love – a form of exaltation that is historically specific, and to which Freud gives us the clue, in the short note I spoke to you about the other day, in which he says that in the modern period the emphasis of the libido is on the object rather than on the instinct (which is in itself something that poses an important question, one that, with your permission, I will be introducing you to, one that requires you to spend a few sessions on something in German history whose form I referred to the other day in connection with Hamlet, namely, the *Minne*, or, in other words, a certain theory and practice of courtly love – and why wouldn't we spend some time on that given the time we give to ethnographic research? – especially if I assure you that it concerns certain traces within us of the object relation that are unthinkable without these historical antecedents), under certain conditions of sublimation, then, it is conceivable for such a step to be taken. After all, a whole corpus of tales stands for something from a fantasmic, if not from a strictly historical point of view; moreover, there are a great many stories in the newspapers that are relevant. All of which leads to the conclusion that it is not impossible for a man to sleep with a woman knowing full well that he is to be bumped off on his way out, by the gallows or anything else (all this, of course, is located under the rubric of passionate excesses, a rubric that raises a lot of other questions); it is not impossible that this man coolly accepts such an eventuality on his leaving – for the pleasure of cutting up the lady concerned in small pieces, for example.

The latter is the other case that one can envisage, and the annals of criminology furnish a great many cases of the type. It is something that obviously changes the facts of the situation, and at the very least the demonstrative value of Kant's example.

I have outlined then two cases that Kant doesn't envisage, two forms of transgression beyond the limits normally assigned to the pleasure principle in opposition to the reality principle given as a criterion, namely, excessive object sublimation and what is commonly known as perversion. Sublimation and perversion are both a certain relationship of desire that attracts our attention to the possibility of formulating, in the form of a question, a different criterion of another, or even of the same, morality, in opposition to the reality principle. For there is another register of morality that takes its direction from that which is to be found on the level of *das Ding;* it is the register that makes the subject hesitate when he is on the point of bearing false witness against *das Ding*, that is to say, the place of desire, whether it be perverse or sublimated.

3

We are only stumbling along here, following the paths of analytical good sense, which isn't, in fact, a very different good sense of the common or garden kind. What one finds at the level of *das Ding* once it is revealed is the place of the *Triebe*, the drives. And I mean by that the drives that, as Freud showed, have nothing at all to do with something that may be satisfied by moderation – that moderation which soberly regulates a human being's relations with his fellow man at the different hierarchical levels of society in a harmonious order, from the couple to the State with a capital S.

We must return now to the meaning of sublimation as Freud attempts to define it for us.

He attaches sublimation to the *Triebe* as such, and that's what makes its theorization difficult for psychoanalysts.

Please forgive me if I don't today read given passages of Freud that might perhaps bore you and that I will take up at the right moment, when you will understand the value of going in one direction or another, of confirming if we are really aligned with Freudian theory. But I don't believe I can hold the interest of most of you here without explaining what my aim is or where I'm taking you.

Sublimation, Freud tells us, involves a certain form of satisfaction of the *Triebe*, a word that is improperly translated as "instincts," but that one should translate strictly as "drives" (*pulsions*) – or as "drifts" (*dérives*), so as to mark the fact that the *Trieb* is deflected from what he calls its *Ziel*, its aim.

Sublimation is represented as distinct from that economy of substitution in which the repressed drive is usually satisfied. A symptom is the return by means of signifying substitution of that which is at the end of the drive in the form of an aim. It is here that the function of the signifier takes on its full meaning, for it is impossible without reference to that function to distinguish the return of the repressed from sublimation as a potential mode of satisfaction of the drive. It is a paradoxical fact that the drive is able to find its aim elsewhere than in that which is its aim – without its being a question of the signifying substitution that constitutes the overdetermined structure, the ambiguity, and the double causality, of the symptom as compromise formation.

The latter notion has never failed to cause problems for theoreticians and analysts alike. What can this change of aim mean? It is a matter of aim and not strictly speaking of object, although, as I emphasized last time, the latter soon enters into consideration. Don't let us forget that Freud points out early on that it is important not to confuse the notion of aim with that of object.

And there is a special passage that I will read you at the appropriate moment, but I will give you the reference right away. If I remember correctly, in *Einführung des Narzissmus* Freud emphasizes the difference that exists between sublimation and idealization as far as the object is concerned. The fact is that idealization involves an identification of the subject with the object, whereas sublimation is something quite different.

To those who know German I suggest you read a little article by Richard Sterba that appeared in *Internationale Zeitschrift* in 1930, "Zur Problematik der Sublimierungslehre" ["On the Problematic of the Doctrine of Sublimation"]; it summarizes the difficulties that analysts found in the notion at the time – that is after an essential article by Bernfeld on the subject and also one by Glover in the *International Journal of Psychoanalysis* of 1931, "Sublimation, Substitution and Social Anxiety."

This article in English will cause you much more difficulty. It's very long and difficult to follow because it literally parades the standard of sublimation across all the notions known to analysis at that time in order to see how one might apply it to this or that level of the theory. The result of this survey is surprising. It gives rise to a review of the whole of psychoanalytic theory from one end to the other, but it clearly shows, at least, the extraordinary difficulty that exists in using the notion of sublimation in practice without giving rise to contradictions, and this text is riddled with them.

I would like to try now to show you in what way we are going to posit sublimation, if only so as to be able to allow you to appreciate its functioning and value.

The satisfaction of the *Trieb* is, then, paradoxical, since it seems to occur elsewhere than where its aim is. Are we going to be satisfied with saying, like Sterba for example, that, in effect, the aim has changed, that it was sexual before and that now it is no longer? That is, by the way, how Freud describes it. Whence one has to conclude that the sexual libido has become desexualized. And that's why your daughter is dumb.

Are we going to be satisfied with the Kleinian register, which seems to me to contain a certain though partial truth, and speak of the imaginary solution of a need for substitution, for repair work with relation to the mother's body?

These formulae will provoke anyone who is not content with verbal solutions – that is, solutions without real meaning – into questioning more closely what sublimation is all about.

You should sense immediately which direction I intend to take. The sublimation that provides the *Trieb* with a satisfaction different from its aim – an aim that is still defined as its natural aim – is precisely that which reveals the true nature of the *Trieb* insofar as it is not simply instinct, but has a relationship to *das Ding* as such, to the Thing insofar as it is distinct from the object.

We have to guide us the Freudian theory of the narcissistic foundations of the object, of its insertion in the imaginary register. The object that specifies directions or poles of attraction to man in his openness, in his world, and that interests him because it is more or less his image, his reflection – precisely that object is not the Thing to the extent that the latter is at the heart of the libidinal economy. Thus, the most general formula that I can give you of sublimation is the following: it raises an object – and I don't mind the suggestion of a play on words in the term I use – to the dignity of the Thing.

That is significant, for example, in relation to something that I alluded to at the limit of our discussion, something I will get to next time, the sublimation of the feminine object. The whole theory of the *Minne* or of courtly love has, in effect, been decisive. Although it has completely disappeared nowadays from the sociological sphere, courtly love has nevertheless left traces in an unconscious that has no need to be called "collective," in a traditional unconscious that is sustained by a whole literature, a whole imagery, that we continue to inhabit as far as our relations with women are concerned.

This mode was created deliberately. It was by no means a creation of the popular soul, of that famous great soul of the blessed Middle Ages, as Gustave Cohen used to say. The rules of polite conduct were articulated deliberately in a small literary circle and, as a result, the celebration of the object was made possible – the absurdity of which I will show you in detail; a German writer who is a specialist of this medieval German literature has used the expression "absurd *Minne.*" This moral code instituted an object at the heart of a given society, an object that is nevertheless completely natural. Don't imagine they made love in those days any less than we do.

The object is elevated to the dignity of the Thing as we define it in our Freudian topology, insofar as it is not slipped into but surrounded by the network of *Ziele*. It is to the degree that this new object is raised to the function of the Thing at a certain historical moment that one is able to explain a phenomenon which, from a sociological point of view, has always struck those who considered it as frankly paradoxical. We will certainly not be able to exhaust the totality of signs, rites, themes and exchange of themes, especially of literary themes, that have constituted the substance and effective influence of this human relation, which has been defined in different terms according to the times and places of its occurrence – courtly love, *Minne,* and all the other forms. Just remember that the circle of male and female *précieux* at the beginning of the seventeenth century is the last manifestation of the phenomenon in our own cycle.

That is nevertheless not the last word on the subject, for it is not enough to say, "They did that" or "That's how it is," for the matter to be solved, for the object to come and play the required role. I am not concerned only with giving you the key to that historical event; what I seek in the end, thanks to that distant affair, is both to get a better grasp of something that has happened to us, relative to the Thing, as the result of a collective education that remains to be defined and is called art, and to understand how we behave on the level of sublimation.

The definition I gave you doesn't close the debate, first, because I must confirm and illustrate it for you, and, second, because I have to show you that, if the object is to become available in that way, something must have occurred at the level of the relation of the object to desire; it is quite impossible to explain it correctly without reference to what I had to say last year on the subject of desire and its behavior.

4

I will end today with a little fable in which I would like you just to see an example, albeit a paradoxical and demeaning one, that is yet significant for what goes on in sublimation. Since we have remained today on the level of the object and the Thing, I wanted to show you what it means to invent an object for a special purpose that society may esteem, valorize, and approve.

I draw on my memories for this fable, that you can, if you like, place in the psychological category of collecting. Someone who recently published a work on collectors and those sales thanks to which collectors are presumed to get rich, has long asked me to give him some ideas on the meaning of collecting. I didn't do it because I would have had to tell him to come to my seminar for five or six years.

There's a lot to say on the psychology of collecting. I am something of a collector myself. And if some of you like to think that it is in imitation of Freud, so be it. I believe my reasons are very different from his. I have seen the remains of Freud's collections on Anna Freud's shelves. They seemed to me to have to do with the fascination that the coexistence of [. . .][1] and of Egyptian civilization exercised over him at the level of the signifier rather than for the enlightened taste of what is called an object.

What is called an object in the domain of collecting should be strictly distinguished from the meaning of object in psychoanalysis. In analysis the object is a point of imaginary fixation which gives satisfaction to a drive in any register whatsoever. The object in collecting is something entirely different, as I will show in the following example, which reduces collecting to its most rudimentary form. For one usually imagines that a collection is composed of a diversity of elements, but it is not necessarily true at all.

During that great period of penitence that our country went through under Pétain, in the time of "Work, Family, Homeland" and of belt-tightening, I

[1] This ellipsis is there in the French edition.

once went to visit my friend Jacques Prévert in Saint-Paul-de-Vence. And I saw there a collection of match boxes. Why the image has suddenly resurfaced in my memory, I cannot tell.

It was the kind of collection that it was easy to afford at that time; it was perhaps the only kind of collection possible. Only the match boxes appeared as follows: they were all the same and were laid out in an extremely agreeable way that involved each one being so close to the one next to it that the little drawer was slightly displaced. As a result, they were all threaded together so as to form a continuous ribbon that ran along the mantlepiece, climbed the wall, extended to the molding, and climbed down again next to a door. I don't say that it went on to infinity, but it was extremely satisfying from an ornamental point of view.

Yet I don't think that that was the be all and end all of what was surprising in this "collectionism," nor the source of the satisfaction that the collector himself found there. I believe that the shock of novelty of the effect realized by this collection of empty match boxes – and this is the essential point – was to reveal something that we do not perhaps pay enough attention to, namely, that a box of matches is not simply an object, but that, in the form of an *Erscheinung*, as it appeared in its truly imposing multiplicity, it may be a Thing.

In other words, this arrangement demonstrated that a match box isn't simply something that has a certain utility, that it isn't even a type in the Platonic sense, an abstract match box, that the match box all by itself is a thing with all its coherence of being. The wholly gratuitous, proliferating, superfluous, and quasi absurd character of this collection pointed to its thingness as match box. Thus the collector found his motive in this form of apprehension that concerns less the match box than the Thing that subsists in a match box.

Whatever you do, however, you don't find that in a random way in any object whatsoever. For if you think about it, the match box appears to be a mutant form of something that has so much importance for us that it can occasionally take on a moral meaning; it is what we call a drawer. In this case, the drawer was liberated and no longer fixed in the rounded fullness of a chest, thus presenting itself with a copulatory force that the picture drawn by Prévert's composition was designed to make us perceive.

So now, that little fable of the revelation of the Thing beyond the object shows you one of the most innocent forms of sublimation. Perhaps you can even see something emerge in it that, goodness knows, society is able to find satisfaction in.

If it is a satisfaction, it is in this case one that doesn't ask anything of anyone.

January 20, 1960

IX

On creation *ex nihilo*

THE WONDERS OF PSYCHOANALYSIS
THAT WHICH IN THE REAL SUFFERS FROM THE SIGNIFIER
THE FABLE OF THE POT AND THE VASE
INTRODUCTION TO CATHARISM
THE DRIVE, AN ONTOLOGICAL NOTION

I will take up my discussion of the function I attribute to the Thing in the definition of sublimation with an amusing anecdote.

After leaving you the other day, I was conscious-stricken as I often am when I feel that I haven't exhausted the bibliography on a subject I am treating, and I looked up that very afternoon two articles by Melanie Klein that are referred to by Glover. They have been collected in *Contributions to Psychoanalysis*

The first of the articles, "Infant Analysis," of 1923, contains some very important things on sublimation and on the secondary phenomenon of inhibition – that is to say, on how, in Klein's conception, functions in the child that are sufficiently libidinalized through sublimation are subsequently subjected to an effect of inhibition.

I am not going to spend time on this, for it is to the very conception of sublimation that I want to draw your attention; all the misunderstandings that follow derive from the lack of insight into this problem.

It was the second, 1929 article, entitled "Infantile Anxiety Situations Reflected in a Work of Art and in the Creative Impulse," that I regretted not having looked at. It is short, but as sometimes happens, it gave me the satisfaction of fitting my purposes like a glove.

1

The first part is a discussion of the musical composition of Ravel based on a scenario by Colette, *L'Enfant et les Sortilèges*. I read it with pleasure, which was by no means guaranteed, since it speaks of the work in German and English translations.

Melanie Klein is amazed that the work of art follows so closely a child's fantasms concerning the mother's body, those concerning primitive aggression and the counteraggression it feels. In short, it is a quite long and agreeable statement of those features in the imagination of the creator of the work, and especially of the composer, that are in remarkable accordance with the primordial and central field of the psychic structure as indicated by the Kleinian fantasms derived from child analysis. And it is striking to perceive their convergence with the structural forms revealed in the work of art – not that all of this is fully satisfying for us, of course.

The second part of the article is more remarkable; it is this part that is amusing. Here it is a question of a reference to the article of an analyst called Karin Mikailis, who under the title "Empty Space" narrates a case history which has a certain piquancy. According to the four pages that summarize it, a striking limit case is involved. But it isn't described in such a way that one can offer a certain diagnosis or know if it should be described as melancholic depression or not.

The case concerns a patient whose life is briefly sketched out and who is called Ruth Kjar. She was never a painter, but at the center of the lived experience of her crises of depression this woman always complained of what she called an empty space inside her, a space she could never fill.

I won't bother you with the episodes of her life. In any case, helped by her psychoanalyst, she gets married, and once she is married things go well at first. Yet after a short period of time, we find a recurrence of the attacks of melancholia. And here we come to the wonder of the case. We find ourselves, in effect, in the domain of those wonders of psychoanalysis that works of this kind bring out, although not without a certain naive satisfaction.

For a reason that isn't made clear, the walls of the young couple's house are covered with the paintings of the brother-in-law, who is a painter, including one room in particular. Then at a given moment, the brother-in-law, who is talented, although we have no means of verifying this, sells one of his paintings, which he takes down from wall and carries away. It leaves an empty space on the wall.

It turns out that this empty space plays a polarizing and precipitating role in the attacks of melancholic depression that start up again at this point in the life of the patient. She recovers from them in the following way. One fine day she decides to "daub a little"[1] on the wall, so as to fill up that damned empty space that has come to have for her such a crystallizing power, and whose function we would like to know more about in her case, with a better clinical description. So as to fill up that empty space in imitation of her brother-in-law, she tries to paint a painting that is as similar to the others as possible. She goes to an artists' supply shop to look for colors that are the same as those of her brother-in-law's palette, and she begins to work with an enthusiasm that to me seems characteristic of the beginning of a phase tending

---

[1] In English in the original.

toward depression. And out of this there emerges a work of art.

The amusing part of the story is that when the thing is shown to the brother-in-law and the patient's heart is beating with anxiety as she waits for the connoisseur's verdict, he almost flies into a rage. "You will never make me believe that it is you who painted that," he tells her. "It's the work of an artist, not just an experienced artist, but a mature one. The devil take your story. Who could it possibly be?" They are unable to convince him, and he continues to swear that if his sister-in-law painted that, then he can conduct a Beethoven symphony at the Royal Chapel, even though he doesn't know a note of music.

This tale is narrated with a lack of critical distance at the hearsay involved, which cannot fail to inspire some reservations. Such a miracle of technique is after all worth subjecting to some fundamental questions. But it is not very important from our point of view. Melanie Klein finds confirmation of a structure that seems to her illustrated admirably there. And you cannot fail to see how that structure coincides with the central plan I use to present a topological diagram of the way in which the question of what we call the Thing is raised.

As I said before, the Kleinian doctrine places the mother's body there, and she locates the phases of all sublimation there, including such miraculous sublimations as that of this spontaneous accession – one might call it an illumination – of a novice to the most expert forms of pictorial technique. Mrs. Klein finds her theory confirmed – and that no doubt explains her lack of astonishment – by the series of subjects painted by her patient with the purpose of filling up the empty space. First, there is a nude negress, then a very old woman with all the signs of the weight of years, of disillusion, of the inconsolable resignation of extremely advanced age, and the series ends with the rebirth, the reemergence into the light of day, of the image of her own mother at the height of her beauty. As a result of which, we have according to Melanie Klein, Q.E.D., all we need to understand the motivation of the whole phenomenon.

The amusing thing here is surely what we are told concerning the topology in which the phenomena of sublimation are situated. But you must sense that we are left a little in the dark concerning its very possibilities.

I am trying to give you the information about sublimation required if we are to account for its relation to what we are calling the Thing – in its central position as far as the constitution of the reality of the subject is concerned. How can we define it more precisely in our topology?

The little example from last time borrowed from the psychology of collecting – an example that you would be wrong to hope exhausts the subject, although it does allow us to go quite a long way in the right direction – illustrates, in brief, the transformation of an object into a thing, the sudden elevation of the match box to a dignity that it did not possess before. But it is a thing that is not, of course, the Thing.

If the Thing were not fundamentally veiled, we wouldn't be in the kind of relationship to it that obliges us, as the whole of psychic life is obliged, to encircle it or bypass it in order to conceive it. Wherever it affirms itself, it does so in domesticated spheres. That is why the spheres are defined thus; it always presents itself as a veiled entity.

Let's say today that if the Thing occupies the place in the psychic constitution that Freud defined on the basis of the thematics of the pleasure principle, this is because the Thing is that which in the real, the primordial real, I will say, suffers from the signifier – and you should understand that it is a real that we do not yet have to limit, the real in its totality, both the real of the subject and the real he has to deal with as exterior to him.

In effect, the first relation that is constituted in the subject in the psychic order, which is itself subject to homeostasis or the law of the pleasure principle, involves flocculation, the crystallization into signifying units. A signifying organization dominates the psychic apparatus as it is revealed to us in the examination of a patient. Whereupon we can say in a negative way that there is nothing between the organization in the signifying network, in the network of *Vorstellungsrepräsentanzen*, and the constitution in the real of the space or central place in which the field of the Thing as such presents itself to us.

It is precisely in this field that we should situate something that Freud presents, on the other hand, as necessarily corresponding to the find itself, as necessarily being the *wiedergefundene* or refound object. Such is for Freud the fundamental definition of the object in its guiding function, the paradox of which I have already demonstrated, for it is not affirmed that this object was really lost. The object is by nature a refound object. That it was lost is a consequence of that – but after the fact. It is thus refound without our knowing, except through the refinding, that it was ever lost.

We come once again upon a fundamental structure, which allows us to articulate the fact that the Thing in question is, by virtue of its structure, open to being represented by what I called earlier, in connection with boredom and with prayer, the Other thing.

And that is the second characteristic of the Thing as veiled; it is by nature, in the refinding of the object, represented by something else.

You cannot fail to see that in the celebrated expression of Picasso, "I do not seek, I find," that it is the finding *(trouver)*, the *trobar* of the Provençal troubadours and the *trouvères*, and of all the schools of rhetoric, that takes precedence over the seeking.

Obviously, what is found is sought, but sought in the paths of the signifier. Now this search is in a way an antipsychic search that by its place and function is beyond the pleasure principle. For according to the laws of the pleasure principle, the signifier projects into this beyond equalization, homeostasis, and the tendency to the uniform investment of the system of the self as such; it provokes its failure. The function of the pleasure principle is, in effect, to lead the subject from signifier to signifier, by generating as many signifiers as are required to maintain at as low a level as possible the tension that regulates the whole functioning of the psychic apparatus.

We are thus led to the relation between man and this signifier – something that will allow us to take another step forward.

If the pleasure regulates human speculation with the law of the lure right through the immense discourse that isn't simply made up of what it articulates but also of all its action – insofar as it is dominated by that search which leads it to find things in signs – how then can the relation of man to the signifier, to the extent that he can manipulate it, put him in relationship with an object that represents the Thing? We thus come to the question of what man does when he makes a signifier.

2

As far as the signifier is concerned, the difficulty is to avoid leaping on the fact that man is the artisan of his support system.

For many years now I have habituated you to the notion, the primary and dominant notion, that the signifier as such is constituted of oppositional structures whose emergence profoundly modifies the human world. It is furthermore the case that those signifiers in their individuality are fashioned by man, and probably more by his hands than by his spirit.

And here we encounter linguistic usage that, at least in connection with sublimation in the sphere of art, never hesitates to speak of creation. We must now, therefore, consider the notion of creation with all it implies, a knowledge of the creature and of the creator, because it is central, not only for our theme of the motive of sublimation, but also that of ethics in its broadest sense.

I posit the following: an object, insofar as it is a created object, may fill the function that enables it not to avoid the Thing as signifier, but to represent it. According to a fable handed down through the chain of generations, and that nothing prevents us from using, we are going to refer to what is the most primitive of artistic activities, that of the potter.

Last time I spoke to you about a match box; I had my reasons and we will come back to it. It will also perhaps enable us to explore further our dialectic of the vase. But the vase is simpler. It was certainly born before the match box. It has always been there; it is perhaps the most primordial feature of human industry. It is certainly a tool, a utensil that allows us to affirm unambiguously a human presence wherever we find it. This vase which has always been there, and which has long been used to make us conceive the mysteries of creation by means of parables, analogies and metaphors, may still be of use to us.

To have confirmation of the appropriation of the vase for this purpose, look up what Heidegger affirms when he writes about *das Ding*. He's the last in a long line to have meditated on the subject of creation; and he develops his dialectic around a vase.

I will not be concerned here with the function of *das Ding* in Heidegger's approach to the contemporary revelation of what he calls Being and that is linked to the end of metaphysics. You can all of you easily go to the volume entitled *Essays and Lectures* and to the article on *das Ding*. You will see the function Heidegger assigns it of uniting celestial and terrestrial powers around it in an essential human process.

Today I simply want to stick to the elementary distinction as far as a vase is concerned between its use as a utensil and its signifying function. If it really is a signifier, and the first of such signifiers fashioned by human hand, it is in its signifying essence a signifier of nothing other than of signifying as such or, in other words, of no particular signified. Heidegger situates the vase at the center of the essence of earth and sky. It unites first of all, by virtue of the act of libation, by its dual orientation – upwards in order to receive and toward the earth from which it raises something. That's the function of a vase.

This nothing in particular that characterizes it in its signifying function is that which in its incarnated form characterizes the vase as such. It creates the void and thereby introduces the possibility of filling it. Emptiness and fullness are introduced into a world that by itself knows not of them. It is on the basis of this fabricated signifier, this vase, that emptiness and fullness as such enter the world, neither more nor less, and with the same sense.

This is the moment to point to the fallacious opposition between what is called concrete and what is called figurative. If the vase may be filled, it is because in the first place in its essence it is empty. And it is exactly in the same sense that speech and discourse may be full or empty.

That's a question that we took up at a certain conference at Royaumont, where I insisted on the fact that a mustard pot possesses as essence in our practical life the fact that it presents itself as an empty mustard pot. This comment, that must at the time have passed for a *concetto* or conceit, will find its explanation in the argument I am developing here. Go as far as your fantasy allows you in this direction. I don't, in fact, mind if you recognize in the name of Bornibus, which is one of the most familiar and opulent forms taken by a mustard pot, a divine name, since it is Bornibus who fills those pots.

We are limited to this – we are, so to speak, bound by Bornibus.[2]

The example of the mustard pot and the vase allows us to introduce that around which the central problem of the Thing has revolved, to the extent that it is the central problem of ethics, namely, if a reasonable power created the world, if God created the world, how is it that whatever we do or don't do, the world is in such bad shape?

The potter makes a pot starting with a clay that is more or less fine or refined; and it is at this point that our religious preachers stop us, so as to make us hear the moaning of the vase in the potter's hand. The preacher makes it talk in the most moving of ways, even to the point of moaning, and makes it ask its creator why he treats it so roughly or, on the contrary, so gently. But what is masked in this example of creationist mythology – and strangely enough by those who use the example of the vase, which is so familiar in the imagery of the act of creation (I told you that they are always writers who work at the borderline between religion and mythology, and there's a good reason for that) – is the fact that the vase is made from matter. Nothing is made from nothing.

The whole of ancient philosophy is articulated around that point. If Aristotelian philosophy is so difficult for us to think, that is because it must be thought in a style that never omits the fact that matter is eternal, and that nothing is made from nothing. In consideration of which, it remains mired in an image of the world that never permitted even an Aristotle – and it is difficult to imagine in the whole history of human thought a mind of such power – to emerge from the enclosure that the celestial surface presented to his eyes, and not to consider the world, including the world of interhuman relations, the world of language, as included in eternal nature, which is fundamentally limited.

Now if you consider the vase from the point of view I first proposed, as an object made to represent the existence of the emptiness at the center of the real that is called the Thing, this emptiness as represented in the representation presents itself as a *nihil*, as nothing. And that is why the potter, just like you to whom I am speaking, creates the vase with his hand around this emptiness, creates it, just like the mythical creator, *ex nihilo*, starting with a hole.

Everyone makes jokes about macaroni, because it is a hole with something around it, or about canons. The fact that we laugh doesn't change the situation, however: the fashioning of the signifier and the introduction of a gap or a hole in the real is identical.

I remember that one evening when I was dining at the home of a descen-

---

[2] Bornibus is the trade name of a well-known French manufacturer of mustard. The pun at the end of this sentence depends on a play of words between Bornibus and "se borner," "to limit oneself."

dant of one of those royal bankers who welcomed Heinrich Heine to Paris just over a century ago, I astonished him by telling him – he remains astonished up to this day, and is still clearly not ready to get over it – that modern science, the kind that was born with Galileo, could only have developed out of biblical or judaic ideology, and not out of ancient philosophy or the Aristotelian tradition. The increasing power of symbolic mastery has not stopped enlarging its field of operation since Galileo, has not stopped consuming around it any reference that would limit its scope to intuited data; by allowing free rein to the play of signifiers, it has given rise to a science whose laws develop in the direction of an increasingly coherent whole, but without anything being less motivated than what exists at any given point.

In other words, the vault of the heavens no longer exists, and all the celestial bodies, which are the best reference point there, appear as if they could just as well not be there. Their reality, as existentialism puts it, is essentially characterized by facticity; they are fundamentally contingent.

It is also worth noting that in the end what is expressed for us in the energy / matter equivalence is that one final day we may find that the whole texture of appearance has been rent apart, starting from the gap we have introduced there; the whole thing might just disappear.

The introduction of this fabricated signifier that is the vase already contains the notion of creation *ex nihilo*. And the notion of the creation *ex nihilo* is coextensive with the exact situation of the Thing as such. It is effectively relative to this that through the ages, and especially those ages that are closest to us, those that have formed us, the articulation or the balance of the moral problem is situated.

A passage in the Bible that is marked by a tone of gay optimism tells us that when the Lord completed his famous six-day creation, at the end he contemplated the whole and saw that it was good. You could say the same thing of the potter when he has made his vase – it's good, it's right, it holds together. In other words, it's always fine from the side of the work.

Yet everybody knows what may emerge from a vase or what can be put in one. And it is obvious that the optimism is in no way justified by the way things function in the human world, nor by what is born of its works. Thus it is around the question of the benefit or the cost of a work that the crisis of consciousness has crystallized, which in the West at least was in the balance for centuries and which ended in the period I referred to the other day, when I quoted a classic passage from Luther – a man who long tormented Christian consciousness,[3] to the point of affirming that no merit should be attributed to any work.

[3] This is one of the occasions when the single French word "conscience" implies both "consciousness" and "conscience."

It is by no means a heretical position without validity; there are good grounds for such a position. So as to orient you in the flood of sects that consciously or unconsciously broke away over the question of evil, the simple tripartition which emerges from the example of the vase, as we articulated it, is excellent.

In his troubled search for the source of evil, man finds himself faced with the choice of these three because there are no others.

There is the work, and this is the position of renunciation which other bodies of traditional wisdom than our own have adopted. Every work is of and by itself harmful, and it engenders the consequences that it gives rise to, that is to say, at least as many negative as positive ones. This position is formally expressed in Taoism, for example, to the point where it is barely tolerated for one to use a vase as a spoon – the introduction of the spoon into the world is already the source of a whole flood of dialectical contradictions.

Then there is matter. We find ourselves here faced with those theories that you have, I assume, heard something about, the theories of the sect called the Cathars – a name whose origin is unknown to us.

This is something I need to develop a little.

3

I am not going to give you a lecture on Catharism, but I will mention where you can easily find a good bibliography on the subject in a book that you have no doubt heard of, namely, *Love and the Western World* by Denis de Rougement. It's not the best book on the subject, nor the most profound, but it's fun to read.

I reread the whole thing in the revised edition, and on a second reading I disliked it less than I had expected. I even liked it. You will find expressed there in connection with the author's particular theory all kinds of facts which enable us to understand the profound crisis that Cathar ideology, or rather theology, represents in the development of Western man's thought, since it is Western man who is at issue here – although the author does show that the questions involved probably had their origin at the limit of what we usually call the West, a term that I have no particular fondness for, and that one would be wrong to see as the center of my thought.

In any case, at a certain point in the collective life of Europe, the question was asked as to what was wrong with the creation as such. It was asked by people about whom it is very difficult for us to know exactly what they thought, or what at a deeper level the religious and mystical movement we call the Cathar heresy, in effect, represented. One can even say that it is the only example in history in which a temporal power proved to be so efficient that it succeeded in eliminating almost all traces of the trial. Such was the *tour de force* realized by the holy Catholic church of Rome. We are reduced to seeking documents in out-of-the-way corners and few of them are very satisfying. The Inquisition's trial transcripts have vanished, and all we have are a few indirect testimonies here and there. A Dominican father tells us, for example, that the Cathars were good people, deeply Christian in their way of life and exceptionally pure in their morals.

I'm willing to believe that their morals were of an exceptional purity, since they had basically to desist from any act that might in any way favor the perpetuation of the world, considered as execrable and bad in its essence. The practice of perfection thus consisted essentially in seeking to achieve death in the most advanced state of detachment, which was a sign of reintegration into an Edenic world characterized by purity and light, the true world of the original good Creator, whose creation had been sullied by the intervention of the bad Creator or Demiurge. The latter had introduced that horrible element, generation, as well as corruption, which is to say transformation.

It is from the Aristotelian perspective of the transformation of matter into another matter, which engenders itself, that the perpetuity of matter became the site of evil.

The solution, as you see, is simple. It has a certain coherence, if it doesn't have all the rigor one would like.

One of the rare solid documents that we have on the enterprise, for we do not really know what was the basic doctrine of the Cathars, is a late work, which is, therefore, likely to provoke some doubt. It was discovered in 1939 and was published with the name the *Book of Two Principles*. It is easy to find under the title *Cathar Writings,* a fine book edited by René Nelli.

Evil is in matter. But evil can be elsewhere as well. The question remains open. And it is no doubt an indispensable key if one is to understand what happened historically to moral thought on the topic of evil. Evil may be not only in works, not only in execrable matter – from which the whole subsequent ascetic task will consist in turning away, without, however, entering the world we call mystic, and which might just as well be called mythic or indeed illusory – evil may be in the Thing.

It may be in the Thing insofar as it is not the signifier that guides the work or insofar as it is not the matter of the work either, but only insofar as, at the heart of the myth of the creation on which the whole issue depends, it maintains the presence of the human factor. And it should be noted parenthetically that whatever you do – even if you don't give a tinker's cuss for the Creator – it is nevertheless true that you think of the notion of evil and interrogate it in creationist terms. The Thing is, in effect, involved insofar as it is defined by the fact that it defines the human factor – although, as we know, the human factor escapes us.

In this connection the human factor will not be defined otherwise than in the way that I defined the Thing just now, namely, that which in the real suffers from the signifier.

Note the following: Freudian thought directs us to raise the problem of what it is exactly that one finds at the heart of the functioning of the pleasure principle, namely, a beyond of the pleasure principle, and very probably that which the other day I called a fundamentally good or bad will. It is, of course, true that all kinds of traps and temptations present themselves to your thinking, such as the question of whether what we call man – as if it were so easy to define man – is fundamentally good or bad. But it's not a question of that; it is rather a question of the whole. The fact is man fashions this signifier and introduces it into the world – in other words, we need to know what he does when he fashions it in the image of the Thing, whereas the Thing is characterized by the fact that it is impossible for us to imagine it. The problem of sublimation is located on this level.

That is why I have chosen the history of the *Minne* as a point of departure. I began there because it is of exemplary value, and because the word is unambiguous in German. The *Minne* is quite distinct from *Liebe*, whereas in French we only have the word "amour," love.

The problem posed for the author referred to is that of the link that may exist between the highly profound and secret heresy which began to dominate Europe from the end of the eleventh century on – although we don't know how far back things actually went – and the appearance, articulation, establishment, of a whole moral code, of a whole ethic, a whole way of life, that is called courtly love.

I am not forcing things in saying that once one has examined all the historical, social, political, and economic evidence, and applied all the available modes of interpretation of the superstructure, our contemporary historians are unanimous in giving up on the question. Nothing offers a completely satisfying explanation of the success of this extraordinary fashion at a period which was not, believe me, so mild or civilized – on the contrary. Society was just emerging from the first feudal period, which in practice can be summed up as being dominated across a large area of geographical space by the manners of bandits; and then one suddenly finds codes that regulate the relations between man and woman that have all the characteristics of a stupefying paradox.

Given the time, I am not even going to begin my discussion today. You should nevertheless be aware of what I shall be talking about next time. It will have to do with the ambiguous and enigmatic problem of the feminine object.

Don't imagine that it is something exclusive to me; I will not attempt to exercise my feeble powers of investigation on the subject. But the fact is that this object of praise, of service, of devotion, and of all kinds of sentimental, stereotyped behavior on the part of the defender of courtly love relative to the Lady, leads one commentator to say that they all seemed to have been praising the same person. And it is a fact that is calculated to leave us with a question mark. The Romance scholar in question is Mr. André Morin, a Professor in the Department of Literature at the *Université de Lille,* to whom we also owe a fine anthology of *Minnesang* published by Aubier.

The creation involved is a function of an object about which we naturally wonder: what was the exact role played by creatures of flesh and blood who were indeed involved in the matter? We have no trouble in naming the ladies and people who were at the center of the spread of this new style of behavior and of existence at the moment when it emerged. We know the first stars of this veritable social epidemic as well as we know Mr. Sartre or Miss de Beauvoir. Eleanor of Aquitaine is not a mythical figure, and nor is her daughter, the Countess of Champagne.

The important point will be to see how certain of the enigmas that historians raise in this connection may be resolved as a function of the doctrine that I am expounding here, the analytical doctrine. To what extent does it allow us to explain the phenomenon as a work of sublimation in its purest sense?

You will see in detail how it was possible to give an object, which in this case is called the Lady, the value of representing the Thing. So as to give you an idea of the path we will follow to the moment when I leave you in February, note that this will allow me to go on and show the subsequent developments of that construction relative to the feminine object, including the problematic character that it still possesses for us today. We will consider it in terms of the analytical structure.

Beyond the February break, my aim is to allow you to calculate at its true worth the originality of the Freudian contribution.

The idea of creation is cosubstantial with your thought. You cannot think, no one can think, except in creationist terms. What you take to be the most familiar model of your thought, namely, evolutionism, is with you, as with all your contemporaries, a form of defense, of clinging to religious ideals, which prevents you from seeing what is happening in the world around you. But it is not because you, like everyone else, whether you know it or not, are caught up in the notion of creation, that the Creator is in a clear position for you.

It is obvious that God is dead. That is something Freud expresses from one end of his myth to the other; since God derives from the fact that the Father is dead, that clearly means we have all noticed that God is dead. And that is why Freud reflects so intensely on the subject. But at the same time, because it was the originary dead Father that God releases, he, too, was dead from the beginning. The question of the Creator in Freud is, therefore, attached nowadays to that which continues to function on that level.

That is the goal of our inquiry this year; the form of the question concerning what the Thing is all about has to be addressed by us. It is something that Freud considers in his psychology of the drive, for the *Trieb* can in no way be limited to a psychological notion. It is an absolutely fundamental ontological notion, which is a response to a crisis of consciousness that we are not necessarily obliged to identify, since we are living it.

However we live it, in any case, the intention of what I am trying to expound before you is to attempt to make you aware of it.

January 27, 1960

X

Marginal comments

GNOMIC PROPOSITIONS
ART, RELIGION, SCIENCE
ON THE SUBJECT OF SPITZ
ANAMORPHOSIS AND ARCHITECTURE
THE PRIMACY OF THE *ES*

I am not this morning in the state of readiness I consider necessary for me to conduct my seminar in the usual manner. And this is especially the case, given the point we have reached, when I particularly want to be able to present you with some very precise formulas. You will thus allow me to put it off until next time.

The break caused by my absence of two weeks comes at a bad time, since I would have liked to go beyond what I announced last time that I would be dealing with – after having dealt with it, of course.

1

Courtly love is, in effect, an exemplary form, a paradigm, of sublimation. We only have essentially the documentary testimony of art, but we still feel today the ethical ramifications.

If on the subject of courtly love, apart from the lively archaeological interest in the matter, we still only have the documentary testimony of art in a form that is almost dead, it is obvious that its ethical ramifications are still felt in the relations between the sexes.

The long-lasting influence of the effects of a phenomenon that one might think is little more than an issue of aesthetics is thus of a kind to make us aware of the importance of sublimation – something that psychoanalysis has specifically foregrounded.

I would like to be at the top of my form in order to show you how the question has been posed historically, and how it is posed from the point of view of method, for I believe that there again we are in a position to throw some light on admitted difficulties that historians, Romance scholars, philologists, and various specialists who have approached the problem have encountered. They apparently recognize that they have in no way managed to reduce the phenomenon of courtly love in its historical emergence to an identifiable form of conditioning.

The recognition of the fact is common, and I would say almost uniform. One encounters a paradoxical phenomenon, one that is almost taken for granted; in every example of this kind scholars have often been led to examine influences – something that in many cases is only a way of displacing the problem. They tell us that the origin of the problem is to be found in the transmission of something that happened somewhere else. Yet we still need to know how that happened somewhere else. But in the event that is precisely what gets lost.

In this case, the recourse to influences is far from having illuminated the problem. We will try to approach the problem at its very center, and we will see that Freudian theory is of a kind to shed a certain light there. Thus in this way I take up the problem not only for its value as example but also for its value relative to method.

To start out from this very specific point doesn't mean that everything that concerns sublimation is to be considered from the perspective developed here, namely, from the point of view of the man / woman relation, of the couple. I do not claim to reduce sublimation to that, nor even to center it on that. I believe on the contrary that to start out from this example is essential in order to arrive at a general formula, whose beginnings we can find in Freud, if we know where to look for it – and I don't mean search for this or that detail.

If I proceed sometimes by emphasizing one of Freud's sentences, an isolated formula, or, I was about to say, some gnomic proposition, then I am very conscious of making that gnomic proposition work for me. When I give you a formula such as "The desire of man is the desire of the Other," it is a gnomic formula, although Freud didn't seek to present it as such. But he does so from time to time without doing it on purpose. Thus I once quoted a very short formula which brought together the respective mechanisms of hysteria, obsessional neurosis and paranoia with three forms of sublimation, art, religion and science. At another point he relates paranoia to scientific discourse. These clues will help us articulate in all its generality the formula in which we will in the end order the function of sublimation with reference to the Thing.

This Thing is accessible in very elementary examples, which are almost of the type of the classic philosophical demonstration, including a blackboard and a piece of chalk. I referred last time to the schematic example of the vase, so as to allow you to grasp where the Thing is situated in the relationship that places man in the mediating function between the real and the signifier. This Thing, all forms of which created by man belong to the sphere of sublimation, this Thing will always be represented by emptiness, precisely because it cannot be represented by anything else – or, more exactly, because it can only be represented by something else. But in every form of sublimation, emptiness is determinative.

I will point out right away three different ways according to which art, religion and the discourse of science turn out to be related to that; I will point this out by means of three formulas that I don't say I will retain at the end, when we have completed our journey together.

All art is characterized by a certain mode of organization around this emptiness. I don't believe that that is a vain formula, in spite of its generality, in guiding those who are interested in explaining the problems of art; and I believe I have the means of illustrating that to you in a variety of striking ways.

Religion in all its forms consists of avoiding this emptiness. We can illustrate that in forcing the note of Freudian analysis for the good reason that Freud emphasized the obsessional traits of religious behavior. Yet although the whole ceremonial phase of the body of religious practices, in effect, enters into this framework, we can hardly be fully satisfied with this formula. A phrase like "respecting this emptiness" perhaps goes further. In any case, the emptiness remains in the center, and that is precisely why sublimation is involved.

As for our third term, the discourse of science, to the extent that it finds its origin in our tradition in the discourse of wisdom or of philosophy, the term Freud uses in connection with paranoia and its relation to psychic reality, the term, *Unglauben*, finds its full meaning there.

I emphasized this fact in passing in a recent Seminar; *Unglauben* is not the negation of the phenomenology of *Glauben*, of belief. Freud never returned to the subject in a comprehensive and definitive way, yet it nevertheless runs throughout his work, and he gives extreme importance to this function in the *Entwurf*. The phenomenology of belief remained for him an obsession to the end; thus *Moses and Monotheism* is constructed in its entirety in order to explain the fundamental phenomena of belief.

More profound and more dynamically significant for us is the phenomenon of unbelief. It is not the suppression of belief, but it has to do with man's relationship to the world and to truth that is specific to man, a relationship he inhabits.

In this connection you would be wrong to trust in summary oppositions or to think that history has known sensational turning points, such as the supposed passage from the theocratic age to so-called humanist forms of liberation of the individual and of reality. The conception of the world is not decisive here. On this occasion, it has nothing to do with something resembling a *Weltanschauung* – and certainly not mine. I am only pointing the way here, I am only trying to help you orientate yourself in the bibliography of significant works on the subject, works by specialist who in their different fields are equipped with some talent for analysis. I advise you to look up the work of an historian, Lucien Febvre, who is the author of the widely accessible, *The Problem of Unbelief in the Sixteenth Century*. It is a work that enables you to see how the thoughtful use of historical methods allows us to pose more precisely the question of the forms of development of thinking on the subject of problems of faith.

If you have the time and you would like to read something amusing, you should read a little book by the same author that is supplementary but not secondary, not a little boat bobbing in the wake of a ship; it is called *Concerning the Heptameron*. The author of the *Heptameron* is Marguerite de Navarre, whom, I hope, you will not mix up with Queen Margot, the wife of Henry IV. She is not just a libertine author, but turns out to have written a treatise that is mystical in kind. But that is not something which excites the astonishment of the historian.

He tries to show us what the collections of tales that go under the title of the *Heptameron* might mean in the context of the time and of the psychology of their author. And he does it in such a way as to allow us to read that work with not so much a more informed eye as an eye that doesn't censure the text or, in particular, the reflections of each of the characters after each of the tales that are supposed to be true, and that certainly are for the most part. The thoughts of the respondents that belong to the register of moral and even formal religious reflection are usually censured because one assumes at the beginning that they are no more than the accompanying sauce. But that is something it is important not to get wrong – in any dish it is the sauce that is the essential ingredient. Lucien Febvre teaches us how to read the *Heptameron*. Yet if we knew how to read, we wouldn't need him.

As far as unbelief is concerned, it is from our point of view a place in discourse that is to be conceived precisely in relation to the Thing – the Thing is repudiated or foreclosed in the proper sense of *Verwerfung*.

In the same way that in art there is a *Verdrängung*, a repression of the Thing, and in religion there is probably a *Verschiebung* or displacement, it is strictly speaking *Verwerfung* that is involved in the discourse of science. The discourse of science repudiates the presence of the Thing insofar as from its point of view the ideal of absolute knowledge is glimpsed, that is, something that posits the Thing while it pays no attention to it. As everyone knows, this point of view has historically proved in the end to be a failure.

The discourse of science is determined by this *Verwerfung*, and, in the light of my formula that what is foreclosed in the symbolic reappears in the real, this is probably why it leads to a situation in which, at the end of physics, it is something as enigmatic as the Thing that is glimpsed.

I will postpone until next time a discussion of my paradigm of courtly love, an example of sublimation in art whose vital effects we still come across. We will take note of them after I come back from my trip; we will take a sampling of these traces, of the indisputable effects of the primary signifying construction that is determinative in the phenomenon of courtly love. And we will attempt to recognize in contemporary phenomena something that can only be explained through recourse to such an origin.

Since I am engaged in marginal commentary today, let me point out in passing that you would be wrong to think that this concept of the Thing to which I am giving a new development this year wasn't, in fact, immanent in our discussions of previous years.

Moreover, since there are those who question certain characteristics of my style, let me remind you for example of the expression "The Freudian Thing" that was the title of something I wrote, and it wouldn't be a bad idea for you to look it up. That text and that title surprised because if one starts to analyze my intentions from a philosophical point of view, one comes to relate them to a concern that was very popular at one time, namely, the resistance to reification. Of course, I never said anything about reification. But intentions can always be wrapped around a discourse. It is clear that if I chose such a title, I did so deliberately. If you reread the text, you will see that I am essentially speaking of the Thing. And I speak about it in a way that was evidently the cause of the undoubted discomfort the text provoked at the time. The fact is I sometimes make the Thing itself speak.

2

I would like now to make sure that today's meeting might be of some use to those who have travelled some distance to get here.

Given the point we have reached in my Seminar, it seems likely that some of you may have questions to ask me or answers to give, so as to suggest the meaning for them of some element or other in my argument.

I know that it is never easy to break the silence in a crowd, to ring one's little bell, so to speak. I will, therefore, give you the opportunity to ask me a written question. The only disadvantage there is that I am free to read it as I see fit.

At the same time we are going to do something unexpected that strikes me as a good idea. Some of you attended the scientific meeting of our Society yesterday. I don't know how it ended because I had to leave after having responded at some length to the lecturers, people for whom I have the greatest affection, and after I had expressed my deep interest in their work. They are here today and I would like to ask Smirnov for some clarification on the subject of Spitz's "No and Yes."[1]

[1] The words in quotation marks here and in the following paragraph are in English in the original.

Why did you not tackle the "Yes"? [Mr. Smirnov's answer.]

Let me explain to those who do not know the text that it is a book belonging to a series of investigations founded on the direct observation of newborn babies or more precisely of infants, that is to say, up to the point of the appearance of articulated language as such. Within this dimension, Spitz claims to find the "No" as a "pattern," as a semantic form in a certain number of gestures and expressions, and primarily in "rooting" – that is to say, in the oscillating gesture of the head that the infant makes in its approach to the breast. The word is very difficult to translate into French, but there is a correlative in the English text in the word "snout," which clearly indicates what is involved.

I am far from being critical of Spitz. I intend rather to defend him. I don't mean he is right, but the work is good and sharply articulated. And I would fault you with failing to have brought out the fact that the phenomenon is analogous to what occurs in traumatic neurosis – it is, he says, the last memory before the emergence of the catastrophic reaction.

I embarrassed you by asking you to comment on Spitz's other works, namely, his fiction on *The Primal Cavity* or at the very least his references to the screen of the dream.

Spitz doesn't on the whole elaborate on the fact that a form of reaction deriving from an earlier stage may be used in a critical situation. That seems to be a very useful idea, however, something that should always be emphasized. I think you made the point, unless it was Laplanche.

Spitz is reduced to having a mechanism as passive as that of traumatic neurosis intervene. He thus implies some preceding frustration of the infant. He considers the act of "rooting" to be a trace which remains inscribed after something like the refusal or withdrawal of the breast that immediately precedes it. It is surprising that he expresses it in an isolated form, on the basis of a given case, and not in general.

[Statements by Mr. Smirnov and Laplanche; a question from Mr. Audouard: "Why do you speak to us about the Thing instead of simply speaking about mediation?"]

To answer you briefly right away, I note that you have always been attentive to the note of what one might call Hegelian reinterpretations of analytical experience. We are concerned here with the Freudian experience as an ethics, which is to say, at its most essential level, since it directs us towards a therapeutic form of action that, whether we like it or not, is included in the register or in the terms of an ethics. And the more we deny this, the more it is the case. Experience demonstrates this: a form of analysis that boasts of its highly scientific distinctiveness gives rise to normative notions that I characterize by evoking the curse Saint Matthew utters on those who make the bundles heavier when they are to be carried by others. Strengthening the categories of affective normativity produces disturbing results.

It is clear that we put the accent on the irreducible element in the instinct, on that which appears at the limit of a mediation and that reification is unable to encompass. But in encircling that something whose limits we explore, we are encircling the empty image.

The deliberate intention to emphasize this notion has never been absent from what I have said thus far. If you look up the texts I referred you to on this subject, you will see that there is no ambiguity. That Hegelian radicalism that was rashly attributed to me somewhere by a contributor to *Les Temps Modernes* should in no way be imputed to me. The whole dialectic of desire that I developed here, and that I was beginning at the very moment the rash individual was writing that particular sentence, is sharply distinguished from such Hegelianism. It is even more marked this year. The inevitable character seems to me to be especially marked in the effect of sublimation.

Mr. X: The formula for sublimation that you have given us is to raise the object to the dignity of the Thing. This Thing doesn't exist to start with, because sublimation is going to bring us to it. The question I have is, therefore, isn't this Thing not really a thing, but on the contrary a Non-Thing, and isn't it through sublimation that one comes to see it as being the Thing (. . .)?

What you are saying strikes me as on the right track; it's obvious you follow my presentation of these questions without difficulty. Something is offered to us as analysts, if we follow the sum of our experience and if we know how to evaluate it. You state that the attempt at sublimation tends in the end to realize the Thing or to save it. It's true and it's not true. There's an illusion there.

3

Neither science nor religion is of a kind to save the Thing or to give it to us, because the magic circle that separates us from it is imposed by our relation to the signifier. As I have told you, the Thing is that which in the real suffers from this fundamental, initial relation, which commits man to the ways of the signifier by reason of the fact that he is subjected to what Freud calls the pleasure principle, and which, I hope it is clear in your minds, is nothing else than the dominance of the signifier – I, of course, mean the true pleasure principle as it functions in Freud.

In brief, it is the effect of the influence of the signifier on the psychic real that is involved, and it is for this reason that the activity of sublimation is not purely and simply senseless in all its forms – one responds with whatever is at hand.

I wanted to have here today, so as to be able to show it to you at the end of the Seminar, an object that to be understood, if not to be described, demands a long commentary on the history of art. That one managed to construct such an object and to find pleasure in it requires that we make a significant detour.

I will describe it to you. It is an object that embodies an anamorphosis. I assume that many of you know what that is. It is any kind of construction that is made in such a way that by means of an optical transposition a certain form that wasn't visible at first sight transforms itself into a readable image. The pleasure is found in seeing its emergence from an indecipherable form.

Such a thing is extremely widespread in the history of art. Just go to the Louvre; you will see Holbein's painting of *The Ambassadors* and at the feet of one of the two men, who is just as well built as you or I, you will see an enigmatic form stretched out on the ground. It looks roughly like fried eggs. If you place yourself at a certain angle from which the painting itself disappears in all its relief by reason of the converging lines of its perspective, you will see a death's head appear, the sign of the classic theme of *vanitas*. And this is found in a proper painting, a painting commissioned by the ambassadors in England, who must have been very pleased with his work; and what was at the bottom must have amused them a lot, too.

This phenomenon is datable. It was in the sixteenth and seventeenth centuries that things reached this point of heightened interest and even of fascination. In a chapel built by order of the Jesuits in Descartes's time, there existed a whole wall some eighteen meters long that represented a scene from the life of the saints or a nativity scene, and that was completely unreadable from any point in the room, but if one entered by a certain corridor, you can see for a brief moment the extraordinarily dispersed lines come together and perceive the body of the scene.

The anamorphosis I wanted to bring here is much less voluminous. It belongs to the collector I have already referred to. It is formed of a polished cylinder that has the function of a mirror, and around it you put a kind of bib or flat surface on which there are also indecipherable lines. When you stand at a certain angle, you see the image concerned emerge in the cylindrical mirror; in this case it is a beautiful anamorphosis of a painting of the crucifixion copied from Rubens.

This object could never have been produced, never have had a necessary meaning without a whole preceding development. There is behind it the whole history of architecture as well as that of painting, their combination and the history of this combination.

To put it briefly, primitive architecture can be defined as something organized around emptiness. That is also the authentic impression that the forms of a cathedral like Saint Mark's give us, and it is the true meaning of all architecture. Then subsequently, for economic reasons, one is satisfied with painting images of that architecture, one learns to paint architecture on the walls of architecture; and painting, too, is first of all something that is organized around emptiness. Since it is a matter of finding once more the sacred emptiness of architecture in the less marked medium of painting, the attempt is made to create something that resembles it more and more closely, that is to say, perspective is discovered.

The following stage is paradoxical and quite amusing; it shows how one strangles oneself with one's own knots.

From the moment when perspective was discovered in painting, a form of architecture appears that adopts the perspectivism of painting. Palladio's art, for example, makes this very obvious. Go and see Palladio's theater in Vicenze, a little masterpiece of its kind that is in any case instructive and exemplary. Neoclassical architecture submits itself to the laws of perspective, plays with them, and makes them its own. That is, it places them inside of something that was done in painting in order to find once again the emptiness of primitive architecture.

From that point on one is entangled in a knot which seems to flee increasingly from the meaning of this emptiness. And I believe that the Baroque return to the play of forms, to all manner of devices, including anamorphosis, is an effort to restore the true meaning of artistic inquiry; artists use the discovery of the property of lines to make something emerge that is precisely there where one has lost one's bearings or, strictly speaking, nowhere.

Rubens' painting that suddenly appears in the place of the unintelligible image reveals what is at issue here. At issue, in an analogical or anamorphic form, is the effort to point once again to the fact that what we seek in the illusion is something in which the illusion as such in some way transcends itself, destroys itself, by demonstrating that it is only there as a signifier.

And it is this which lends primacy to the domain of language above all, since with language we only ever have to do with the signifier in all cases. That is why in raising the problems of the relationship of art to sublimation, I will begin with courtly love. One finds there texts which show in an exemplary way its conventional side, in the sense that language always involves artifice relative to anything intuitive, material or lived.

This phenomenon is all the more striking since we see it develop at a period of uninhibited fucking. I mean that they didn't attempt to hide it, didn't mince their words.

The coexistence of two styles on the subject is the remarkable thing.

You introduce the idea of the Thing and the Non-Thing. It is, if you like, true that the Thing is also the Non-Thing. In reality, the Non- as such is certainly not individualized in a significant way. Exactly the same problem is posed by the Freudian notion of *Todestrieb*, whereas Freud tells us at the same time that there is no negation in the unconscious.

We don't make a philosophy out of it. I remind you of the notion that I modified the other day, so as not to give the impression that I don't accept my responsibilities: when I talk about the Thing, I am certainly talking about something. But I am, of course, talking operationally, with reference to the place that it occupies in a certain logical stage of our thought and of our conceptualization, with reference to its function in what concerns us.

Yesterday evening I referred to and denounced the substitution for Freud's whole classic topology of the term "ego" – something that is particularly regrettable in someone as deeply immersed in analytical thought as Spitz.

It is indeed difficult to recognize in that concept the essential function with which analytical experience began, that was its shock value as well as its echo and suite. Let us not forget that Freud, in effect, immediately countered it with the invention of the term *das Es*. That primacy of the *Es* is now completely forgotten.

To some extent, the *Es* is not sufficiently emphasized by the way it is presented in the texts of the second topic. It is to remind us of the primordial and primary character of this intuition in our experience at the level of ethics that this year I am calling a certain zone of reference "the Thing."

Mr. Laplanche: I would like to ask a further question on the relationship of the pleasure principle to the play of the signifier.

This relationship is founded on the fact that the pleasure principle basically involves the sphere of investment, *Besetzung*, and its *Bahnungen*, and it is facilitated by the *Vorstellungen* and even more by what Freud calls the *Vorstellungsrepräsentanzen* – a term that appears very early, before the article on the *Unconscious*. Each time a state of need arises, the pleasure principle tends to provoke a reinvestment in its content – in inverted commas, that is, since at this metapsychological level clinical practice is not involved – an hallucinated reinvestment of what had previously been a satisfying hallucination.

The diffuse energy of the pleasure principle tends toward this reinvestment of representation. The intervention of the reality principle can only therefore be a radical one; it is never a second stage. Naturally, there is no adaptation to reality that doesn't involve a phenomenon of tasting, of sampling, by means of which the subject manages to monitor, one might almost say with his tongue, that which enables him to be sure that he isn't dreaming.

This is what constitutes the originality of Freud's thought and no one, moreover, has been mistaken about that. It is both paradoxical and provocative. Before Freud no one has ever dared articulate the functioning of the psychic apparatus in that way. He describes it on the basis of his experience of the irreducible element he saw emerge at the core of hysterical substitutions; the first thing that poor, defenseless man can do when he is tortured by need is to begin to hallucinate his satisfaction, and after that he can only monitor the situation. Fortunately, he more or less makes at the same time the gestures required to attach himself to the zone in which this hallucination coincides with the real in an approximative form.

If the basic texts are to be respected, that's the miserable beginning from which the whole dialectic of experience is articulated in Freudian terms. That's what I told you when I discussed the relationship between the pleasure principle and the signifier.

Thus the *Vorstellungen* have right from the beginning the character of a signifying structure.

February 3, 1960

XI

Courtly love as anamorphosis

ON THE HISTORY AND ENDS OF ART
THE SUBLIMATION OF THE FATHER
ON THE SUBJECT OF BERNFELD
THE VACUOLE AND THE INHUMAN PARTNER
NEGOTIATING THE DETOUR

Why is this example of anamorphosis on this table?[1] It is here to illustrate my ideas.

Last Time I sketched out the meaning or the goal of art in the usual sense we give that term – the fine arts, for example. I'm not the only psychoanalyst to have been interested in that. I've already mentioned Ella Sharpe's article on the subject of sublimation, an article that starts out with the cave walls of Altamira, which is the earliest decorated cave to have been discovered. Perhaps what we described as the central place, as the intimate exteriority or "extimacy," that is the Thing, will help us to shed light on the question or mystery that remains for those who are interested in prehistoric art, namely, its site as such.

1

It is surprising that an underground cavern was chosen. Such a site only creates obstacles to the viewing that one assumes is presupposed by the creation and observation of the striking images which decorate the walls. The production of images and their viewing could not have been easy given the forms of lighting available to primitive men. Yet in the beginning those paintings that we take to be the earliest productions of primitive art were thrown up on the walls of a cavern.

One could call them tests in both senses of the word, subjective and objective. Tests no doubt for the artist, for, as you know, these images are often painted over each other; it's as if in a consecrated spot it represented, for each subject capable of undertaking such an exercise, the opportunity to draw or project afresh what he needed to bear witness to, and to do so moreover over what had already been done before. That suggests the idea of something

---

[1] For a description of an anamorphosis in the form of an object, see page 135.

like the updating of a certain creative potential. Tests also in the objective sense, for these images cannot fail to seize us as being deeply linked both in a tight relationship to the world – and by that I mean to the very subsistence of populations that seem to have been composed chiefly of hunters – and to something that in its subsistence appears as possessing the character of a beyond of the sacred – something that we are precisely trying to identify in its most general form by the term, the Thing. I would say it is primitive subsistence viewed from the perspective of the Thing.

There is a line which runs from that point to the other end, infinitely closer to us, in the exercise of anamorphosis, probably around the beginning of the seventeenth century. And I pointed out the interest that exercises of this kind had for the constructive thought of artists. I tried to make you understand briefly how the genesis of this tradition might be sketched.

In the same way that the exercise on the wall consists in fixing the invisible inhabitant of the cavern, we see the link forged between the temple, as a construction around emptiness that designates the place of the Thing, to the figuration of emptiness on the walls of this emptiness itself – to the extent that painting progressively learns to master this emptiness, to take such a tight hold of it that painting becomes dedicated to fixing it in the form of the illusion of space.

I am moving fast and I just throw out these crumbs so that you can put them to the test of whatever you may subsequently read on the subject.

Before the systematic establishment of geometrical laws of perspective formulated at the end of the fifteenth and the beginning of the sixteenth centuries, painting passed through a stage in which various artifices made it possible to structure space. The double band that appears in the sixth and seventh centuries on the walls of Santa Maria Maggiore is one way of treating certain stereognoses. But let's leave that aside. The important thing is that at a given moment one arrives at illusion. Around it one finds a sensitive spot, a lesion, a locus of pain, a point of reversal of the whole of history, insofar as it is the history of art and insofar as we are implicated in it; that point concerns the notion that the illusion of space is different from the creation of emptiness. It is this that the appearance of anamorphoses at the end of sixteenth and the beginning of the seventeenth centuries represents.

I spoke last time of a Jesuit convent; it was a mistake. I checked in Baltrusaïtis's excellent dictionary of anamorphoses, and it is a convent of the Minim Friars in Rome as well as in Paris. I don't know why I also placed Holbein's *Ambassadors* in the Louvre, when the painting is in the National Gallery in London. You will find in Baltrusaïtis's book a subtle study of that painting and of the skull that emerges when, having passed in front of it, you leave the room by a door located so that you see it in its sinister truth, at the very moment when you turn around to look at it for the last time.

Thus, as I say, the interest of anamorphosis is described as a turning point when the artist completely reverses the use of that illusion of space, when he forces it to enter into the original goal, that is to transform it into the support of the hidden reality – it being understood that, to a certain extent, a work of art always involves encircling the Thing.

This also allows us to approach a little closer to the unanswered question on the ends of art: is the end of art imitation or non-imitation? Does art imitate what it represents? If you begin by posing the question in those terms, you are already caught in the trap, and there is no way out of remaining in the impasse in which we find ourselves between figurative and so-called abstract art.

We can only sense the aberration that is articulated in the unyielding position of the philosopher; Plato places art at the lowest level among human works, since for him everything that exists only exists in relation to the idea, which is the real. Everything that exists is already no more than an imitation of a more-than-real, of a surreal. If art imitates, it is shadow of a shadow, imitation of an imitation. You can, therefore, see the vanity of the work of art, of the work of the brush.

That's a trap one must not enter. Of course, works of art imitate the objects they represent, but their end is certainly not to represent them. In offering the imitation of an object, they make something different out of that object. Thus they only pretend to imitate. The object is established in a certain relationship to the Thing and is intended to encircle and to render both present and absent.

Everybody knows this. At the moment when painting turns once again upon itself, at the moment when Cézanne paints his apples, it is clear that in painting those apples, he is doing something very different from imitating apples – even though his final manner of imitating them, which is the most striking, is primarily oriented toward a technique of presenting the object. But the more the object is presented in the imitation, the more it opens up the dimension in which illusion is destroyed and aims at something else. Everyone knows that there is a mystery in the way Cézanne paints apples, for the relationship to the real as it is renewed in art at that moment makes the object appear purified; it involves a renewal of its dignity by means of which these imaginary insertions are, one might say, repetitively restated. The fact is, as has been noted, such insertions cannot be detached from the efforts of earlier artists to realize the ends of art in their own way.

Obviously, the notion of historicity should not be used here without great caution. The expression "history of art" is highly misleading. Every appearance of this way of proceeding consists in overthrowing the illusory operation so as to return to the original end, which is to project a reality that is not that of the object represented. In the history of art, on the other hand, by virtue of the necessity that supports it, there is only substructure. The relation of the artist to the time in which he appears is always a contradictory one. It is against the current, in opposition to reigning norms – including, for example, political norms, or indeed, systems of thought – that art attempts to operate its miracle once more.

With the anamorphosis I have here, we find ourselves faced with a game that may seem futile to you, when you think of the sophisticated operational techniques required for the success of such a little artifact. And yet how can one not be touched or even moved when faced with this thing in which the image takes a rising and descending form? When faced with this sort of syringe which, if I really let myself go, would seem to me to be a kind of apparatus for taking a blood sample, a blood sample of the Grail? But don't forget that the blood of the Grail is precisely what is lacking.

The argument I have been developing thus far in my lecture should be interpreted only in a metaphorical way. I have only been following this line of argument because I want to discuss today that form of sublimation which appeared at a certain moment in the history of poetry, and which interests us in an exemplary way in connection with something that Freudian thought has placed at the center of our interest in the economy of the psyche, namely, Eros and eroticism.

I just wanted to point it out to you at the beginning: you might almost structure around this anamorphosis the ideas I am sketching out for you on the subject of the ethics of psychoanalysis. It is something that is wholly founded on the forbidden reference that Freud encountered at the terminal point of what in his thought one might call the Oedipus myth.

2

It is remarkable that the experience of what goes on in the neurotic caused Freud to leap to the level of the poetic creation of art, to the drama of Oedipus, insofar as it is something datable in the history of culture. You will see this when we take up *Moses and Monotheism*, which I asked you to read during our break. There is in Freud no distance from the facts of the Judeo-Greek experience, and I mean by that those that characterize our culture in its most modern everyday life.

It is equally striking that Freud couldn't fail to pursue his reflection on the origins of morality to the point of examining Moses' action. When you read the astonishing work that is *Moses and Monotheism*, you will see that Freud cannot help revealing the duplicity of his reference, of the reference that I have declared to you over the years to be the essential reference, namely, the No / Name-of-the-Father in its signifying function.

From a formal point of view, Freud makes recourse to paternal power for a structuring purpose that appears to be a sublimation. He emphasizes, in the same text in which he leaves at a distance the primordial trauma of the murder of the father – and without worrying about the contradiction – that this sublimation emerges at a given historical date against the background of a visible, evident fear that she who engenders is the mother. There is, he tells us, genuine progress in spirituality in affirming the function of the father, namely, of him of whom one is never sure. This recognition implies a whole mental elaboration. To introduce as primordial the function of the father represents a sublimation. But, Freud asks, how can one conceive of this leap, this progress, since, in order to introduce it, it was necessary that something appear that imposes its authority and its reality from outside?

He himself underlines the impasse constituted by the fact that sublimation exists, but that such sublimation can only be motivated historically by means of the myth to which it has recourse. At that point the function of myth becomes evident. In truth, this myth is nothing other than something that is inscribed in the clearest of terms in the spiritual reality of our time, namely, the death of God. It is as a function of the death of God that the murder of the father which represents it in the most direct way is introduced by Freud as a modern myth.

It is a myth that has all the properties of a myth. That is to say that it doesn't explain anything, anymore than any other myth. As I pointed out in citing Lévi-Strauss and especially in referring to that which buttresses his own formulation of the issue, myth is always a signifying system or scheme, if you like, which is articulated so as to support the antimonies of certain psychic relations. And this occurs at a level which is not simply that of individual anguish and which is not exhausted either in a construction presupposing the collectivity, but which assumes its fullest possible dimension.

We suppose that it concerns the individual and also the collectivity, but there is no such opposition between them at the level involved. For it is a matter here of the subject insofar as he suffers from the signifier. It is in this passion of the signifier that the critical point emerges, and its anguish is no more than an intermittent emotion that plays the role of an occasional signal.

Freud brought to the question of the source of morality the invaluable significance implied in the phrase *Civilization and Its Discontents* or, in other words, the breakdown by means of which a certain psychic function, the superego, seems to find in itself its own exacerbation, as the result of a kind of malfunctioning of the brakes which should limit its proper authority. It remains to be seen how within this breakdown in the depths of the psychic life the instincts may find their proper sublimation.

But to begin with, what is the possibility we call sublimation? Given the time at our disposal, I am not in a position to take you through the virtually absurd difficulties that authors have encountered every time they have tried to give a meaning to the term "sublimation." I would nevertheless like one of you to go to the *Bibliothèque Nationale*, look up Bernfeld's article in volume VIII of *Imago* entitled "Bemerkungen über Sublimierung," ["Observations on Sublimation"], and give us a summary of it here.

Bernfeld was a particularly powerful mind of the second generation, and in the end the weaknesses of his articulation of the problem of sublimation are of a kind that will prove illuminating. He is first of all quite troubled by Freud's reference to the fact that the operations of sublimation are always ethically, culturally, and socially valorized. This criterion, external to psychoanalysis, certainly creates a difficulty, and on account of its extra-psychological character clearly merits to be emphasized and criticized. But as we will see, this character causes less difficulty than at first appears.

On the other hand, the contradiction between the *Zielablenkung* side of the *Strebung*, of the *Trieb* or drive, and the fact that that takes place in a domain which is that of the object libido, also poses all kinds of problems for Bernfeld – problems that he resolves with the extreme clumsiness which characterizes everything that has so far been said on the analysis of sublimation.

According to him, at the point he reached around 1923–1924, we must start from the part of the instinct that may be employed for the ends of the ego, for the *Ichziele*, in order to define sublimation. And he goes on to give examples whose naiveté is striking. He refers to a certain little Robert Walter, who like many children tries his hand at poetry even before puberty. And what does he tell us on the subject? That to be a poet is an *Ichziel* for the boy. It is in relation to that choice fixed very early that everything that follows will be judged, namely, the way in which at the onset of puberty the upheaval of his libidinal economy, which is clinically perceptible although quite confused in this case, will be seen to be gradually integrated into the *Ichziel*. In particular, his activity as a little poet and his fantasms, which were quite separate at the beginning, come to be progressively coordinated.

Bernfeld thus assumes the primordial, primitive character of the goal set by the child to become a poet. And a similar argument is to be found in the other, equally instructive examples he gives us – some of which concern the function of the *Verneinungen*, of the negations that occur spontaneously among groups of children. He was, in effect, very interested in this question in a publication devoted to the problems of youth for which he was responsible at the time.

The important point to note on the subject is the following, and it is something that is to be found in all formulations of the problem, including Freud's. Freud points out that once the artist has carried out an operation on the level of sublimation, he finds himself to be the beneficiary of his operation insofar as it is acclaimed after the fact; it brings in its wake in the form of glory, honor, and even money, those fantasmic satisfactions that were at the origin of the instinct, with the result that the latter finds itself satisfied by means of sublimation.

That is all well and good as long as we assume that the already established function of poet exists on the outside. It seems to be taken for granted that especially among those whom Bernfeld calls eminent men, a little child might choose to become a poet as an ego goal. It is true that he hastens to add parenthetically that, in using the expression "hervorragender Mensch," eminent man, he is divesting it as much as possible of all connotations of value – something that is very strange as soon as one starts to talk of eminence. To be frank, the dimension of the eminent personality cannot be eliminated. And we see that, in fact, in *Moses and Monotheism* it isn't eliminated by Freud, but thrust into the foreground.

What needs to be justified is not simply the secondary benefits that individuals might derive from their works, but the originary possibility of a function like the poetic function in the form of a structure within a social consensus.

Well now, it is precisely that kind of consensus we see born at a certain historical moment around the ideal of courtly love. For a certain highly restricted circle, that ideal is to be found at the origin of a moral code, including a whole series of modes of behavior, of loyalties, measures, services, and exemplary forms of conduct. And if that interests us so directly, it is because its central point was an erotics.

3

What interests us here very probably emerged in the middle or at the beginning of the eleventh century, and continued into the twelfth or even, in Germany, to the beginning of the thirteenth. The phenomenon in question is courtly love, its poets and singers, who were known as "troubadours" in the South, as "trouvères" in the North of France, and as "Minnesänger" in the Germanic realm – England and parts of Spain were only involved at second hand. These games were linked to a very precise poetic craft and emerged at that moment, only to be eclipsed subsequently to the point where the following centuries only retained a somewhat dim memory of them.

At the high point, which stretches from the beginning of the eleventh century to the first third of the thirteenth, the very special technique of these courtly love poets played a highly important role. It is difficult for us today to evaluate precisely the importance of that role, but certain circles – in the courtly love sense, court circles, aristocratic circles – that occupied an elevated position in society were certainly influenced markedly.

The question as to whether there were, in fact, formal lessons in love has been raised. The way in which Michel de Nostre-Dame, otherwise known as Nostradamus, represents at the beginning of the fifteenth century the way in which juridical power was exercised by the Ladies – whose extravagant Languedocian names he cites – cannot fail to excite a thrill in us at its strangeness. This is something that was faithfully reproduced by Stendhal in *On Love*, an admirable work on the subject, and one that is very close to the interest displayed by the romantics in the resurgence of the poetry of courtly love, which was called Provençal at the time, but which was, properly speaking, from the region of Toulouse or indeed from the Limousin.

The existence and operations of these tribunals devoted to the casuistry of love and evoked by Michel de Nostre-Dame are open to debate and often debated. Nevertheless, we do have certain texts, including especially the work by Andreas Capellanus that Rénouart discovered and published in 1917. The shortened title is *De Arte Amandi*, which thus makes it a homonym of Ovid's treatise – a work that was passed down to posterity by the clergy.

This fourteenth-century manuscript that Rénouart discovered in the *Bibliothèque Nationale* gives us the text of judgments handed down by Ladies, who are well-known historical figures and include Eleanor of Aquitaine. She was successively – and this "successively" involved a great degree of personal involvement in the unfolding drama – the wife of Louis VII the Younger and Henry Plantagenet, whom she married when he was Duke of Normandy and who subsequently became King of England, with all that that involved relative to claims made on French territory. Then there was her daughter, who married a certain Henry I, Count of Champagne, and still others who were historical figures. In Capellanus's work they are all said to have participated in tribunals devoted to the casuistry of love, and such tribunals all presuppose perfectly coded points of reference that are by no means vague, but imply ideals to be pursued, of which I will give you some examples.

It doesn't matter whether we take them from the Southern French domain or the German domain except as far as the signifier is concerned, which in the former case is the "langue d'oc" and in the latter the German language – this is after all a poetry written in the vernacular. Except for the signifier, then, the terms overlap, repeat each other; both involve the same system. They are organized around diverse themes, the first of which is mourning, and even mourning unto death.

As one of those put it who at the beginning of the nineteenth century in Germany formulated its characteristics, the point of departure of courtly love is its quality as a scholastics of unhappy love. Certain terms define the register according to which the Lady's values are attained – a register indicated by the norms which regulate the exchanges between the partners of the strange rite, namely, reward, clemency, grace or *Gnade*, felicity. So as to imagine the extremely rarified and complex organization concerned, think of the seventeenth-century Map of Love *(Carte du Tendre)*, although what one finds there is a far more pallid version; the *précieuses*, too, at another historical moment placed the emphasis on a certain social art of conversation.

With courtly love things are all the more surprising because they emerge at a time when the historical circumstances are such that nothing seems to point to what might be called the advancement of women or indeed their emancipation. To give you an idea of the situation, I would just refer to the story of the Countess of Comminges, the daughter of a certain William of Montpellier, that took place at the time of the full flowering of courtly love.

There was a certain Peter of Aragon, who was King of Aragon and was ambitious to extend his power north of the Pyrenees in spite of the obstacle raised at the time by the first historical campaign of the north against the south, namely, in the form of the Albigensian crusade and Simon de Montfort's victories over the Counts of Toulouse. By reason of the fact that the lady in question was the natural heir upon the death of her father of the county of Montpellier, Peter of Aragon wanted her. She was, however, already married, and seems to have been someone who was not cut out to involve herself in sordid intrigues. She was of a highly reserved personality, not far from sainthood in the religious sense of the word, since it was at Rome that she ended her days with a reputation for saintliness. Political intrigue and the pressure of the noble Lord Peter of Aragon forced her to leave her husband. Papal intervention obliged the latter to take her back, but on her father's death, everything happened in accordance with the will of the powerful Lord. She was repudiated by her husband, who was used to such things, and she married Peter of Aragon, who proceeded to mistreat her to such a degree that she fled. And that is why she finished her days in Rome under the protection of the Pope, who turned out to be on occasion the only protector of persecuted innocence.

The style of this story simply shows the effective position of woman in feudal society. She is, strictly speaking, what is indicated by the elementary structures of kinship, i.e., nothing more than a correlative of the functions of social exchange, the support of a certain number of goods and of symbols of power. She is essentially identified with a social function that leaves no room for her person or her own liberty, except with reference to her religious rights.

It is in this context that the very curious function of the poet of courtly love starts to be exercised. It is important to recall his social situation, which is of a kind to throw a little light on the fundamental idea or graphic style that Freudian ideology can give to a fashion whose function the artist manages in a way to delay.

Satisfactions of power are involved, Freud tells us. That is why it is all the more remarkable to emphasize that in the whole collection of *Minnesange*, there are numerous poets who occupy positions that are not inferior to those of emperor, king, or prince. There are, in fact, 126 *Minnesange* in the *Manes* manuscript collection, which was in the *Bibliothèque Nationale* in Paris at the beginning of the nineteenth century, and which Heinrich Heine used to go and pay homage to, as if to the very beginnings of German poetry. But after 1888, as the result of negotiations I know nothing about, but that were certainly justified, it was given back to the Germans and is now in Heidelberg.

The first of the troubadours was a certain Guillaume de Poitiers, the seventh Count of Poitiers and ninth Duke of Aquitaine. Before he devoted himself to his early poetic activities in the sphere of courtly love poetry, he appears to have been a formidable brigand of the kind that, goodness knows, every right-minded feudal nobleman of the period seems readily to have been. In a number of historical situations that I won't go into, he can be seen to have behaved in conformity with the norms of the most barbarous practice of ransom. That was the kind of service one could expect from him. Then, from a particular moment on, he became the poet of that singular form of love.

I urge you right away to read those specialized works that contain a thematic analysis of the veritable love ritual which was involved. The question is, How should we situate it as analysts?

I will just mention in passing a book that is somewhat depressing in the way it solves problems by neatly avoiding them, although it is full of material and quotations, namely, *The Joy of Love* by Pierre Perdu, which was published by Plon. Another work of a very different type, since it deals less with courtly love than its historical relations, is also worth reading, and that is the nice little collection of Benjamin Perret, which, without explaining very well what it's about, he has called *The Anthology of Sublime Love*. Then there is René Nelli's book, published by Hachette, *Love and the Myths of the Heart*, in which I find a certain philogenic moralism along with a lot of facts. And finally you have Henry Corbin's *The Creative Imagination* from Flammarion; however, it goes much further than the limited domain that interests us today.

I am not going to expatiate on the obvious themes of this poetry, both for lack of time and because you will find them in the examples in which I will show what might be called their conventional origin. On this subject all the historians agree: courtly love was, in brief, a poetic exercise, a way of playing with a number of conventional, idealizing themes, which couldn't have any real concrete equivalent. Nevertheless, these ideals, first among which is that of the Lady, are to be found in subsequent periods, down to our own. The influence of these ideals is a highly concrete one in the organization of contemporary man's sentimental attachments, and it continues its forward march.

Moreover, march is the right word because it finds its point of origin in a certain systematic and deliberate use of the signifier as such.

A great deal of effort has been expanded to demonstrate the relationship between this apparatus or organization of the forms of courtly love and an intuition that is religious in origin, mystical for example, and that is supposed to be located somewhere in the center that is sought, in the Thing, which comes to be exalted in the style of courtly love. Experience has shown that this whole effort is condemned to failure.

On the level of the economy of the reference of the subject to the love object, there are certain apparent relationships between courtly love and foreign mystical experiences, Hindu or Tibetan, for example. As everyone knows, Denis de Rougemont made a great deal of this, and that is why I told you to read Henry Corbin's book. There are nevertheless serious difficulties and even critical impossibilities involved, if only because of dates. The themes in question among certain Moslem poets from the Iberian peninsula, for example, appear after Guillaume de Poitier's poetry.

Of interest to us from a structural point of view is the fact that an activity of poetic creation was able to exercise a determining influence on manners at a time – and subsequently in its historical consequences – when the origin and the key concepts of the whole business had been forgotten. But we can only judge the function of this sublimated creation in features of the structure.

The object involved, the feminine object, is introduced oddly enough through the door of privation or of inaccessibility. Whatever the social position of him who functions in the role, the inaccessibility of the object is posited as a point of departure. Some of those involved were, in fact, servants, *sirvens*, at their place of birth; Bernard de Ventadour was, for example, the son of a servant at Ventadour castle, who was also a troubadour.

It is impossible to serenade one's Lady in her poetic role in the absence of the given that she is surrounded and isolated by a barrier.

Furthermore, that object or *Domnei*, as she is called – she is also frequently referred to with the masculine term, *Mi Dom*, or my Lord – this Lady is presented with depersonalized characteristics. As a result, writers have noted that all the poets seem to be addressing the same person.

The fact that on occasion her body is described as *g'ra delgat e gen* – that means that plumpness was part of the sex appeal of the period, *e gen* signifying graceful – should not deceive you, since she is always described in that way. In this poetic field the feminine object is emptied of all real substance. That is what made it easy subsequently for a metaphysical poet such as Dante, for example, to choose a person whom we definitely know existed – namely, little Beatrice whom he fell for when she was nine years old, and who stayed at the center of his poetry from the *Vita Nuova* to *The Divine Comedy* – and to make her the equivalent of philosophy or indeed, in the end, of the science of the sacred. That also enabled him to appeal to her in terms that are all the more sensual because the person in question is close to allegory. It is only when the person involved is transformed into a symbolic function that one is able to speak of her in the crudest terms.

Here we see functioning in the pure state the authority of that place the instinct aims for in sublimation. That is to say, that what man demands, what he cannot help but demand, is to be deprived of something real. And one of you, in explaining to me what I am trying to show in *das Ding*, referred to it neatly as the vacuole.

I don't reject the word, although its charm derives from the virtual reference to histology. Something of that order is, in effect, involved, if we indulge in that most risqué of reveries associated with contemporary speculation that speaks of communication in connection with transmission inside organic structures – transmission that functions pseudopodically. Of course, there is no communication as such. But if in a monocellular organism such communication were organized schematically around the vacuole, and concerned the function of the vacuole as such, we could, in fact, have a schematic form of what concerns us in the representation.

Where, in effect, is the vacuole created for us? It is at the center of the signifiers – insofar as that final demand to be deprived of something real is essentially linked to the primary symbolization which is wholly contained in the signification of the gift of love.

In this connection I was struck by the fact that, in the terminology of courtly love, the word *domnei* is used. The corresponding verb is *domnoyer*, which means something like "to caress," "to play around." *Domnei*, in spite of the fact that its first syllable in French is an echo of the word "don," gift, is, in fact, unrelated to it. It is related instead to the *Domna*, the Lady, or in other words, to her who on occasion dominates.

That has its amusing side. And one should perhaps explore historically the quantity of metaphors that exist around the term "donner," to give, in courtly love. Can "donner" be situated in the relationship between the partners as something that is predominantly on one side or the other? It has perhaps no other cause than the semantic confusion produced in connection with the term *domnei* and the use of the word *domnoyer*.

The poetry of courtly love, in effect, tends to locate in the place of the Thing certain discontents of the culture. And it does so at a time when the historical circumstances bear witness to a disparity between the especially harsh conditions of reality and certain fundamental demands. By means of a form of sublimation specific to art, poetic creation consists in positing an object I can only describe as terrifying, an inhuman partner.

The Lady is never characterized for any of her real, concrete virtues, for her wisdom, her prudence, or even her competence. If she is described as wise, it is not because she embodies an immaterial wisdom or because she represents its functions more than she exercises them. On the contrary, she is as arbitrary as possible in the tests she imposes on her servant.

The Lady is basically what was later to be called, with a childish echo of the original ideology, "cruel as the tigers of Ircania." But you will not find the extreme arbitrariness of the attitude expressed any better than among the authors of the period themselves, Chrétien de Troyes, for example.

4

Having brought out the artifices embodied in the construction of courtly love and before proceeding to show you to what extent these artifices have proved to be so durable, thus complicating still the relations between men and the service of women, I would like to say one other thing. The object in front of us, our anamorphosis, will also enable us to be precise about something that remains a little vague in the perspective adopted, namely, the narcissistic function.

You are aware that the mirror function, which I thought it necessary to present as exemplary of the imaginary structure, is defined in the narcissistic relation. And the element of idealizing exaltation that is expressly sought out in the ideology of courtly love has certainly been demonstrated; it is fundamentally narcissistic in character. Well now, the little image represented for us by this anamorphosis permits me to show you which mirror function is involved.

It is only by chance that beyond the mirror in question the subject's ideal is projected. The mirror may on occasion imply the mechanisms of narcissism, and especially the diminution of destruction or aggression that we will encounter subsequently. But it also fulfills another role, a role as limit. It is that which cannot be crossed. And the only organization in which it participates is that of the inaccessibilty of the object. But it's not the only thing to participate in that.

There is a whole series of motifs, which constitute the presuppositions or organic givens of courtly love. There is, for example, the fact that the object is not simply inaccessible, but is also separated from him who longs to reach it by all kind of evil powers, one of the names for which, in the charming Provençal language, is *lauzengiers*. The latter are the jealous rivals, but also the slanderers.

Another essential theme is that of the secret. It embodies a certain number of misapprehensions, among which is the idea that the object is never given except through an intermediary called the *Senhal*. It is something also found in Arab poetry in connection with similar themes, where the same curious rite always strikes commentators, since the forms are sometimes highly significant. In particular, at a certain point in his poems, the extraordinary Guillaume de Poitiers calls the object of his aspirations *Bon vezi*, which means "Good neighbor." As a result of which, historians have abandoned themselves to all kinds of conjectures and have been unable to come up with anything better than the name of a Lady who, it is known, played an important role in his personal history, a forward woman apparently, whose estates were close to Guillaume's.

What is for us much more important than the reference to the neighbor, who is supposedly the Lady whom Guillaume de Poitiers occasionally played naughty games with, is the relationship between the expression just referred to and the one Freud uses in connection with the first establishment of the Thing, with its psychological genesis, namely, the *Nebenmensch*. And he designated thereby the very place that from the point of view of the development of Christianity, was to be occupied by the apotheosis of the neighbor.

In brief, I wanted to make you realize today, first, that it is an artificial and cunning organization of the signifier that lays down at a given moment the lines of a certain asceticism, and, second, the meaning we must attribute to the negotiation of the detour in the psychic economy.

The detour in the psyche isn't always designed to regulate the commerce between whatever is organized in the domain of the pleasure principle and whatever presents itself as the structure of reality. There are also detours and obstacles which are organized so as to make the domain of the vacuole stand out as such. What gets to be projected as such is a certain transgression of desire.

And it is here that the ethical function of eroticism enters into play. Freudianism is in brief nothing but a perpetual allusion to the fecundity of eroticism in ethics, but it doesn't formulate it as such. The techniques involved in courtly love – and they are precise enough to allow us to perceive what might on occasion become fact, what is properly speaking of the sexual order in the inspiration of this eroticism – are techniques of holding back, of suspension, of *amor interruptus*. The stages courtly love lays down previous to what is mysteriously referred to as *le don de merci*, "the gift of mercy" – although we don't know exactly what it meant – are expressed more or less in terms that Freud uses in his *Three Essays* as belonging to the sphere of foreplay.

Now from the point of view of the pleasure principle, the paradox of what might be called the effect of *Vorlust*, of foreplay, is precisely that it persists in opposition to the purposes of the pleasure principle. It is only insofar as the pleasure of desiring, or, more precisely, the pleasure of experiencing unpleasure, is sustained that we can speak of the sexual valorization of the preliminary stages of the act of love.

Yet we can never tell if this act or fusion is a matter of mystical union, of distant acknowledgment of the Other or of anything else. In many cases, it seems that a function like that of a blessing or salutation is for the courtly lover the supreme gift, the sign of the Other as such, and nothing more. This phenomenon has been the object of speculation that has even gone as far as identifying this blessing with that which in the *consolamentum* orders the relations between the highest ranks of initiates among the Cathars. In any case, before reaching that point, the stages of the erotic technique are carefully distinguished and articulated; they go from drinking, speaking, touching, which is in part identified with what are known as services, to kissing, and the *osculum*, which is the final stage before that of the union in *merci*.

All that has come down to us in such an enigmatic form that, in order to explain it, the attempt has been made to relate it to Hindu or even Tibetan erotic practices, since it seems that the latter have been codified in the most precise way and constitute a disciplined asceticism of pleasure from which a kind of lived substance may emerge for the subject. It is only on the basis of extrapolation that it is supposed something analogous was effectively practiced by the troubadours. Personally, I don't believe a word of it. Moreover, without assuming an identity between the practices taken from different cultural spheres, I do believe the influence of this poetry has been decisive for us.

Following the notable failure of the different attempts to explain in terms of influence the emergence of this particular kind of idealizing cult of the feminine object in our culture, I am struck most by the fact that a number of the most ascetic and most paradoxical of the texts utilized in the discourse of courtly love are taken over from Ovid's *Art of Love*.

Ovid wrote in a sparkling verse form a little treatise for libertines in which one learns for example, in which neighborhoods of Rome one can meet the prettiest little whores. And he develops his theme in a poem in three parts that ends with the direct evocation of what can only be called the game of the two-backed beast. In the midst of all that one also comes across formulas such as *Arte regendus Amor*, "Love must be ruled by Art." And then, ten centuries later, with the help of those magic words, a group of poets starts to introduce all that word for word into a veritable operation of artistic incantation.

One also reads *Militiae species amor est*, "Love is a kind of military service" – which means for Ovid that the ladies of Rome aren't as easy as all that. And then in the discourse of chivalry, in a form that is nicely outlined in *Don Quixote*, such terms begin to resonate so as to evoke an armed militia devoted to the defense of women and children.

You can certainly understand the importance I attribute to such well-attested analogies, for it is clear that in the priesthood itself, Ovid's *Ars Amandi* had not been forgotten; Chrétien de Troyes even translated it. It is through these kinds of revivals that one is able to understand what the function of the signifier means. And I would like to make my boldest assertion today at this point in affirming that courtly love was created more or less as you see the fantasm emerge from the syringe that was evoked just now.

That doesn't mean that something fundamental isn't involved, however; otherwise it would be inconceivable that André Breton could celebrate in this day and age *l'Amour fou,* "the madness of love," as he puts it in terms dictated by his concerns, or by his interest in the relationship to what he calls "objective chance." That is a strange signifying configuration, since who, a century or so from now, on reading these things in their context, will understand that objective chance means things that occur and are all the richer in meaning because they take place somewhere where we are unable to perceive either rational, or causal, or any other kind of order, that can justify their emergence in the real?

In other words, it is once again in the place of the Thing that Breton has the madness of love emerge.

As I take leave of you today and remind you that we will meet again three weeks from now, I would like to conclude with four lines from a poem, which, thanks to my memory, came to mind this morning. They are from another surrealist poet, Paul Eluard. They are in their poetic context exactly at that frontier or limit which in my own words I am attempting to enable us to localize and feel:

> Against this dilapidated sky, these panes of fresh water,
> Which face will appear and, like a sonorous shell,
> Announce that the night of love has turned to day,
> Open mouth joined to a mouth that is closed?[2]

February 10, 1960

[2] *Capitale de la Douleur*

XII

A critique of Bernfeld

REACTION FORMATION AND SUBLIMATION
THE PRECOCIOUSNESS OF SUBLIMATION
BETWEEN FREUDIAN AESTHETICS AND ETHICS
SUBLIMATION AND IDENTIFICATION
A CURIOSITY

Let us not forget that this year I resolved that this seminar would be a real seminar.

This is all the more essential because we have among us not a few people capable of contributing, including someone whom I can call our friend. That is Pierre Kaufmann, who is an *assistant* at the Sorbonne. He has been following what goes on at this seminar for a long time now, and has been attentive to its work in the most useful of ways. Perhaps some of you follow his philosophical chronicle that appears in *Combat* on Thursdays. He has several times discussed my teaching, on the occasion of the Royaumont Conference, for example, or quite recently when he was good enough to give an account of work that was useful to an author such as Henri Lefebvre – he had complained of a deficiency of some kind in my teaching on the basis of the mere sight of a part of it or of an article.

In any case, four weeks ago I referred to a little article by Bernfeld. It was the "Bemerkungen über Sublimierung," which appeared in *Imago* in 1922. Mr. Kaufmann was good enough to show an interest in it, and our discussion progressed to the point where he brought me something which appeared to me to be both suggestive and promising enough for me to encourage him to develop it as far as time and interest permitted. He will thus present the thoughts that were inspired by Bernfeld's article and the further developments it inspired in him.

Please note especially that on a number of occasions in this presentation very interesting allusions will be made – I can only call them allusions, when I think of all that Mr. Kaufmann has added relative to the sources of the matter he was dealing with in the field of psychology at the moment when he became interested in it. In France, as in the English-speaking countries, we are quite ignorant of a whole, extremely rich German tradition, which shows that Freud, in fact, was the object of readings that were careful and extensive, or, in a word, immense.

On many points, we have a lot to learn about things that even Mr. Kaufmann hasn't yet formulated completely or published. You will get some idea of that today.

I now give him the floor and thank him in advance for what he has prepared for us. [Mr. Kaufmann's talk followed.]

1

What emerges from your talk is the frequent obscurity of Bernfeld's theory or at least of the application of it he attempts to give to the case under consideration. The result is quite ambiguous and gives rise to a problem. It is, in short, Bernfeld's thesis that one can only talk of sublimation when there is a transfer of energy from the object libido to the *Ichziele*.

The *Ichziele* are preexistent, and there is sublimation when libidinal energy is reinvigorated, updated, as the child enters the phase of puberty. A part of the energy is transferred from the aims of pleasure to the aims of the *Ichgerechte*, which are in conformity with the ego. And although the Freudian distinction between *Verdrängung* and *Sublimierung* is maintained, it is nevertheless only at the moment when *Verdrängung* appears that *Sublimierung* is perceptible. For example, it is only when the love of the child for the person Melitta is felt as a process of repression that that which is not completely obscured by the force of the latter is able to pass to the level of sublimation. Thus for him there is a kind of synchrony between the two processes. Let's say that Bernfeld is only able to grasp sublimation when he has the immediate correlative of repression.

Mr. Kaufmann: . . . Although he says that there is some ambiguity in the *Three Essays*, he nevertheless adds that it is clear that sublimation is distinguished from reaction formation by the non-repressed character of the libido.

Dr. Lacan: In reality, the greatest ambiguity reigns in the *Three Essays on the Theory of Sexuality* on the subject of the relations between spiritual reaction and *Sublimierung*. The problem begins with the text on pages 78 and 79 of the *Gesammelte Werke*. At that time this articulation of the problem caused a great many difficulties for the commentators. People wondered, depending on the different passages, whether Freud turns *Sublimierung* into a particular form of reaction formation or whether, on the contrary, reaction formation isn't to be located within a form in which *Sublimierung* would have a broader significance.

The only important thing to remember is the little sentence to be found at the bottom of note 79, which concludes the whole paragraph on reaction formation and sublimation. It makes a distinction that hasn't been further developed, as Bernfeld quite properly notes: "There may be sublimations by means of other, simpler mechanisms."

To summarize, the way of analyzing the economy of energy sources in the poetic activity of the young boy called Robert leaves an obvious residue that Bernfeld himself points to on page 339 as follows: "Aus dem Rest der Melitta geltenden Objektlibido entwickeln sich Stimmungen." – Melitta is the girl he loves. And then on page 340, Bernfeld writes: "Die Energie, mit der die tertiare Bearbeitung vollzogen wird, ist nun unbezweifelbar unverdrängte Objektlibido." There's where the problem lies if we make the phenomenon of sublimation dependent on the distinction between *Libidoziel, Ichziele, Lustziele*. And Sterba, too, in an article that appeared the previous year comes up against the same problem. If everything depends on the redirection of the energy from one sphere to another, or a certain set of aims which undergoes a profound disturbance at the time of puberty, then when Bernfeld identifies that crucial point which seems so important to him in the poetic production of the boy, he is led expressly to refer the poetic vocation to the *Ichziele*. And he resolves the question by saying that to become a poet is an aim of the ego, which was manifested very early in the boy in question. These precocious activities are, in Bernfeld's eyes, only to be distinguished by the fact that they reflect what he has learned at school in a diffuse and non-personalized way, as a result of which all the productions of the time are marked with the sign "of little value." They only seem to become interesting from the moment when the person concerned feels himself to be dramatically engaged in his activities.

I am emphasizing factors that present the author in the most favorable of lights. But in a more or less fleeting way, how many children are there who during the latency period don't engage in poetic activity periodically? Freud was in a good position to observe it in one of his children. There is a problem there that is different from that of cultural transmission or imitation. The problem of sublimation has to be posed early, but we don't for that reason have to limit ourselves to individual development. The reason why there are poets, why a poetic vocation may suggest itself early to a young human being, cannot simply be solved as with Bernfeld by considering genetic development and the new characteristics that appear at the moment when sexuality becomes an issue in an obvious way.

To fail to recognize that sexuality is there from the beginning in the young child, and is an even greater factor during the phase that precedes the latency period, is to fly in the face of the whole Freudian enterprise and discovery. If so much insistence has been placed on the pregenital sources of sublimation, it is for that reason. The problem of sublimation is raised long before the moment when the division between the aims of the libido and the aims of the ego are clear, apparent, and accessible on the level of consciousness.

If I may be permitted to emphasize here something that I have taught you, I would say that the term I use in the effort to articulate sublimation in relation to what we have to deal with, *das Ding*, or what I call the Thing, refers to a decisive place around which the definition of sublimation must be articulated – even before *I* was born, and, obviously, therefore, before the *Ichziele*, the aims of the *I* appear.

The same remark applies to the comparison you have made between the use I make of the image of the Thing and what Simmel does with it.

There is in Simmel something of interest to me, since he has the notion not only of distanciation but also of an object that cannot be attained. But it is nevertheless an object. On the other hand, what cannot be attained in the Thing is precisely the Thing – i.e., it's not an object. And the difference is a radical one that has to do with the appearance between his time and mine of the difference that is the Freudian unconscious.

Simmel comes close to something that you have interpreted as an apprehension of anality, but he is unable to grasp it fully precisely because of that fundamental difference.

Mr. Kaufmann: . . . As far as Bernfeld is concerned, the problem is merely made more confusing if the notion of value is introduced into the analysis of sublimation. He says, for example, that on the level of analysis one shouldn't distinguish between the work of an artist and a stamp collection. . . .

Dr. Lacan: Not only between a collection of works of art and a stamp collection, but between an art collection, and, in a given child or patient, a collection of dirty bits of paper. He resists introducing criteria that are alien to the criteria of psychic development.

The last part of the article has to do with an effort to articulate sublimation on to his curious experiment with groups of young people.

The verification of the size of the penis is in his eyes the essential significant element of that period when children engage in reciprocal exhibitionism. According to him there is here a conflict between the ego and the object libido. On the one hand, the ego exhibits itself narcissistically as the most handsome, strongest and biggest. Another part is opposed to the ego because it goes in the direction of genital excitation.

In the history of the association involved, that is for him the decisive side of the internal or esoteric ceremony of the group. It is from that point on that according to him one can talk of sublimation in their group activity.

The problematic character of all his needs to be emphasized, especially if one adds that, among those who consider themselves to be the strongest and boldest, this exhibitionism is accompanied by collective masturbation.

Mr. Kaufmann: . . . In short, Bernfeld was out of luck. He treated sublimation in connection with the ideal ego just before Freud was in a position to inform him of the nature of this ideal ego, and, in particular, of the need to take into consideration the relation to the other.

Dr. Lacan: You are an optimist. Those who have written on the subject afterwards also don't seem to have profited from the introduction of the ideal ego. Just read them, including in the end the "Observations on Sublimation" and the article "Neutralisation and Sublimation," which appeared in *Analysis Studies;* you won't find there the least attempt to articulate sublimation on to the ideal ego. And that's as far as we've got, that's the point we are starting from here.

2

I would like to thank you for your presentation today. So as to highlight what we have learned, I hope you will allow me to quote the sentence that expresses the essence of Bernfeldian theory: "Those components of the whole that are instinctive emotion and that are held together under the pressure of repression may be sublimated. Thus the particular qualities of these components enable the ego function to be supported through the reinforcement of ego instincts that are currently threatened."

That's the definition to which he holds and which includes the two extremes you refer to. That is, either the ego is strong, and those whose ego instincts are precociously powerful form an aristocracy, an elite – and it is futile for him to say parenthetically that no emphasis is placed on value, given that it is after all impossible to avoid such an emphasis. Or the ego instincts are threatened and have to call for the assistance furnished by the drives, to the extent, that is, that they can escape recuperation. That's the position Bernfeld reaches.

It is, I assume, clear to you all that what I am concerned with this year is situated somewhere between a Freudian ethics and a Freudian aesthetics. Freudian aesthetics is involved because it reveals one of the phases of the function of the ethics. And it really is surprising that it hasn't been given greater prominence, given that in another form the subject has preoccupied psychoanalysis – Jones, for example, is always talking about the moral complacency which is in a way that which ethics makes use of in order to render the Thing inaccessible to us, when it already was inaccessible from the beginning.

I am trying to show you how Freudian aesthetics, in the broadest meaning of the term – which means the analysis of the whole economy of signifiers – reveals that the Thing is inaccessible. That needs to be placed right at the start of the problem, so as to be able to articulate its consequences, and especially the question of idealization. In any case, you saw last time, in connection with the sublimation involved in the moral code of courtly love, the beginnings of the emergence of an ideal type.

By way of conclusion, I would like to introduce a word whose full meaning will be apparent later on. Insofar as we distinguish in the sphere of ethics between two levels that are already there in classical thinkers – and that is discussed in a passage of *De Officiis* to which I shall refer you later – the question is whether the *summum bonum* should be articulated according to *honestas*, that is the style of the *honnête homme* – and which must, therefore, be articulated as a certain form of organization, a certain life style that is located in relation to the initial sublimation – or according to *utilitas*, a concept that is at the basis of the utilitarianism, with which I began by posing the problem of ethics this year, and whose true essence I propose to show.

March 2, 1960

SUPPLEMENTARY NOTE

A CURIOUS CASE OF SUBLIMATION

I have for you today something curious and amusing. But I believe that we analysts are perhaps alone in being in a position to situate things properly.

Last time when Mr. Kaufmann had finished talking about Bernfeld's article, I stated that the problem we face is that of establishing the link between sublimation and identification. Before we leave the subject of sublimation as I have outlined it for you around the notion of the Thing – and it may still seem enigmatic and veiled for very good reasons – I would like to present you with a text, as it were as a note, on the subject of what might be called the paradoxes of sublimation.

Sublimation is not, in fact, what the foolish crowd thinks; and it does not on all occasions necessarily follow the path of the sublime. The change of object doesn't necessarily make the sexual object disappear – far from it; the sexual object acknowledged as such may come to light in sublimation. The crudest of sexual games can be the object of a poem without for that reason losing its sublimating goal.

In short, I don't think it a waste of time for me to read you a piece of evidence from the file of courtly love that even the specialists themselves literally don't know what to do with; they can't make head or tail of it.

There aren't two poems like this in the literature of courtly love. It's a *hapax*, a single occurrence. It appears in the work of one of the most subtle and polished of the troubadours, whose name is Arnaud Daniel, and who is famous for his extraordinarily rich formal inventiveness, most notably in the poetic form of the sestina, which I don't have time to go into here; however, you should at least know the name.

Arnaud Daniel wrote a poem on the oddest of those relations of service that I told you about between the lover and his Lady; it is a whole poem that is distinguished by the fact that, much to the delight of a number of startled writers, it breaches the boundaries of pornography to the point of scatology.

The poem is concerned with a case that seems to be presented as a question to be resolved in terms of the moral casuistry of courtly love. The case involves a Lady, called *Domna* Ena in the poem, who orders her knight to put his mouth to her trumpet – an expression that is quite unambiguous in the text; and the order is designed to test the worthiness of his love, his loyalty and his commitment.

So as not to make you wait any longer then, I will read the poem – in French because I don't think that any of you can understand that lost language which is the *langue d'oc*, a language that nevertheless has its style and its value. The poem is in stanzas of nine lines with a single rhyme, which changes with every stanza.

> Though Lord Raimond, in agreement with Lord Truc Malec, defends Lady Ena and her orders, I would grow old and white before I would consent to a request that involves so great an impropriety. For so as "to put his mouth to her trumpet," he would need the kind of beak that could pick grain out of a pipe. And even then he might come out blind, as the smoke from those folds is so strong.
>
> He would need a beak and a long, sharp one, for the trumpet is rough, ugly and hairy, and it is never dry, and the swamp within is deep. That's why the pitch ferments upwards as it continually escapes, continually overflows. And it is not fitting that he who puts his mouth to that pipe be a favorite.
>
> There will be plenty of other tests, finer ones that are worth far more, and if Lord Bernart withdrew from that one, he did not, by Christ, behave like a coward if he was taken with fear and fright. For if the stream of water had landed on him from above, it would have scalded his whole neck and cheek, and it is not fitting also that a lady embrace a man who has blown a stinking trumpet.
>
> Bernart, I do not agree in this with the remarks of Raimon de Durfort, in saying that you were wrong; for even if you had blown away gladly, you would have encountered a crude obstacle, and the stench would soon have smitten you, that stinks worse than dung in a garden. You should praise God, against whomsoever seeks to dissuade you, that he helped you escape from that.
>
> Yes, he escaped from a great peril with which his son also would have been reproached and all those from Cornil. He would have done better to go into exile than to have blown in that funnel between spine and mount pubic, there where rust colored substances proceed. He could never have been certain that she would not piss all over his snout and eyebrows.
>
> Lady, may Bernart never venture to blow that trumpet without a large bung to stop up the penile hole; then only could he blow without peril.

This quite extraordinary document opens a strange perspective on the deep ambiguity of the sublimating imagination. One should first note that all the poetic works of the *trouvères* and *troubadours* have not come down to us, and that we only find some of Arnaud Daniel's poems in two or three manuscripts. Yet this poem, whose literary merit goes far beyond what a translation is able to reveal, not only was not lost but is to be found in some twenty manuscripts. We have other texts which show that two other *trouvères*, Trumalec and Raymond de Durfort, participated in this debate, arguing on the other side, but I won't go into that.

We find ourselves here faced with a sudden reversal, a strange reaction. Heaven knows that Arnaud Daniel went a long way in the direction of lending the greatest subtlety to the pact between lovers. Doesn't he push desire to the extreme point of offering himself in a sacrifice that involves his own annihilation? Well, he is the very same one who turns out to have written a poem, however reluctantly, on a subject that must have concerned him in some way for him to have taken so much trouble with it.

The idealized woman, the Lady, who is in the position of the Other and of the object, finds herself suddenly and brutally positing, in a place knowingly constructed out of the most refined of signifiers, the emptiness of a thing in all its crudity, a thing that reveals itself in its nudity to be the thing, her thing, the one that is to be found at her very heart in its cruel emptiness. That Thing, whose function certain of you perceived in the relation to sublimation, is in a way unveiled with a cruel and insistent power.

It is nevertheless difficult not to note echoes of this elsewhere, for the oddness involved is not without precedents. Remember, for example, the origin of the flute evoked in Longus's pastoral romance. Pan pursues the nymph Syrinx, who runs away from him and disappears among the reeds. In his rage, he cuts down the reeds, and that, Longus tells us, is the origin of the flute with pipes of unequal length – Pan wanted, the subtle poet adds, to express in that way the fact that his love was without equal. Syrinx is transformed into the pipe of Pan's flute. Now on the level of derision that is to be found in the strange poem that I brought to your attention here, we find the same structure, the same model of an emptiness at the core, around which is articulated that by means of which desire is in the end sublimated.

I wouldn't tell all if I didn't add to the file, in case it proves useful, that Dante places Arnaud Daniel in Canto XIV of his *Purgatory* in the company of sodomites. I haven't been able to pursue the particular genesis of this poem beyond that.

I am now going to ask Madame Hubert to speak. She will be talking to you about a text that is frequently referred to in analytic literature, namely, Sperber's article entitled "On the Influence of Sexual Factors on the Origin and Development of Language," but it also touches on all kinds of problems relative to what we have to say about sublimation.

In his article on the theory of symbolism – an article on which I wrote a commentary in our journal but which, I have heard, is not particularly accessible to a reader – Jones expressly singles out the Sperber article. If, he says,

Sperber's theory is true, if we must consider certain forms of primitive work, agricultural work, in particular, the relations between man and the earth, as the equivalent of the sexual act, features whose traces are, as it were, retained in the meaning we give that primitive relation, then can this be explained by the process of symbolization? Jones says no. In other words, given the conception he has of the function of the symbol, he considers that what is involved is by no means a symbolic transposition, neither can it be registered as a sublimation effect. The sublimation effect is to be taken in its liberality, in its authenticity. The copulation between the ploughman and the earth is not a symbolization but the equivalent of a symbolic copulation.

It is worth taking the time to reflect on that, and in my article I draw certain consequences to which I will return. Sperber's text appeared in the first issue of *Imago*, and it is perhaps even more difficult to find than the others. But so that it may receive its due, Mrs. Hubert has been good enough to concentrate on it, and she will tell us today what it contains.

March 9, 1960

THE PARADOX OF
JOUISSANCE

XIII

The death of God

ON SEXUAL SYMBOLISM
FROM THE *NUMEN* TO MOSES'S MESSAGE
THE GREAT MAN AND HIS MURDER
FREUD'S CHRISTOCENTRISM
JOUISSANCE AND DEBT

If I wanted you to be acquainted with Sperber's article, it is because it is coupled to our sublimation train.

1

I will not engage in a serious critique of the text, for I hope that after several years of following my teaching here, most of you have found something irritating in the way in which Sperber proceeds. Though his goal is undoubtedly interesting, his mode of demonstration has its weaknesses. To refer to the fact that words with an original sexual meaning started to take on a series of meanings increasingly remote from their primitive meaning, as a way of proving the common sexual origin in a sublimated form of fundamental human activities, is to adopt an approach whose demonstrable value seems to me to be eminently refutable from the point of view of common sense.

That words whose meaning was originally sexual spread out so as to overlay meanings that are very remote doesn't mean as a consequence that the whole field of meaning is overlaid in that way. That doesn't mean that all the language we use is in the end reducible to the key words it contains, words whose valorization is considerably facilitated by the fact that one accepts as proven what is, in fact, most questionable, namely, the notion of a root or radical, and what in human language would be its constitutive link to sense.

This emphasis placed on roots and radicals in languages making use of inflections raises particular problems that are far from being applicable to human language universally. What would be the case with Chinese, for example, where all the signifying units are monosyllabic? The notion of a root is highly tenuous. In fact, what is involved is an illusion that is linked to the development of language, of the use of the language system, which can only seem very suspect to us.

That doesn't mean that Sperber's remarks concerning the use of words with what might be called sexual roots in Indo-European languages are of no interest. But they can hardly satisfy us from the perspective in which I believe you have been trained and formed by me, a perspective which involves distinguishing properly the function of the signifier or the creation of signification through the metonymic and metaphoric use of signifiers.

That's where the trouble begins. Why are those zones in which sexual signification spreads outward, why are those rivers through which it ordinarily flows – and, as you have seen, in a direction that isn't just random – specially chosen, so that in order to reach them one uses words that already have a given usage in the sexual sphere? Why is it precisely in connection with a half-failed act of pruning, with an act of cutting that is blocked, thwarted, messed up, that one should evoke the presumed origin of the word and find it in the hole drilling activities of work in its most primitive of forms, with the meaning of sexual operation, of phallic penetration? Why does one resurrect the metaphor "fuck" in connection with something that is "fucked up?" Why is it the image of the vulva that surfaces to express a number of different acts, including those of escaping, of fleeing, of cutting and running (*se tailler*), as the German term in the text has often been translated?

I have, in fact, tried to find confirmation of the historical moment when that nice little expression, *se tailler* (to cut and run), in the sense of "to flee" or "to escape," first appeared. I haven't had time to find out, and I didn't discover it in the dictionaries and other sources that I have at my disposal. It is true that I don't have in Paris the dictionaries that give the popular meanings of words. I would like someone to do some research on the topic.

Thus, why in our everyday life do we find that in our metaphors a certain type of meaning is involved, certain signifiers that are marked by their primitive use in connection with the sexual relation? Why, for example, do we use some slang expression that had originally a sexual significance in order to evoke metaphorically situations that have nothing to do with sex? The metaphorical usage involved is employed to obtain a certain modification.

But if it were only a question of showing how in the normal diachronic development of linguistic usage sexual references are used in a certain metaphorical sense – that is, if I were only concerned with providing another example of certain aberrations of psychoanalytic speculation – I wouldn't have presented you with the Sperber text. If it is still interesting, it is because of what is to be found on its horizon, something that isn't demonstrated there, but which in its intention it strives for, and that is the radical relationship that exists between the first instrumental relations, the earliest techniques, the principal actions of agriculture, such as that of opening the belly of the earth, or again the principal actions in the making of a vase that I have previously emphasized, and something very precise, namely, not so much the sexual act as the female sexual organ.

It is insofar as the female sexual organ or, more precisely, the form of an opening and an emptiness, is at the center of all the metaphors concerned, that the article is of interest and is valuable in focusing our thought, for it is obvious that there is a gap in the text, a leap beyond the supposed reference.

One takes note of the fact that the use of a term that originally meant "coitus" is capable of being extended virtually infinitely, that the use of a term that originally meant "vulva" is capable of generating all kinds of metaphorical uses. And it is in this way that it began to be supposed that the vocalization presumed to accompany the sexual act gave men the idea of using the signifier to designate either the organ, and especially the female organ, in a noun form, or the act of coitus in a verbal form. The priority of the vocal use of the signifier among men is thus supposed to find its origin in the chanted calls that are assumed to be those of primitive sexual relations among humans, in the same way that they are among animals and especially birds.

The idea is very interesting. But you can sense right away the difference that exists between the more-or-less standardized cry that accompanies an activity and the use of a signifier that detaches a given articulatory element, that is to say, either the act or the organ. We don't find the signifying structure as such here; nothing implies that the oppositional element which forms the structure of the use of signifiers – and is already fully developed in the *Fort-Da* from which we took our original example – is given in the natural sexual call. If the sexual call can be derived from a temporal modulation of the act whose repetition may involve the fixation of certain elements of vocal activity, it still cannot give us even the most primitive structuring element of language. There is a gap there.

Nevertheless, the interest of the article is in making us see the way in which what is essential in the development of our experience and in Freud's doctrine may be conceived, that is to say, that sexual symbolism in the ordinary sense of the word may polarize at its point of origin the metaphorical play of the signifier.

That's all I have to say on the subject today, with the understanding that I may return to it later.

2

I wondered how I should take up the thread of our discussions, how I should start out again today.

As the result of conversations I have had with some of you, I said to myself that there would be some value in my giving you an idea of the lectures, comments, and conversations in which I engaged in Brussels. The fact is, when I have something to communicate to you, it is always related to the line of thought I am pursuing, and even when I take it out into the world, I do little more than take it up more or less at the point I have reached.

But to suppose that you already know implicitly what I said up there, which isn't the case, would be to take too great a leap forward. It is, in fact, important that the issues raised not be ignored.

That may seem to you to be an unconventional way of proceeding, but given the distance we still have to go, I don't have time to indulge in professorial scruples. Mine is not a professor's role. I don't even like to put myself in the teaching situation, since a psychoanalyst who speaks to an initiated audience is in the position of a propagandist. If I agreed to talk at the Catholic University of Brussels, I did so in a spirit of mutual assistance; it was in order to support the presence and the activities of those who are our friends and colleagues in Belgium. This concern is not for me the primary one, of course, but it is a secondary one.

I thus found myself in front of an audience that was very large and of which I had a very good impression, summoned there by the Catholic University. And that alone is enough to explain my motivation for speaking to them of what Freud has to say about the function of the Father.

As you might expect from me, I didn't mince my words or censor my language. I didn't attempt to attenuate Freud's position on religion. Moreover, you know what my position is concerning the so-called religious truths.

It is perhaps worthwhile to be more precise on the subject for once, although I believe I have made it clear enough. Whether from personal conviction or in the name of a methodological point of view, the so-called scientific point of view – a point of view that is by the way reached by people who otherwise consider themselves to be believers, but who in a certain sphere assume they are required to put aside their religious point of view – there is a paradox involved in practically excluding from the debate and from analysis things, terms, and doctrines that have been articulated in the field of faith, on the pretext that they belong to a domain that is reserved for believers.

You once heard me make a series of remarks on a passage from Saint Paul's Epistle to the Romans in connection with the theme that it is the Law which causes sin. And you saw that, thanks to an artifice I could have done without, namely, the substitution of the term the Thing for what the text calls sin, I was able to achieve a very precise formulation of what I had to say at the time on the subject of the knot of the Law and desire. Well, that particular example was not chosen by chance – it belonged to a certain order of effectiveness in relation to a special case, and by means of a kind of sleight of hand it was unusually helpful in leading to something I needed at the time to bring to your attention.

We analysts, who claim to go beyond certain conceptions of prepsychology relative to the phenomena of our own field or who approach human realities without prejudice, do not have to believe in these religious truths in any way, given that such belief may extend as far as what is called faith, in order to be interested in what is articulated in its own terms in religious experience – in the terms of the conflict between freedom and grace, for example.

A notion as precise and articulate as grace is irreplaceable where the psychology of the act is concerned, and we don't find anything equivalent in classic academic psychology. Not only doctrines, but also the history of choices, that is, of heresies that have been attested to in this sphere, and the succession of emotional outbursts that have motivated a certain number of directions taken in the concrete ethics of generations, all belong to our sphere of inquiry; they, so to speak, demand all of our attention in their own register and mode of expression.

It is not enough that certain themes be raised only by those who believe they believe – after all, how can we know? – for the whole field to be reserved for them alone. If we accept that they truly believe, then they are not beliefs for them but truths. What they believe in, whether they believe they believe in it or they don't – nothing is more ambiguous than belief – one thing is certain, they believe they know. The knowledge in question is like any other, and for this reason it falls into the field of inquiry that we should conduct on all forms of knowledge; and such is the case, because as analysts we believe that there is no knowledge which doesn't emerge against a background of ignorance.

That is the reason why we accept as such the idea of other forms of knowledge than the kind that is founded scientifically.

It was not useless, then, for me to confront an audience that represents an important sector of the public. Whether or not I may have caused an ear or two to prick up is problematic; the future alone will reveal that. Moreover, it won't have the same impact on a very different audience, like you.

Freud himself took an unequivocal position on the subject of religious experience. He said that everything of that kind that implied a sentimental approach meant nothing to him; it was literally a dead letter for him. Yet if we in this assembly have the position on the letter that we do, that doesn't solve a thing; however dead it might be, that letter was nevertheless definitely articulated. Well now, faced with people who are supposed not to be able to dissociate themselves from a certain message concerning the function of the Father – given that it is at the heart of the experience defined as religious – I had no discomfort in affirming that as far as that matter was concerned, "Freud had what it took," as I put it in a subtitle that was found a little startling.

You only have to open the little book entitled *Moses and Monotheism* that Freud cogitated over for some ten years, for after *Totem and Taboo* he thought of nothing but that, of Moses and the religion of his fathers. And if it weren't for the article on the *Spaltung* of the ego, one might say that the pen fell from his hands at the end of *Moses and Monotheism*. Contrary to what has been suggested to me over the last few weeks in connection with Freud's intellectual production toward the end of his life, I don't at all think that there was a decline. Nothing seems to me to be more firmly articulated in any case and more in conformity with all Freud's previous thought than this work.

It bears on the monotheistic message as such; and for him there is no doubt that it contains an uncontestable weight of superior value over any other. The fact that Freud was an atheist doesn't make any difference. For the atheist that Freud was, if not necessarily for all atheists, the goal of the radical core of this message was of decisive value. On the left of this message, there are some things that are henceforth outdated, obsolete; they no longer hold beyond the manifestation of the message. On the right, things are quite different.

The situation is quite clear from the spirit of Freud's argument. That doesn't mean that there is nothing at all outside of monotheism, far from it. He doesn't give us a theory of the gods, but enough is said concerning the ambiance that is usually connoted by "pagan," a late connotation linked to its retreat to the milieu of the peasantry. In that pagan ambiance at the time when it was flourishing, the *numen* rises up at every step, at the corner of every road, in grottoes, at crossroads; it weaves human experience together, and we can still see traces of it in a great many fields. That is something that contrasts greatly with the monotheistic profession of faith.

The numinous rises up at every step and, conversely, every step of the numinous leaves a trace, engenders a memorial. It didn't take much for a new temple to be erected, for a new religion to be established. The numinous proliferates and intervenes on all sides in human experience; it is, moreover, so abundant that something in the end must be manifested through man; its power cannot be overcome.

It is to this immense envelopment and at the same time to a degradation that the genre of the fable bears witness. Ancient fables are full of meanings that remain richly rewarding, but we have trouble realizing that they could have been compatible with something like a faith in the gods, because, whether they are heroic or vulgar, they are shot through with a kind of riotousness, drunkenness, and anarchy born of divine passions. The laughter of the Olympians in the *Iliad* sufficiently illustrates this on the heroic plane. There's a lot to be said about this laughter. From the pen of the philosophers, on the other hand, we have the other side of this laughter, of the derisory character of the adventures of the gods. It is difficult for us to conceive this.

In opposition to this we have the monotheistic message. How is it possible? How did it rise to this level? The way in which Freud articulates it is crucial if we are to appreciate the level at which its progress is to be situated.

For him everything is founded on the notion of Moses the Egyptian and of Moses the Midianite. I believe that an audience of people like you, eighty per cent of whom are psychoanalysts, should know this book by heart.

Moses the Egyptian is the Great Man, the legislator, the politician, the rationalist, the one whose path Freud claims to discover with the historical appearance in the fourteenth century B.C. of the religion of Akhenaton – something that has been attested by recent discoveries. This religion promotes a unitarianism of energy, symbolized by the sun from which it radiates and spreads out across the earth. This first attempt at a rationalist vision of the world, which is presupposed in the unitarianism of the real, in the substantive unification of the world centered on the sun, failed. Hardly had Akhenaton disappeared, when religious ideas of all kinds begin to multiply again, especially in Egypt; the pandemonium of the gods returns to take charge once more and utterly wipes out the reform. One man keeps the flame of this rationalist cause alight, Moses the Egyptian; it is he who chooses a small group of men and leads them through the test that will make them worthy to found a community based on his principles. In other words, someone wanted to create socialism in a single country, except, of course, there was in addition no country but just a bunch of men to carry the project through.

That's Freud conception of the true Moses, the Great Man; and what we need to know is how his message has come down to us.

You will perhaps respond that this Moses was after all a bit of a magician. How otherwise did he produce the swarms of locusts and frogs? But that was his business. It's not an essential question from the point of view that concerns us here, that of his place in religion. Let's leave the question of magic aside, although it doesn't seem to have hurt him with anyone.

On the other hand, there is Moses the Midianite, the son-in-law of Jethro, whom Freud also calls the one from Sinai, from Horeb, and Freud teaches us that this one was confused with the other. It is this one who claims to have heard the decisive word emerge from the burning bush, the word that cannot be eluded, as Freud eludes it: "I am," not as the whole Christian gnosis has attempted to interpret it, "he who is" – thereby exposing us to difficulties relative to the concept of being that are far from being over, and which have perhaps contributed to compromising exegesis – but "I am what I am." Or, in other words, a God who introduces himself as an essentially hidden God.

This hidden god is a jealous God. He seems to be very difficult to dissociate from the one who, according to the Bible, proclaims in that same ambiance of fire which makes him inaccessible the famous ten commandments to the assembled people, who are required to remain at a certain distance. Given that these commandments turn out to be proof against anything – and by that I mean that whether or not we obey them, we still cannot help hearing them – in their indestructible character they prove to be the very laws of speech, as I tried to show you.

Moses the Midianite seems to pose a problem of his own – I would like to know whom or what he faced on Sinai and on Horeb. But after all, since he couldn't bear the brilliance of the face of him who said "I am what I am," we will simply say at this point that the burning bush was Moses's Thing, and leave it there. In any case, we still have to calculate the consequences of that revelation.

By what means is the problem resolved for Freud? He considers that Moses the Egyptian was assassinated by his little people, who were less docile than ours relative to socialism in a single country. And then these people went on to devote themselves to all kinds of paralyzing observances at the same time that they caused trouble for countless neighbors – for we shouldn't overlook what is, in effect, the history of the Jews. One only has to read a little into these ancient works to realize that they knew all about colonial ambition in Canaan. They even managed to induce neighboring populations to have themselves circumcised on the quiet, and then they profited from the paralysis that that operation between your legs causes for a time, in order to wipe them out. But I don't mention that simply to record grievances about a stage of the religion that is now far behind us.

Having said that, however, it's clear that Freud doesn't for a moment doubt that the major interest of Jewish history is that of being the bearer of the message of one God.

And that's where things stand. We have the dissociation between the rationalist Moses and the inspired, obscurantist Moses, who is scarcely ever discussed. But basing his argument on the examination of historical evidence, Freud finds no other path adapted to the transmission of the rationalist Moses' message than that of darkness; in other words, this message is linked through repression to the murder of the Great Man. And it is precisely in this way, Freud tells us, that it could be transmitted and maintained in a state of efficacy that can be historically measured. It's so close to the Christian tradition that it's really remarkable; it is because the primordial murder of the Great Man reemerges in a second murder that in a sense translates and brings it to light, the murder of Christ, that the monotheistic message is completed. It is because the secret malediction of the murder of the Great Man – which itself only draws its power from the fact that it echoes the inaugural murder of humanity, that of the primitive father – it is because this event emerges into the light of day, that what, in the light of Freud's text, we are obliged to call Christian redemption may be accomplished.

That tradition alone pursues to the end the task of revealing what is involved in the primitive crime of the primordial law.

How after that can one avoid taking note of the originality of Freud's position relative to all that is to be found in the field of the history of religions? The history of religions consists essentially of establishing the common denominator of religiosity. We stake out the religious region in man within which we are required to include religions as different as one from Borneo, Confucianism, Taoism, and the Christian religion. It's not without its difficulties, although, when one sets out to produce typologies, there's no reason why one shouldn't end up with something. And this time, one ends up with a classification of the imaginary, which is in opposition to that which characterizes the origin of monotheism, and which is integrated into the primordial commandments insofar as they are the laws of speech: "Thou shalt not make a carved image of me," and so as to avoid that risk altogether, "Thou shalt not make any image at all."

And since I have happened to talk to you about the primitive sublimation of architecture, let me say that the problem of the temple that was destroyed without trace remains. To which symbolic order, to which set of precautions, to which exceptional circumstances did it appeal for everything to be destroyed, everything down to the remotest corner that might have made possible the reappearance, on the sides of a vase – and it wouldn't have been difficult – of images of animals, plants, and all those forms that were outlined on the walls of the cave? This temple was, in effect, only supposed to be the cover of what was at its center, of the Ark of union, that is the pure symbol of the pact, of the tie that bound him who said "I am what I am," and gave the commandments, to the people who received them, so that among all peoples it might be distinguished as the one that had wise and intelligent laws. How was this temple to be constructed so as to avoid all the traps of art?

It's a question that cannot be answered by any document, by any material image. I simply leave it open.

3

What is involved here is discussed by Freud in *Moses and Monotheism* in connection with the business of the moral law. He thoroughly integrates it there into the adventure which, as he writes in his text, only found its further development and its fulfillment in the Judeo-Christian story.

As far as other religions are concerned – he vaguely defines these as Oriental, thereby alluding apparently to a whole range that includes Buddhism, Lao-Tseu, and others – he affirms, with a boldness that one can only wonder at, that they are all nothing more than the religion of the Great Man. Thus things there remained stuck halfway, more or less aborted, without reaching the point of the primitive murder of this Great Man.

I am far from agreeing with all that. Yet in the history of the avatars of

Buddhism, one can find a great many things which, legitimately or not, can be made to illustrate Freud's theory; in other words, it is because they did not push the development of the drama through to the end that they stayed where they are. But it is, needless to say, odd to find this strange Christo-centrism in Freud's writings. There must have been a reason for him to have slipped into it almost without realizing it.

In any case, we find ourselves brought back to following the path to the end.

So that something like the order of the law may be transmitted, it has to pass along the path traced by the primordial drama articulated in *Totem and Taboo*, that is to say, the murder of the father and its consequences, the murder at the origin of culture of the figure about whom one can say nothing, a fearful and feared as well as dubious figure, an all-powerful, half-animal creature of the primal horde, who was killed by his sons. As a result of which – and the articulation here is important – an inaugural pact is established that is essential for a time to the institution of that law, which Freud does his best to tie to the murder of the father and to identify with the ambivalence that is thus at the basis of the relations between son and father or, in other words, involves the return of love once the act is accomplished.

All the mystery is in that act. It is designed to hide something, namely, that not only does the murder of the father not open the path to *jouissance* that the presence of the father was supposed to prohibit, but it, in fact, strengthens the prohibition. The whole problem is there; that's where, in fact as well as in theory, the fault lies. Although the obstacle is removed as a result of the murder, *jouissance* is still prohibited; not only that, but the prohibition is reinforced.

This fault that denies is thus sustained, articulated, made visible by the myth, but at the same time it is also camouflaged by it. That is why the important feature of *Totem and Taboo* is that it is a myth, and, as has been said, perhaps the only myth that the modern age was capable of. And Freud created it.

It is important to grasp what is embodied in this fault. Everything that passes across it is turned into a debt in the Great Book of debts. Every act of *jouissance* gives rise to something that is inscribed in the Book of debts of the Law. Furthermore, something in this regulatory mechanism must either be a paradox or the site of some irregularity, for to pass across the fault in the other direction is not equivalent.

Freud writes in *Civilization and Its Discontents* that everything that is transferred from *jouissance* to prohibition gives rise to the increasing strengthening of prohibition. Whoever attempts to submit to the moral law sees the demands of his superego grow increasingly meticulous and increasingly cruel.

Why isn't it the same in the other direction? It is a fact that it isn't the case at all. Whoever enters the path of uninhibited *jouissance*, in the name of the rejection of the moral law in some form or other, encounters obstacles whose power is revealed to us every day in our experience in innumerable forms, forms that nevertheless perhaps may be traced back to a single root.

We are, in fact, led to the point where we accept the formula that without a transgression there is no access to *jouissance*, and, to return to Saint Paul, that that is precisely the function of the Law. Transgression in the direction of *jouissance* only takes place if it is supported by the oppositional principle, by the forms of the Law. If the paths to *jouissance* have something in them that dies out, that tends to make them impassable, prohibition, if I may say so, becomes its all-terrain vehicle, its half-track truck, that gets it out of the circuitous routes that lead man back in a roundabout way toward the rut of a short and well-trodden satisfaction.

That is the point that our experience leads us to, on condition that we are guided by Freud's articulation of the problem. Sin needed the Law, Saint Paul said, so that he could become a great sinner – nothing, of course, affirms that he did, but so that he could conceive of the possibility.

Meanwhile, what we see here is the tight bond between desire and the Law. And it is in the light of this that Freud's ideal is an ideal tempered with civility that might be called patriarchal civility, in the full idyllic sense. The father is as sentimental a figure as you can imagine, the kind of figure suggested by the humanitarian ideal that resonates in Diderot's bourgeois dramas, or indeed in the figures that are the favorites of eighteenth-century engravings. That patriarchal civility is supposed to set us on the most reasonable path to temperate or normal desires.

Yet what Freud is proposing through his myth is, in spite of its novelty, not something that wasn't from a certain point of view a response to a demand. The demand to which it was, in fact, a response is not difficult to see.

The myth of the origin of the Law is incarnated in the murder of the father; it is out of that that the prototypes emerged, which we call successively the animal totem, then a more-or-less powerful and jealous god, and, finally, the single God, God the Father. The myth of the murder of the father is the myth of a time for which God is dead.

But if for us God is dead, it is because he always has been dead, and that's what Freud says. He has never been the father except in the mythology of the son, or, in other words, in that of the commandment which commands that he, the father, be loved, and in the drama of the passion which reveals that there is a resurrection after death. That is to say, the man who made incarnate the death of God still exists. He still exists with the commandment which orders him to love God. That's the place where Freud stops, and he stops at the same time – the theme is developed in *Civilization and Its Discontents* – at the place that concerns the love of one's neighbor, which is something that appears to be insurmountable for us, indeed incomprehensible.

I will attempt to explain why next time. I just wanted to emphasize the fact today that there is a certain atheistic message in Christianity itself, and I am not the first to have mentioned it. Hegel said that the destruction of the gods would be brought about by Christianity.

Man survives the death of God, which he assumes, but in doing so, he presents himself before us. The pagan legend tells us that at the moment when the veil of the temple was rent on the Aegean Sea, the message resounded that "The great Pan is dead." Even if Freud moralizes in *Civilization and Its Discontents,* he stops short at the commandment to love thy neighbor. It is to the heart of this problem that his theory of the meaning of the instinct brings us back. The relationship of the great Pan to death was, then, a stumbling block for the psychologism of his current disciples.

That's why my second lecture in Brussels turned on the question of love of one's neighbor. It was another theme I had in common with my audience. What I did, in fact, come up with, I will allow you to judge next time.

March 16, 1960

XIV

Love of one's neighbor

A SPECIAL GOD
FOOL AND KNAVE
THE TRUTH ABOUT TRUTH
WHY *JOUISSANCE* IS EVIL[1]
SAINT MARTIN
KANTIAN TALES

You know that last time I picked up my discussion with you by connecting it to my lecture to the Catholics.

Don't imagine that that was an easy way out. I didn't merely serve up again what I had to say in Brussels; I didn't tell them half of what I told you.

What I laid out last time concerning the death of God the Father will lead us to another question today, one that will show you Freud situating himself directly at the center of our true experience. For he doesn't attempt to evade the issue by making generalizations about the religious function in man. He is concerned with the way in which it manifests itself to us, that is to say, in the commandment which is expressed in our civilization in the form of the love of one's neighbor.

1

Freud confronts this commandment directly. And if you take the time to read *Civilization and Its Discontents,* you will see that that is where he begins, where he remains throughout, and where he ends up. He talks of nothing but that. What he has to say on the subject should under normal circumstances make our ears ring and set our teeth on edge. But that doesn't happen. It's a funny thing, but once a text has been in print for a certain period of time, it allows the transitory vertigo that is the vital source of its meaning to evaporate.

So I will try to reanimate the meaning of Freud's lines today. And since that will lead me toward some pretty potent notions, all I can do is ask language, what Freud would call *logos*, to lend me a measured tone.

God, then, is dead. Since he is dead, he always has been. I explained to

---

[1] It should be borne in mind throughout the following discussion that "le mal" in French includes the ideas both of "evil" and of "suffering."

you Freud's theory on the topic, namely, the myth expressed in *Totem and Taboo*. It is precisely because God is dead, has always been dead, that it was possible to transmit a message via all those beliefs which made him appear to be still alive, resurrected from the emptiness left by his death in those noncontradictory gods whom Freud indicates proliferated above all in Egypt.

The message in question is that of a single God who is both the Lord of the universe and the dispenser of the light that warms life and spreads the brightness of consciousness. His attributes are those of a thought which regulates the order of the real. It is Akhenaton's God, the God of the secret message that the Jewish people bears by reason of the fact that, by assassinating Moses, it reenacted the archaic murder of the father. That, according to Freud, is the God to whom the sentiment, of which only a few are capable, is addressed, namely, *amor intellectualis Dei*.

Freud also knows that, although that love is articulated now and then in the thought of such exceptional men as the famous polisher of lenses who lived in Holland, it is nevertheless not of such great importance; it didn't prevent the construction in the same period of Versailles, a building whose style proves that the Colossus of Daniel with the feet of clay was still standing upright, as is still the case, although it had collapsed a hundred times.

No doubt a science has been erected on the fragile belief I was discussing, namely, the one that is expressed in the following terms, which always reappear at the horizon of our aims: "The real is rational, the rational is real."

It's a strange thing that if the science in question has made use of the belief, it has nevertheless remained subservient, remained in the service of the colossus I just referred to, the one that has collapsed a hundred times and is still there. The fervent love that a solitary individual like Spinoza or Freud may feel for the God of the message has nothing to do with the God of the believers. Nobody doubts that, and especially the believers themselves, who, whether Jews or Christians, have never failed to cause Spinoza trouble.

But it is odd to see that for some time now, since it became known that God was dead, the believers involved practice ambiguity. By referring to the dialectical God, they are seeking an alibi for the crisis of confidence in their faith. It is a paradoxical fact, which hadn't occurred before in history, that the torch of Akhenaton functions nowadays as an alibi for the disciples of Ammon.

And I don't say this to slander the historical role played by the God of the believers, the God of the Judeo-Christian tradition. That the message of Akhenaton's God was preserved in the tradition of the latter made it worthwhile for Moses the Egyptian to be confused with the Midianite, with the Moses whose Thing, speaking from the burning bush, affirmed himself to be a special God – not the only God, note, but a special God, compared to whom all the others don't count. I don't want to emphasize more than necessary the line I am pursuing today on this point; it's not, strictly speaking, that it is forbidden to honor other gods, but you musn't do it in the presence of the God of Israel – the distinction is no doubt important for historians.

We who are trying to articulate Freud's thought and experience so as to give them their due weight and importance, we will articulate it in the following form: if this Symptom-God, this Totem-God or taboo, is worthy of our pondering the claim to turn him into a myth, it is because he was the vehicle of the God of truth. It is by means of the former that the truth about God could come to light, namely, that God was really killed by men, and that once the thing was reenacted, the primitive murder was redeemed. Truth found its way via him who the Scriptures no doubt call the Word, but also the Son of Man, thereby admitting the human nature of the Father.

Freud does not overlook the No/Name-of-the-Father. On the contrary, he speaks about it very well in *Moses and Monotheism* – in a contradictory way clearly, if you fail to take *Totem and Taboo* for what it is, namely, a myth; and he says that in human history the recognition of the function of the Father is a sublimation that is essential to the opening up of a spirituality that represents something new, a step forward in the apprehension of reality as such.

Freud also doesn't overlook – far from it – the real father. It is desirable according to Freud that in the course of the adventure of the subject, there is, if not the Father as God, then at least the Father as good father. I will read you some time the passage in which Freud speaks almost tenderly of the exquisiteness of that virile identification which flows from the love for the father and from his role in the normalization of desire. But that result only occurs in a favorable form as long as everything is in order with the No/Name-of-the-Father, that is to say, with the God who doesn't exist. The resulting situation for this good father is a remarkably difficult one; to a certain extent he is an insecure figure.

We know this only too well in practice. And it is also articulated in the Oedipus myth – although the latter also shows as well that it is preferable for the subject himself to be unaware of these reasons. But he now knows them, and the fact of knowing them is precisely that which has certain consequences in our time.

These consequences are self-evident. They can be seen in common speech and, indeed, in the speech of the analyst. If we want to complete the task we have given ourselves this year, it is only fitting that we articulate them.

Let me note in passing that as the first person to demystify the function of the Father, Freud himself couldn't be a thoroughly good father. I don't want to dwell on it today; it is something we can sense through his biography, and it could be the topic of a special chapter. Suffice it to characterize him as what he was, a bourgeois whose biographer and admirer, Jones, calls "uxorious." As we all know, he wasn't a model father.

There, too, where he was truly the father, the father of us all, the father of psychoanalysis, what did he do but hand it over to the women, and also perhaps to the master-fools? As far as the women are concerned, we should reserve judgment; they are beings who remain rich in promise, at least to the extent that they haven't yet lived up to them. As for the master-fools, that's another story altogether.

2

To the extent that a sensitive subject such as ethics is not nowadays separable from what is called ideology, it seems to me appropriate to offer here some clarification of the political meaning of this turning point in ethics for which we, the inheritors of Freud, are responsible.

That is why I spoke of master-fools. This expression may seem impertinent, indeed not exempt from a certain excess. I would like to make clear here what in my view is involved.

There was a time, an already distant time right at the beginning of our Society, you will remember, when we spoke of intellectuals in connection with Plato's *Meno*. I would like to make a few condensed comments on the subject, but I believe they will prove to be illuminating.

It was noted then that, for a long time now, there have been left-wing intellectuals and right-wing intellectuals. I would like to give you formulas for them that, however categorical they may appear at first sight, might nevertheless help to illuminate the way.

"Fool" (*sot*) or, if you like, "simpleton" (*demeuré*) – quite a nice term for which I have a certain fondness – these words only express approximately a certain something for which the English language and its literature seem to me to offer a more helpful signifier – I will come back to this later. A tradition that begins with Chaucer, but which reaches its full development in the theater of the Elizabethan period is, in effect, centered on the term "fool."[2]

The "fool" is an innocent, a simpleton, but truths issue from his mouth that are not simply tolerated but adopted, by virtue of the fact that this "fool" is sometimes clothed in the insignia of the jester. And in my view it is a similar happy shadow, a similar fundamental "foolery," that accounts for the importance of the left-wing intellectual.

---

[2] In this and subsequent passages, the words "fool" and "knave" along with "foolery" and "knavery" in quotation marks are in English in the original.

And I contrast this with the designation for that which the same tradition furnishes a strictly contemporary term, a term that is used in conjunction with the former, namely, "knave" – if we have the time, I will show you the texts, which are numerous and unambiguous.

At a certain level of its usage "knave" may be translated into French as *valet*, but "knave" goes further. He's not a cynic with the element of heroism implied by that attitude. He is, to be precise, what Stendhal called an "unmitigated scoundrel." That is to say, no more than your Mr. Everyman, but your Mr. Everyman with greater strength of character.

Everyone knows that a certain way of presenting himself, which constitutes part of the ideology of the right-wing intellectual, is precisely to play the role of what he is in fact, namely, a "knave." In other words, he doesn't retreat from the consequences of what is called realism; that is, when required, he admits he's a crook.

This is only of interest if one considers things from the point of view of their result. After all, a crook is certainly worth a fool, at least for the entertainment he gives, if the result of gathering crooks into a herd did not inevitably lead to a collective foolery. That is what makes the politics of right-wing ideology so depressing.

But what is not sufficiently noted is that by a curious chiasma, the "foolery" which constitutes the individual style of the left-wing intellectual gives rise to a collective "knavery."

What I am proposing here for you to reflect on has, I don't deny, the character of a confession. Those of you who know me are aware of my reading habits; you know which weeklies lie around on my desk. The thing I enjoy most, I must admit, is the spectacle of collective knavery exhibited in them – that innocent chicanery, not to say calm impudence, which allows them to express so many heroic truths without wanting to pay the price. It is thanks to this that what is affirmed concerning the horrors of Mammon on the first page leads, on the last, to purrs of tenderness for this same Mammon.

Freud was perhaps not a good father, but he was neither a crook nor an imbecile. That is why one can say about him two things which are disconcerting in their connection and their opposition. He was a humanitarian – who after checking his works will contest that? – and we must acknowledge it, however discredited the term might be by the crooks on the right. But, on the other hand, he wasn't a simpleton, so that one can say as well, and we have the texts to prove it, that he was no progressive.

I am sorry but it's a fact, Freud was in no way a progressive. And as far as this is concerned, there are even some extraordinarily scandalous things in his writings. From the pen of one of our guides, the little optimism manifested for the perspectives opened by the masses is certainly apt to shock, but it is indispensable for us to remember that, if we want to know where we stand.

You will see in what follows the usefulness of such remarks, which may appear crude.

One of my friends and patients had a dream which bore the traces of some yearning or other stimulated in him by the formulations of this seminar, a dream in which someone cried out concerning me, "But why doesn't he tell the truth about truth?"

I quote this, since it is an impatience that I have heard expressed by a great many in other forms than dreams. The formula is true to a certain extent – I perhaps don't tell the truth about truth. But haven't you noticed that in wanting to tell it – something that is the chief preoccupation of those who are called metaphysicians – it often happens that not much truth is left? That's what is so risky about such a pretension. It is a pretension that so easily lands us at the level of a certain knavery. And isn't there also a certain "knavery," a metaphysical "knavery," when one of our modern treatises on metaphysics, under this guise of the truth about truth, lets a great many things by which truly ought not to be let by?

I am content to tell the truth of the first stage and to proceed step by step. When I say that Freud is a humanitarian but not a progressive, I say something true. Let's try to follow the thread and take another true step.

We started out from the truth, which we must take to be a truth if we follow Freud's analysis, that we know God is dead.

However, the next step is that God himself doesn't know that. And one may suppose that he never will know it because he has always been dead. This formula nevertheless leads us to something that we have to resolve here, to something that remains on our hands from this adventure, something that changes the bases of the ethical problem, namely, that *jouissance* still remains forbidden as it was before, before we knew that God was dead.

That's what Freud says. And that's the truth – if not the truth about truth, then at least the truth about what Freud has to say.

As a result, if we continue to follow Freud in a text such as *Civilization and Its Discontents*, we cannot avoid the formula that *jouissance* is evil. Freud leads us by the hand to this point: it is suffering because it involves suffering for my neighbor.

This may shock you, upset certain habits, cause consternation among the happy souls. But it can't be helped; that's what Freud says. And he says it at the point of origin of our experience. He wrote *Civilization and Its Discontents* to tell us this. That's what was increasingly announced, promulgated, publicized, as analytical experience progressed. It has a name; it's what is known as beyond the pleasure principle. And it has effects that are by no means metaphysical; they oscillate between a "certainly not" and a "perhaps."

Those who like fairy stories turn a deaf ear to talk of man's innate tendencies to "evil, aggression, destruction, and thus also to cruelty." And Freud's text goes on: "Man tries to satisfy his need for aggression at the expense of his neighbor, to exploit his work without compensation, to use him sexually without his consent, to appropriate his goods, to humiliate him, to inflict suffering on him, to torture and kill him."[3]

If I hadn't told you the title of the work from which this passage comes, I could have pretended it was from Sade. Moreover, my upcoming lecture will, in effect, concern the Sadean account of the problem of morality.

For the time being, we will stick to Freud. *Civilization and Its Discontents* concerns the effort to rethink the problem of evil once one acknowledges that it is radically altered by the absence of God. This problem has always been avoided by the moralists in a way that is literally calculated to arouse our disgust once we have been alerted to the terms of the experience.

Whoever he might be, the traditional moralist always falls back into the rut of persuading us that pleasure is a good, that the path leading to good is blazed by pleasure. The trap is striking, for it has a paradoxical character that lends it its air of audacity. One is, so to speak, swindled in the second degree; one assumes there is just a hidden drawer, and one is pleased to have found it, but one is screwed even more when one has found it than if one hadn't even suspected its existence. Something that is relatively rare, for everyone can see that there's something fishy.

What does Freud have to say about this? Even before the formulations of *Beyond the Pleasure Principle*, it is evident that the first formulation of the pleasure principle as an unpleasure principle, or least-suffering principle, naturally embodies a beyond, but that it is, in effect, calculated to keep us on this side of it rather than beyond it. Freud's use of the good can be summed up in the notion that it keeps us a long way from our *jouissance*.

Nothing is more obvious in our clinical experience. Who is there who in the name of pleasure doesn't start to weaken when the first half-serious step is taken toward *jouissance*? Isn't that something we encounter directly everyday?

One can understand, therefore, the dominance of hedonism in the moral teachings of a certain philosophical tradition, whose motives do not seem to us to be absolutely reliable or disinterested.

In truth, it isn't because they have emphasized the beneficial effects of pleasure that we criticize the so-called hedonist tradition. It is rather because they haven't stated what the good consisted of. That's where the fraud is.

In the light of this one can understand that Freud was literally horrified by

---

[3] S.E. *XXI*, p. iii.

the idea of love for one's neighbor. One's neighbor in German is *der Nächste*. "Du sollst den Nächsten lieben wie sich selbst" – that's how the commandment, "Thou shalt love thy neighbor as thyself," is expressed in German. Freud underlines the excessive side of this by means of an argument that starts from several different points, which are, in fact, one and the same.

In the first place, the neighbor, whose fundamental nature is, as you have seen, revealed in Freud's writings, is bad. But that's not all there is to it. Freud also says – and it shouldn't make you smile just because it is expressed in a somewhat sparse manner – my love is something precious and I'm not going to give it whole to whomever claims to be what he is, simply because he happened to come by.

Freud makes comments about this that are quite right, moving comments on the subject of what is worth loving. He reveals how one must love a friend's son because, if the friend were to lose his son, his suffering would be intolerable. The whole Arisotelian conception of the good is alive in this man who is a true man; he tells us the most sensitive and reasonable things about what it is worth sharing the good that is our love with. But what escapes him is perhaps the fact that precisely because we take that path we miss the opening on to *jouissance*.

It is in the nature of the good to be altruistic. But that's not the love of thy neighbor. Freud makes us feel this without articulating it fully. We will now attempt, without forcing anything, to do so in his stead.

We can found our case on the following, namely, that every time that Freud stops short in horror at the consequences of the commandment to love one's neighbor, we see evoked the presence of that fundamental evil which dwells within this neighbor. But if that is the case, then it also dwells within me. And what is more of a neighbor to me than this heart within which is that of my *jouissance* and which I don't dare go near? For as soon as I go near it, as *Civilization and Its Discontents* makes clear, there rises up the unfathomable aggressivity from which I flee, that I turn against me, and which in the very place of the vanished Law adds its weight to that which prevents me from crossing a certain frontier at the limit of the Thing.

As long as it's a question of the good, there's no problem; our own and our neighbor's are of the same material. Saint Martin shares his cloak, and a great deal is made of it. Yet it is after all a simple question of training; material is by its very nature made to be disposed of – it belongs to the other as much as it belongs to me. We are no doubt touching a primitive requirement in the need to be satisfied there, for the beggar is naked. But perhaps over and above that need to be clothed, he was begging for something else, namely, that Saint Martin either kill him or fuck him. In any encounter there's a big difference in meaning between the response of philanthropy and that of love.

It is in the nature of the useful to be utilized. If I can do something in less time and with less trouble than someone near me, I would instinctively do it in his place, in return for which I am damned for what I have to do for that most neighborly of neighbors who is inside me. I am damned for having assured him to whom it would cost more time and trouble than me, what precisely? – some measure of ease that only means something because I imagine that, if I had that ease or absence of work, I would make the best possible use of it. But it is far from proven that I would know how to do so, even if I had all the power required to satisfy myself. Perhaps I would simply be bored.

Consequently, by granting others such power, perhaps I am just leading them astray. I imagine their difficulties and their sufferings in the mirror of my own. It is certainly not imagination that I lack; it is, if anything, tenderness, namely, what might be called the difficult way, love for one's neighbor. And here again you may note how the trap of the same paradox occurs to us in connection with the so-called discourse of utilitarianism.

I began my lectures this year with the onerous topic of the utilitarians, but the utilitarians are quite right. They are countered with something that, in effect, only makes the task of countering them much more difficult, with a sentence such as "But, Mr. Bentham, my good is not the same as another's good, and your principle of the greatest good for the greatest number comes up against the demands of my egoism." But it's not true. My egoism is quite content with a certain altruism, altruism of the kind that is situated on the level of the useful. And it even becomes the pretext by means of which I can avoid taking up the problem of the evil I desire, and that my neighbor desires also. That is how I spend my life, by cashing in my time in a dollar zone, ruble zone or any other zone, in my neighbor's time, where all the neighbors are maintained equally at the marginal level of reality of my own existence. Under these conditions it is hardly surprising that everyone is sick, that civilization has its discontents.

It is a fact of experience that what I want is the good of others in the image of my own. That doesn't cost so much. What I want is the good of others provided that it remain in the image of my own. I would even say that the whole thing deteriorates so rapidly that it becomes: provided that it depend on my efforts. I don't even need to ask you to go very far into your patients' experience: if I wish for my spouse's happiness, I no doubt sacrifice my own, but who knows if her happiness isn't totally dissipated, too?

Perhaps the meaning of the love of one's neighbor that could give me the true direction is to be found here. To that end, however, one would have to know how to confront the fact that my neighbor's *jouissance*, his harmful, malignant *jouissance*, is that which poses a problem for my love.

It wouldn't be difficult at this point to take a leap in the direction of the excesses of the mystics. Unfortunately, many of their most notable qualities always strike me as somewhat puerile.

No doubt the question of beyond the pleasure principle, of the place of the unnameable Thing and of what goes on there, is raised in certain acts that provoke our judgment, acts of the kind attributed to a certain Angela de Folignio, who joyfully lapped up the water in which she had just washed the feet of lepers – I will spare you the details, such as the fact that a piece of skin stuck in her throat, etc. – or to the blessed Marie Allacoque, who, with no less a reward in spiritual uplift, ate the excrement of a sick man. The power of conviction of these no doubt edifying facts would vary quite a lot if the excrement in question were that of a beautiful girl or if it were a question of eating the come of a forward from your rugby team. In other words, the erotic side of things remains veiled in the above examples.

That is why I will have to back up a little. We are now on the threshold of exploring something which has after all attempted to break down the doors of the hell within. Its claim to do so is clearly much greater than ours. Yet it is our concern, too. And that is why, in order to show you step by step the ways in which access to the problem of *jouissance* may be envisaged, I will lead you through what someone by the name of Sade has had to say about it.

I would certainly need a couple of months to talk about Sadism. I will not talk about Sade as eroticist, for he is definitely an inferior eroticist. The path of *jouissance* with a woman is not necessarily to subject her to all the acts practiced on poor Justine. On the other hand, in the domain of the articulation of ethical questions, it seems to me that Sade has some very solid things to say, at least in connection with the problem that currently concerns us.

4

Before I take up the question next time, I would like to end today by making you sense this in connection with a contemporary example, namely, Kant's, which I have already devoted some time to – and it's not for nothing that it is contemporary with Sade.

In the example in question Kant claims to prove the weight of the Law, formulated by him as practical reason, as something that imposes itself in purely reasonable terms, that is to say, divorced from all pathological affect, as he puts it, which means with no motive that appeals to the subject's interest. This is a critical exercise that will bring us back to the very center of the problem we are addressing today.

Let me remind you that Kant's example is made up of two little stories. The first concerns the individual who is placed in the situation of being executed on his way out, if he wants to spend time with the lady whom he desires unlawfully – it's not a waste of time to emphasize this, because even the apparently simplest details constitute traps. The other case is that of someone who lives at the court of a despot and who is put in the position of either bearing false witness against someone who, as a result, will lose his life or of being put to death himself if he doesn't do it.

Thereupon, Kant, our dear Kant, tells us in all his innocence, his innocent subterfuge, that in the first case everyone, every man of good sense, will say no. For the sake of spending a night with a woman, no one would be mad enough to accept an outcome that would be fatal to him, since it isn't a question of combat but of death by hanging. For Kant, the answer to the question is not in doubt.

In the other case, whatever the degree of pleasure promised as a result of bearing false witness or whatever the harshness of the penalty following the refusal to bear such witness, one can at least assume that the subject stops to reflect for a moment. One might even conceive that, rather than bear false witness, the subject will envisage accepting his own death in the name of the so-called categorical imperative. In effect, if an assault on the goods, the life, or the honor of someone else were to become a universal rule, that would throw the whole of man's universe into a state of disorder and evil.

Can't we stop here and offer our critique?

The striking significance of the first example resides in the fact that the night spent with the lady is paradoxically presented to us as a pleasure that is weighed against a punishment to be undergone; it is an opposition which homogenizes them. There is in terms of pleasure a plus and a minus. I will not quote the worst examples – in his *Essay on Negative Greatness*, Kant discusses the feelings of the Spartan mother who learns of the death of her son on the field of honor. And the little mathematical calculation Kant makes concerning the pleasure the family derives from the glory, from which one has to deduct the pain felt at the boy's loss, is quite touching. But it is important to note that one only has to make a conceptual shift and move the night spent with the lady from the category of pleasure to that of *jouissance,* given that *jouissance* implies precisely the acceptance of death – and there's no need of sublimation – for the example to be ruined.

In other words, it is enough for *jouissance* to be a form of evil, for the whole thing to change its character completely, and for the meaning of the moral law itself to be completely changed. Anyone can see that if the moral law is, in effect, capable of playing some role here, it is precisely as a support for the *jouissance* involved; it is so that the sin becomes what Saint Paul calls inordinately sinful. That's what Kant on this occasion simply ignores.

Then there is the other example, whose little errors of logic should not, between ourselves, be overlooked. The circumstances involved are somewhat different. In the first case, pleasure *and* pain are presented as a single packet to take or leave, in consideration of which one avoids the risk and gives up *jouissance.* In the second case, there is pleasure *or* pain. It's not insignificant that I underline it, for this choice is destined to produce in you a certain effect of *a fortiori*, as a result of which you may be deceived about the real significance of the question.

What's at issue here? That I attack the rights of another who is my fellow man in that statement of the universal rule, or is it a question of the false witness as such?

And what if I changed the example a little? Let's talk about true witness, about a case of conscience which is raised if I am summoned to inform on my neighbor or my brother for activities which are prejudicial to the security of the state. That question is of a kind that shifts the emphasis placed on the universal rule.

And I who stand here right now and bear witness to the idea that there is no law of the good except in evil and through evil, should I bear such witness?

This Law makes my neighbor's *jouissance* the point on which, in bearing witness in this case, the meaning of my duty is balanced. Must I go toward my duty of truth insofar as it preserves the authentic place of my *jouissance*, even if it is empty? Or must I resign myself to this lie, which, by making me substitute forcefully the good for the principle of my *jouissance*, commands me to blow alternatively hot and cold? Either I refrain from betraying my neighbor so as to spare my fellow man or I shelter behind my fellow man so as to give up my *jouissance*.

March 20, 1960

XV

The *jouissance* of transgression

THE BARRIER TO *JOUISSANCE*
THE RESPECT OF THE IMAGE OF THE OTHER
SADE, HIS FANTASM AND HIS DOCTRINE
METIPSEMUS
FRAGMENTED AND INDESTRUCTIBLE

I announced that I would talk about Sade.

It is not without some vexation that I take up the subject today because of the break for the vacation, which will be a long one.

I would like at least during this lecture to clear up the misunderstanding that might occur because we are dealing with Sade, and it might be thought that that constitutes a wholly external way of looking upon ourselves as pioneers or militants embracing a radical position. Such a view implies that, as a result of our function or profession, we are destined to embrace extremes, so to speak, and that Sade in this respect is our progenitor or precursor, who supposedly opened up some impasse, aberration or aporia, in that domain of ethics we have chosen to explore this year, and that we would be well-advised to follow him.

It is very important to clear up that misunderstanding, which is related to a number of others I am struggling against in order to make some progress here before you.

The domain that we are exploring this year isn't interesting for us only in a purely external sense. I would even say that up to a certain point this field may involve a certain degree of boredom, even for such a faithful audience as you, and it's not to be neglected – it has its own significance. Naturally, since I am speaking to you, I try to interest you; that's part of the deal. But that mode of communication which binds us together isn't necessarily calculated to avoid something that the art of the teacher normally proscribes. When I compare two audiences, if I managed to interest the one in Brussels, so much the better, but it isn't at all in the same way that you here are interested in my teaching.

If I adopt for a moment the point of view of what one finds in the situation, not so much of the young analyst, as of the analyst beginning his practice – and it's such a humanly sensitive and valid position – I would say that it is conceivable that what I am attempting to articulate under the title of the ethics of psychoanalysis comes up against the domain of what might be called analysis's pastoral letter.

Even then I am ascribing to what I am aiming at its noble name, its eternal name. A less flattering name would be the one invented by one of the most unpleasant authors of our time, "intellectual comfort." The question of "How does one proceed?" may, in effect, lead to impatience and even disappointment, when one is faced with the need to approach things at a level, that, it seems, is not that of our technique on the basis of which a great many things are to be resolved – or such at least is the promise. A great many things perhaps, but not everything. And we shouldn't necessarily turn our eyes away from those things that our technique warns us constitute an impasse or even a gap, even if all the consequences of our action are in question.

As for this young person who is beginning his practice as an analyst, I would call what is involved here his skeleton; it will give his action a vertebrate solidarity, or the opposite of that movement toward a thousand forms which is always on the point of collapsing in on itself and of becoming caught up in a circle – something that a certain number of recent explorations give the image of.

It is, therefore, not a bad idea to expose the fact that something may degenerate from the expectation of assurance – which is doubtless of some use in the exercise of one's profession – into a form of sentimental assurance. It is as a result of this that those subjects whom I take to be at a crossroads in their existence turn into prisoners of an infatuation that is the source of both an inner disappointment and a secret demand.

And if we are to make any progress, this is what the perspective of the ethical ends of psychoanalysis, whose significance I am trying to demonstrate here, has to combat. It is something one encounters sooner rather than later.

1

Our path thus far has led us to a point that I will call the paradox of *jouissance*.

The paradox of *jouissance* introduces its problematic into that dialectic of happiness which we analysts have perhaps rashly set out to explore. We have grasped the paradox in more than one detail as something that emerges routinely in our experience. But in order to lead you to it and relate it to the thread of our discussion, I have chosen this time the path of the enigma of its relation to the Law. And this is something that is marked by the strangeness of the way the existence of this Law appears to us, as founded on the Other as I have long taught you.

In this we have to follow Freud; not the individual with his atheistic profession of faith, but the Freud who was the first to acknowledge the value and relevance of a myth that constituted for us an answer to a certain fact that was formulated for no particular reason, but that has wide currency and is fully articulated in the consciousness of our time – though it went unnoticed by the finest minds and even more so by the masses – I mean the fact we call the death of God.

That's the problematic with which we begin. It is there the sign appears that I presented to you in my graph in the form of S (O). Situated as you know in the upper left section, it signifies the final response to the guarantee asked of the Other concerning the meaning of that Law articulated in the depths of the unconscious. If there is nothing more than a lack, the Other is wanting, and the signifier is that of his death.

It is as a function of this position, which is itself dependent on the paradox of the Law, that the paradox of *jouissance* emerges. This I will now try to explain.

We should note that only Christianity, through the drama of the passion, gives a full content to the naturalness of the truth we have called the death of God. Indeed, with a naturalness beside which the approaches to it represented by the bloody combats of the gladiators pale. Christianity, in effect, offers a drama that literally incarnates that death of God. It is also Christianity that associates that death with what happened to the Law; namely, that without destroying that Law, we are told, but in substituting itself for it, in summarizing it, and raising it up in the very movement that abolishes it – thus offering the first weighty historical example of the German notion of *Aufhebung*, i.e., the conservation of something destroyed at a different level – the only commandment is henceforth "Thou shalt love thy neighbor as thyself."

The whole thing is articulated as such in the Gospel, and it is there that we will continue on our way. The two notions, the death of God and the love of one's neighbor, are historically linked; and one cannot overlook that fact unless one attributes to everything that occurred in history in the Judeo-Christian tradition as constitutionally just a matter of chance.

I am aware of the fact that the message of the believers is that there is a resurrection in the afterlife, but that's simply a promise. That's the space through which we have to make our way. It is thus appropriate if we stop in this pass, in this narrow passage where Freud himself stops and retreats in understandable horror. "Thou shalt love thy neighbor as thyself," is a commandment that seems inhuman to him.

Everything he finds objectional is summed up in this phrase. As the examples he cites confirm, it is in the name of the most legitimate $\varepsilon\grave{v}\delta\alpha\iota\mu o\nu\acute{\iota}\alpha$ on all levels that he stops and rightly acknowledges, when he reflects on the commandment's meaning, the extent to which the historical spectacle of a humanity that chose it as its ideal is quite unconvincing, when that ideal is measured against actual accomplishments.

I have already referred to what it is that arouses Freud's horror, arouses the horror of the civilized man he essentially was. It derives from the evil in which he doesn't hestitate to locate man's deepest heart.

I don't really need to emphasize the point where I bring my two threads together to form a knot. Man's rebellion is involved here, the rebellion of *Jederman*, of everyman, insofar as he aspires to happiness. The truth that man seeks happiness remains true. The resistance to the commandment "Thou shalt love they neighbor as thyself" and the resistance that is exercised to prevent his access to *jouissance* are one and the same thing.

Stated thus, this may seem an additional paradox, a gratuitous assertion. Yet don't you recognize there what we refer to in the most routine way each time we see a subject retreat from his own *jouissance?* What are we drawing attention to? To the unconscious aggression that *jouissance* contains, to the frightening core of the *destrudo*, which, in spite of all our feminine affectations and quibbles, we constantly find ourselves confronting in our analytical experience.

Whether or not this view is ratified in the name of some preconceived view of nature, it is nevertheless true that at the heart of everything Freud taught, one finds the following: the energy of the so-called superego derives from the aggression that the subject turns back upon himself.

Freud goes out of his way to add the supplementary notion that, once one has entered on that path, once the process has been begun, then there is no longer any limit; it generates ever more powerful aggression in the self. It generates it at the limit, that is to say, insofar as the mediation of the Law is lacking. Of the Law insofar as it comes from elsewhere, from the elsewhere, moreover, where its guarantor is lacking, the guarantor who provides its warranty, namely, God himself.

To say that the retreat from "Thou shalt love thy neighbor as thyself" is the same thing as the barrier to *jouissance*, and not its opposite, is, therefore, not an original proposition.

I retreat from loving my neighbor as myself because there is something on the horizon there that is engaged in some form of intolerable cruelty. In that sense, to love one's neighbor may be the cruelest of choices.

That, then, is the nicely whetted edge of the paradox I am asserting here. No doubt in order to give it its full weight, one should take it step by step, so that by understanding the way in which that intimate line of demarcation appears, we may not so much know as feel the ups and downs to be found on its path.

We have, of course, long learned to recognize in our analytical experience the *jouissance* of trangression. But we are far from knowing what its nature might be. In this respect our position is ambiguous. Everybody knows that we have restored full civil rights to perversion. We have dubbed it a component drive, thereby employing the idea that it harmonizes with a totality, and at the same time shedding suspicion on the research, which was revolutionary at a certain moment in the nineteenth century, of Krafft-Ebing with his monumental *Psychopathia Sexualis*, or also on the work of Havelock Ellis.

Incidentally, I don't want to fail to give the latter's work the kind of thumbs down I think it deserves. It offers amazing examples of a lack of systematicity – not the failure of a method, but the choice of a failed method. The so-called scientific objectivity that is exhibited in books that amount to no more than a random collection of documents offers a living example of the combination of a certain "foolery" with the sort of "knavery," a fundamental knavery, that I invoked last time as the characteristic of a certain kind of thought known as left-wing, without excluding the possibility of its spreading its stain to other domains. In short, if I recommend reading Havelock Ellis, it is simply in order to show you the difference, not just in results but in tone, that exists between such a futile mode of investigation and what Freud's thought and experience reintroduce into the domain – it's simply a question of responsibility.

We are familiar with the *jouissance* of transgression, then. But what does it consist of? Does it go without saying that to trample sacred laws under foot, laws that may be directly challenged by the subject's conscience, itself excites some form of *jouissance*? We no doubt constantly see the strange development in a subject that might be described as the testing of a faceless fate or as a risk that, once it has been survived by the subject, somehow guarantees him of his power. Doesn't the Law that is defied here play the role of a means, of a path cleared that leads straight to the risk? Yet if the path is necessary, what is the risk that is involved? What is the goal *jouissance* seeks if it has to find support in transgression to reach it?

I leave these questions open for the moment so as to move on. If the subject turns back on his tracks, what is it that guides this backtracking? On this point, we find a more motivated response in analysis; we are told that it is the identification with the other that arises at the extreme moment in one of our temptations. And by extreme here I do not mean it has to do with extraordinary temptations, but with the moment when one perceives their consequences.

We retreat from what? From assaulting the image of the other, because it was the image on which we were formed as an ego. Here we find the convincing power of altruism. Here, too, is the leveling power of a certain law of equality – that which is formulated in the notion of the general will. The latter is no doubt the common denominator of the respect for certain rights – which, for a reason that escapes me, are called elementary rights – but it can also take the form of excluding from its boundaries, and therefore from its protection, everything that is not integrated into its various registers.

And the power of expansion is also seen in what I expressed last time as the utilitarian tendency. At this level of homogenization, the law of utility, as that which implies its distribution over the greatest number, imposes itself in a form that is effectively innovative. It is an enchanting power, scorn for which is sufficiently indicated in the eyes of us analysts when we call it philanthropy, but which also raises the questions of the natural basis of pity in the sense implied by that morality of feeling which has always sought its foundation there.

We are, in effect, at one with everything that depends on the image of the other as our fellow man, on the similarity we have to our ego and to everything that situates us in the imaginary register. What is the question I am raising here, when it seems to be obvious that the very foundation of the law "Thou shalt love thy neighbor as thyself" is to be found there?

It is indeed the same other that is concerned here. Yet one only has to stop for a moment to see how obvious and striking the practical contradictions are – individual, inner contradictions as well as social ones – of the idealization expressed relative to the respect that I formulated for the image of the other. It implies a certain continuity and filiation of problematic effects on the religious law, which is expressed and manifested historically by the paradoxes of its extremes, i.e., the extremes of saintliness, and moreover by its failure on the social level, insofar as it never manages to achieve fulfillment, reconciliation, or the establishment on earth of what is promised by it.

To emphasize the point even more strongly, I will refer directly to something that seems to be opposed to this denunciation of the image, that is to the statement which is always listened to with a kind of more-or-less amused purr of satisfaction, "God made man in his own image." Religious tradition once again reveals more cunning in pointing to the truth than the approach of psychological philosophy imagines.

You can't get away with answering that man no doubt paid God back in kind. The statement in question is of the same inspiration, the same body, as the holy book in which is expressed the prohibition on forging images of God. If this prohibition has a meaning, it is that images are deceitful.

Why is that? Let's go to what is simplest: if these are beautiful images – and goodness only knows that religious images always correspond by definition to reigning canons of beauty – one doesn't notice that they are always hollow images. Moreover, man, too, as image is interesting for the hollow the image leaves empty – by reason of the fact that one doesn't see in the image, beyond the capture of the image, the emptiness of God to be discovered. It is perhaps man's plenitude, but it is also there that God leaves him with emptiness.

Now God's power resides in the capacity to advance into emptiness. All of that gives us the figures of the apparatus of a domain in which the recognition of another reveals itself as an adventure. The meaning of the word *recognition* tends toward that which it assumes in every exploration, with all the accents of militancy and of nostalgia we can invest in it.

Sade is at this limit.

2

Sade is at this limit, and insofar as he imagines going beyond it, he teaches us that he cultivates its fantasm with all the morose enjoyment – I will come back to this phrase – that is manifest in that fantasm.

In imagining it, he proves the imaginary structure of the limit. But he also goes beyond it. He doesn't, of course, go beyond it in his fantasm, which explains its tedious character, but in his theory, in the doctrine he advances in words that at different moments in the work express the *jouissance* of destruction, the peculiar virtue of crime, evil sought for evil's sake, and, in the last instance, the Supreme-Being-in-Evil – a strange reference made by the character of Saint-Fond, who proclaims in *The Story of Juliette* his renewed but not particularly new belief in this God.

This theory is called in the same work the System of Pius VI, the Pope who is introduced as one of the characters in the novel. Taking things even further, Sade lays out a vision of Nature as a vast system of attraction and repulsion of evil by evil. Under these circumstances the ethical stance consists in realizing to the most extreme point this assimilation to absolute evil, as a consequence of which its integration into a fundamentally wicked nature will be realized in a kind of inverted harmony.

I am just pointing to something that appears not as stages of thought in search of a paradoxical formulation, but much more as its wrenching apart, its collapse, in the course of a development that created its own impasse.

Can't one nevertheless say that Sade teaches us, in the order of symbolic play, how to attempt to go beyond the limit, and how to discover the laws of one's neighbor's space as such? The space in question is that which is formed when we have to do not with this fellow self whom we so easily turn into our reflection, and whom we necessarily implicate in the same misrecognitions that characterize our own self, but this neighbor who is closest to us, the neighbor whom we sometimes take in our arms, if only to make love to. I am not speaking here of ideal love, but of the act of making love.

We know well how the images of the self may frustrate our propulsion into that space. Don't we have something to learn about the laws of this space from the man who enters it with his atrocious discourse, given that the imaginary capture by the image of one's fellow man functions as a lure there?

You can see where I am taking you. At the precise point to which I attach our inquiry, I am not prejudging what the other is. I simply emphasize the lures of one's fellow man because it is from this fellow as such that the misrecognitions which define me as a self are born. And I will just stop for a moment and refer to a little fable in which you will recognize my personal touch.

I once spoke to you about a mustard pot. If I draw three pots here, I simply demonstrate that you have a whole row of mustard or jam pots. They stand on shelves and are numerous enough to satisfy your contemplative appetites. Note that it is insofar as the pots are identical that they are irreducible. Thus at this level we come up against the condition of individuation. And that's as far as the problem usually goes, namely, that there is this one, which isn't that one.

Naturally, the affected quality of this little trick doesn't escape me. But do try to understand the truth it hides, like all sophisms. I don't know if you have noticed that the etymology of the French word *même* (self) is none other than *metipsemus*, which makes this *même* in *moi-même* redundant. The phonetic evolution is from *metipsemus* to *même* – that which is most myself in myself, that which is at the heart of myself, and beyond me, insofar as the self stops at the level of those walls to which one can apply a label. What in French at least serves to designate the notion of self or same (*même*), then, is this interior or emptiness, and I don't know if it belongs to me or to nobody.

That's what the use of my sophism signifies; it reminds me that my neighbor possesses all the evil Freud speaks about, but it is no different from the evil I retreat from in myself. To love him, to love him as myself, is necessarily to move toward some cruelty. His or mine?, you will object. But haven't I just explained to you that nothing indicates they are distinct? It seems rather that they are the same, on condition that those limits which oblige me to posit myself opposite the other as my fellow man are crossed.

And here I should make my approach clear. Panic drunkenness, sacred orgy, the flagellants of the cults of Attis, the Bacchantes of the tragedy of Euripides, in short, all that remote Dionysionism lost in a history to which reference has been made since the nineteenth century with the expectation of restoring, beyond Hegel, Kierkegaard and Nietzsche, the vestiges still available to us of the sphere of the great Pan, in an apologetic, utopian and apocalyptic form that was condemned by Kierkegaard and not less effectively by Nietzsche – that's not what I mean when I speak of the sameness (*mêmeté*) of someone else and myself. That is by the way why I finished the seminar before last with the evocation of the statement that is correlative to the rending of the veil of the temple, namely, Great Pan is dead.

I will say no more today. It's not just a question of my prophesying in my turn, but I will take an appointment with you for the time when I will have to try to justify why and from what the Great Pan died, and at the precise moment no doubt that the legend points to.

3

It is Sade's approach that concerns us now, insofar as it points the way to my neighbor's space in connection with what I will call – thereby paraphrasing the title of the work of his that is called *Ideas on the Novel* – the idea of a technique oriented toward a sexual *jouissance* that is not sublimated.

This idea shows us all kinds of lines of divergence, to the point that it gives rise to the idea of difficulty. Consequently, it will be necessary for us to evaluate the scope of the literary work as such. And isn't that quite a detour, which will definitely set us back again, and haven't I been criticized for being slow for some time now?

To finish rapidly with this further refinement, I will need to evoke several directions from which Sade's work may be grasped, if only to indicate the one that I am choosing.

Is this work a form of witness? A conscious or unconscious witness? Don't think in terms of the psychoanalytic unconscious here; I mean by "unconsious" here the fact that the subject Sade wasn't fully aware of the conditions in which he as nobleman found himself, during the period from the beginning of the French Revolution and down through the Terror, which he was to live through only to be banished to the asylum at Charenton, apparently at the will of the First Consul.

In truth, Sade seems to me to have been fully aware of the relationship of his work to the attitudes of the type I called the man of pleasure. The man of pleasure as such bears witness against himself, by publicly confessing the extremes to which he may go. The great joy with which he recalls the emergence of this tradition historically is a clear sign of the point the master always reaches when he doesn't bow his head before the being of God.

There is no reason to hide in any way the realistic side of Sade's atrocities. Their developed, insistent, extravagant character is so obvious and constitutes such a challenge to credibility that the idea that this is an ironic discourse becomes quite plausible. It is nevertheless true that the things involved are commonly found in the works of Suetonius, Dion Cassius and others. Read the *Memoirs on the Great Days in Auvergne* by Esprit Fléchier, if you want to learn what a great Lord at the beginning of the seventeenth century could get up to with his peasants.

We would be quite wrong to think that, in the name of the self-restraint the fascinations of the imaginary impose on our weakness, men are incapable in certain situations of transgressing given limits without knowing what they are doing.

In this connection, Freud helps us out with that absolute lack of subterfuge, that total absence of "knavery" that characterizes him, when he doesn't hesitate to make the point in *Civilization and Its Discontents* that there is nothing in common between the satisfaction a *jouissance* affords in its original state and that which it gives in the indirect or even sublimated forms that civilization obliges it to assume.

In one place he doesn't disguise his view of the fact that those *jouissances* which are forbidden by conventional morality are nevertheless perfectly accessible and accepted by certain people, who live under a given set of conditions and whom he points to, namely, those whom we call the rich – and it is doubtless the case that, in spite of obstacles that are familiar to us, they sometimes make the most of their opportunities.

To make things clear, let me use this passage to make an incidental remark, similar to the remarks Freud makes on the subject, but that are often omitted or neglected. The security of *jouissance* for the rich in our time is greatly increased by what I will call the universal legislation of work. Just imagine what social conflicts were like in times past. Try to find something equivalent nowadays not at the frontiers of our societies, but within them.

And now a point on the value of Sade's work as witness of reality. Shall we investigate its value as sublimation? If we consider sublimation in its most developed form, indeed in the fiercest and most cynical form in which Freud took pleasure in representing it, namely, as the transformation of the sexual instinct into a work in which everyone will recognize his own dreams and impulses, and will reward the artist for having given him that satisfaction by granting the latter a fuller and happier life – and for giving him in addition access to the satisfaction of the instinct involved from the beginning – if we seek to grasp the work of Sade from this perspective, then it's something of a failure.

It's something of a failure, if one thinks of the amount of time poor Sade spent either in prison or interned in special institutions. As for the work itself, at least *The New Justine* along with *The Story of Juliette* had a great deal of success during his lifetime in an underground form, a success of the night, a success of the damned. But I won't insist on that here. If I refer to it, it is so as to cast some light on those sides of Sade that are worth illuminating.

Let us now try to see how we should situate Sade's work. It has been called an unsurpassable body of work, in the sense that it achieves an absolute of the unbearable in what can be expressed in words relative to the transgression of all human limits. One can acknowledge that in no other literature, at no other time, has there been such a scandalous body of work. No one else has done such deep injury to the feelings and thoughts of mankind. At a time when Henry Miller's stories make us tremble, who would dare rival the licentiousness of Sade? One might indeed claim that we have there the most scandalous body of work ever written. Thus, as Maurice Blanchot puts it, "Isn't that a reason for us to be interested in it?"

And we are interested in just that way here. I urge you to make the effort to read the book in which two articles by Blanchot on Lautréamont and Sade are to be found. They constitute a part of the material to be put in our file.

That is certainly saying a lot then. It seems, in fact, as if one cannot conceive of an atrocity that isn't to be found in Sade's catalogue. The assault on one's sensibility is of a kind that is literally stupefying; in other words, one loses one's bearings. As far as this is concerned, one might even say that the effect in question is achieved artlessly, without any consideration for an economy of means, but through the accumulation of details and perepetia, to which is added a whole stuffing of treatises and rationalizations whose contradictions are of particular interest to us and that we can analyze in detail.

It takes a crude mind to assume that the treatises are simply there to make the erotic passages acceptable. Even minds that are far subtler have attributed to such treatises, dubbed digressions, a loss of suggestive tension on the level that the subtler minds in question – I am thinking of Georges Bataille – consider to be that of the works' true value, namely, their power to open up the possibility of the assumption of being on the level of immorality.

That's a mistake. The real problem is something else. It is nothing else but the response of a being, whether reader or writer, at the approach to a center of incandescence or an absolute zero that is physically unbearable. The fact that the book falls from one's hands no doubt proves that it is bad, but literary badness here is perhaps the guarantee of the very badness or *mauvaisité*, as it was still called in the eighteenth century, that is the object of our investigation. As a consequence, Sade's work belongs to the order of what I shall call experimental literature. The work of art in this case is an experiment that through its action cuts the subject loose from his psychosocial moorings – or to be more precise, from all psychosocial appreciation of the sublimation involved.

There is no better example of such a work than the one which I hope some of you at least are addicted to – addicted to in the same sense as "addicted to opium" – namely, the *Songs of Maldoror* by Lautréamont. And it is only fitting if Maurice Blanchot combines the points of view he presents us with on these two authors.

But with Sade the social reference is retained, and he claims to valorize socially his extravagant system, whence his astonishing avowals that suggest incoherence and lead to a multiple contradiction, which one would be wrong to ascribe purely and simply to the absurd. The absurd has recently become a somewhat too convenient category. One respects the dead, but I can't avoid noting the indulgence shown by a certain Nobel Prize winner to all the mumbo jumbo on the topic.[1] That prize is a wonderful universal reward for "knav-

---

[1] The reference is to Albert Camns, who received the Nobel Prize for literature in 1957.

ery"; its honor roll bears the stigmata of a form of abjection in our culture.

By way of conclusion, I will focus on two terms that point to the next stage in our project.

When one approaches that central emptiness, which up to now has been the form in which access to *jouissance* has presented itself to us, my neighbor's body breaks into pieces. Proclaiming the law of *jouissance* as the foundation of some ideally utopian social system, Sade expresses himself in italics in the nice little edition of *Juliette* published recently by Pauvert, though it is still a book that circulates surreptitiously: "Lend me the part of your body that will give me a moment of satisfaction and, if you care to, use for your own pleasure that part of my body which appeals to you."

We find in this formulation of the fundamental law, which expresses the side of Sade's social system that claims to be socially viable, the first considered manifestation of something that we psychaoanlysts have come to know as part object.

But when the notion of part object is articulated in that way, we imply that this part object only wants to be reintegrated into the object, into the already valorized object, the object of our love and tenderness, the object that brings together within it all the virtues of the so-called genital stage. Yet we should consider the problem a little differently; we should notice that this object is necessarily in a state of independence in a field that we take to be central as if by convention. The total object, our neighbor, is silhouetted there, separate from us and rising up, if I may say so, like the image of Carpaccio's San Giorgio degli Schiavone in Venice, in the midst of a charnel house figure.

The second term that Sade teaches us concerns that which appears in the fantasm as the indestructible character of the Other, and emerges in the figure of his victim.

Whether in *Justine* itself or in a certain Sadean posterity that is less than distinguished, namely, that erotic or pornographic posterity, which recently produced one of its finest works, *The Story of O-*, the victim survives the worst of her ordeals, and she doesn't even suffer in her sensual power of attraction, that the author never ceases evoking, as is always the case in such descriptions; she always has the prettiest eyes in the world, the most pathetic and touching appearance. That the author always insists on placing his subjects under such a stereotyped heading poses a problem in itself.

It seems that whatever happens to the subject is incapable of spoiling the image in question, incapable even of wearing it out. But Sade, who is different in character from those who offer us these entertaining little stories, goes further, since we see emerge in him in the distance the idea of eternal punishment. I will come back to this point, because it amounts to a strange contradiction in a writer who wants nothing of himself to survive, who doesn't even want any part of the site of his tomb to remain accessible to men, but wants it instead to be covered with bracken. Doesn't that indicate that he locates in the fantasm the content of the most intimate part of himself, which we have called the neighbor, or in other words the *metipsemus?*

I will finish my lecture today on a point of detail. By what deep attachments is it that a certain relationship to the Other, that we call Sadistic, reveals its true connection to the psychology of the obsessional? – the obsessional, whose defenses take the form of an iron frame, of a rigid mold, a corset, in which he remains and locks himself up, so as to stop himself having access to that which Freud somewhere calls a horror he himself doesn't know.

March 30, 1960

PARENTHESIS
The Death Drive According to Bernfeld

You will not be hearing the continuation of my last lecture today. You will not be hearing it for personal reasons.

The break occasioned by the vacation was used by me to prepare an article for the next issue of our periodical, which is devoted to structure, and it took me back to an earlier period of my thinking. It also broke my rhythm relative to the subject I am exploring with you, namely, the deeper dimension of analytical thought, work and technique that I am calling ethics.

I read over what I said last time, and, believe me, it's not bad at all. It is because I want to stay at that level that I will postpone the continuation until next time.

We have at present reached that barrier beyond which the analytical Thing is to be found, the place where brakes are applied, where the inaccessibility of the object as object of *jouissance* is organized. It is in brief the place where the battlefield of our experience is situated. This crucial point is at the same time the new element psychoanalysis brings, however inaccessible it may be in the field of ethics.

In order to compensate for that inaccessibility, all individual sublimation is projected beyond that barrier, along with the sublimations of the systems of knowledge, including – why not? – that of analytical knowledge itself.

That's something I will probably be obliged to articulate for you next time; that is to say, the last word of Freud's thought, and especially that concerning the death drive, appears in the field of analytical thought as a sublimation.

From this point of view, it seemed to me to be useful, by way of a parenthesis, to give you the background against which this notion might be formulated. In the usual spirit of a seminar, I have, therefore, asked Mr. Kaufmann to summarize for us what the representatives of a good psychoanalytic generation, namely, Bernfeld and his collaborator Freitelberg, thought up on the subject of the meaning of the drive, so as to try to give it its fullest extension in the scientific context of the time, where they believe it should be situated.

As a result, you will learn about a moment in the history of psychoanalytic thought today. You know the importance I attach to such moments, precisely because in their very aporia I often teach you to find an authentic ridge in the land across which we are traveling.

You will see the difficulties encountered by Bernfeld in his attempt to insert the death drive in a theory of energy that is no doubt already dated, but that is definitely that of the context in which Freud was speaking. Mr. Kaufmann has made a great many helpful comments on the common fund of scientific notions from which Freud borrowed some of his terms, terms that we misread simply by taking them as is, and limiting ourselves to Freud's enunciation of them alone. It is, of course, true that their internal coherence gives them their meaning, but knowing from which period discourse they were borrowed is never futile. [Mr. Kaufmann's presentation follows]

I would like to thank Mr. Kaufmann emphatically for having helped us to unravel the chain of reflections represented by these three essential articles of Bernfeld's.

If to some of you – and I hope that such is the case with as few as possible – the whole thing may have seemed to be a mere detour relative to the overall plan of our research, it is certainly not an *hors-d'oeuvre*. If the death drive in Freud encounters in Bernfeld's work the objection that it supposedly teaches us nothing about the phenomenon from within, you will see that it teaches us a lot about the space in which Freud's thought moves. In a word, you have heard enough to know that this dimension is, properly speaking, that of the subject. It is the necessary condition for the natural phenomenon of the instinct in entropy to be taken up at the level of the person, so that it may take on the value of an oriented instinct and is significant for the system insofar as the latter as a whole is situated in an ethical dimension.

We would be wrong to be surprised, otherwise this would be neither the method nor the therapeutic nor indeed ascetic way, of our analytical experience.

April 27, 1960

XVI

The death drive

MARX AND THE PROGRESSIVES
JOUISSANCE, THE SATISFACTION OF A DRIVE
THE SYSTEM OF POPE PIUS VI
CREATIONISM AND EVOLUTIONISM
WOMAN AS *EX NIHILO*

I wouldn't want to begin my seminar today without telling you briefly what I didn't have time to tell you yesterday at the meeting of our Society.

We heard a remarkable paper, given by someone who wasn't trying to revolutionize the field of hysteria, and who wasn't in a position to bring us an immense or original body of experience, since the person involved is only just beginning his career in psychoanalysis; nevertheless, his very complete and, as was noted, perhaps overly rich presentation was extremely well articulated.

That doesn't mean that it was perfect. And if I had felt it necessary to force the issue by intervening after the somewhat premature termination of the discussion, I would certainly have rectified certain points made concerning the relations of the hysteric to the ego ideal and the ideal ego, notably in the element of uncertainty in the linking of these two functions.

But that isn't important. A presentation of the kind in question reveals how the categories that I have been striving to promote in this seminar for years prove to be useful and allow one to articulate things with some precision. They shed a light that is adequate to the limits of our experience. And however much one may take issue with some point of detail or other, you can see the theoretical concepts come alive as if by themselves, and make contact with the level of experience.

We have spoken about the relations between the hysteric and the signifier. In our clincial experience we can feel its presence at every moment, and last night you were presented with what might well be called a well-oiled machine that started working before your very eyes. So many points were presented to the test of experience, but the whole brought you into direct contact with the convergence of the theoretical notions I have given you and the structure that concerns us, namely, a structure that is defined by the fact that the subject is to be situated in the signifier. Directly in front of us, we see appear the "It speaks."[1]

The "It speaks" derived from theory joins everyday clinical experience.

We saw the hysteric come alive in her own sphere, and not by reference to obscure forces that are unevenly divided in a space that is not moreover homogeneous – the latter is typical of a discourse that only claims to be analytical. The reason it can only claim to be analytical is that it alienates itself in all kinds of references to sciences that are altogether worthy in their own domain, but which are often only involved by the theorist so as to mask his clumsiness in moving about in his own sphere.

This is not simply a form of homage paid to the work you heard, nor is it a simple *hors-d'oeuvre* to what I am attempting with you, but a reminder that I am trying with all the means at my disposal, which are simply those of experience, to make the ethical dimension of psychoanalysis come alive before you.

1

I don't claim to do anything more this year than I have done in years past in the form of a progressive development – from the first reference to speech and to language up to the attempt last year to define the function of desire in the economy of our experience – that is guided by Freudian thought.

In this discussion of Freud's thought I do not proceed like a professor. The usual approach of professors to the thought of those who happen to have taught us something in the course of human history generally consists in formulating it in such a way that it can only be seen from its narrowest and most partial side. Hence the impression of taking in deep breaths one always has when one goes directly to the original texts – I am, of course, referring to texts that are worthwhile.

One never goes beyond Descartes, Kant, Marx, Hegel and a few others because they mark a line of inquiry, a true orientation. One never goes beyond Freud either. Nor does one attempt to measure his contribution quantitatively, draw up a balance sheet – what's the point of that? One uses him. One moves around within him. One takes one's bearings from the direction he points in. What I am offering you here is an attempt to articulate the essence of an experience that has been guided by Freud. It is in no way an effort to measure the volume of his contribution or summarize him.

---

[1] "Le ça parle." "Le ça" is the everyday French word Lacan prefers to translate "das Es." That is why "it" seems more appropriate in this particular context than "Id."

That the ethical dimension is the stuff of our experience is revealed to us in the implicit deviations in ethics that appear in the so-called objectifying notions which have been gradually laid down through the different periods of analytical thought. Isn't an implicit ethical notion contained in the concept of the offering that you often see me criticize here? Don't those unformulated, scarcely acknowledged, yet often explicit goals that are expressed in the notion of remaking the subject's ego or of accomplishing through analysis the restructuring of the subject's ego – not to speak of reformation or reform with all its implications in analysis – don't they all imply an ethical dimension? I just want to show you that it doesn't correspond to the reality of our experience, to the real dimensions in which the ethical problem is posed. Freud suggests as much through the particular orientation he has opened up for us.

Thus by leading you on to the ground of the ethics of psychoanalysis this year, I have brought you up against a certain limit that I illustrated through a confrontation, or heightening of the difference by contrast, of Kant and Sade, however paradoxical that may seem. I have led you to the point of apocalypse or of revelation of something called transgression.

This point of transgression has a significant relation to something that is involved in our inquiry into ethics, that is to say, the meaning of desire. And my discussions of previous years have taught you to make a strict distinction between desire and need in Freudian experience, which is also our own daily experience. There is no way one can reduce desire in order to make it emerge, emanate, from the dimension of need. That provides you with the framework in which our research progresses.

Let me come back to something which has a contingent character in the comments I have made to you. In a byway of one of my lectures, I made a paradoxical and even whimsical excursion on the topic of two figures that I set in opposition to one another, those of the left-wing intellectual and the right-wing intellectual.

By using these two terms in a certain register and by setting them up in opposition to each other, I might have seemed to bear witness to that imprudence which encourages indifference on political questions. In brief, it turned out that I was criticized for having emphasized in terms I chose with some care that Freud wasn't a progressive – yet I did go out of my way to say that Freud's ethics in *Civilization and Its Discontents* were humanitarian, which is not exactly to say that he was a reactionary.

The remarks made struck some as dangerous, although their accuracy was not, in fact, challenged. I was surprised that something of the kind was said to me, and especially given the political orientation from which it came. To those who may have been similarly surprised, I would encourage them to take the time to look these things up by reading certain short works – that's always a valuable exercise, if one wants to check up on the movements of one's feelings.

I have brought one such work today. It is the first volume of Karl Marx's *Philosophical Works*, translated by Molitor, and published by Alfred Coste. I encourage those concerned to read, for example, "The Contribution to the Critique of Hegel's Philosophy of Law," or quite simply that curious little work called "The Jewish Question." Perhaps they would get a more precise notion of what Marx would think, if he were alive now, about what is called progressivism; and I mean by that a certain style of ideology, characterized by its generosity and apparently widespread in our bourgeoisie. The way in which Marx would evaluate such progressivism will be apparent to all those who look up those sources I just mentioned; they are a good, healthy standard of a certain kind of intellectual honesty.

Thus, in saying Freud was not a progressive, I didn't at all want to say, for example, that he wasn't interested in the Marxist experience. But it is nevertheless a fact that he wasn't a progressive. I am not imputing things of a political nature to Freud in saying that; it is just that he did not share certain types of bourgeois prejudice.

However, it is also a fact that Freud wasn't a Marxist. I didn't emphasize that because I don't really see the interest or the ramifications of it. I will reserve for later a discussion of the interest that the dimension opened up by Freud might have for Marxism. This point will be much more difficult to introduce, since up to now no one among the Marxists seems to have noticed particularly – if it is true that Marxists still exist – the meaning embodied in the experience opened up by Freud.

Marx takes up the tradition of a thought that culminated in the work which was the object of his perspicacious comments, namely, Hegel's *Philosophy of Law* – a work that articulates something that, as far as I know, we are still immersed in, namely, the foundation of the State, of the bourgeois State, which lays down the rules of a human organization founded on need and reason. Marx makes us see the biased, partial and incomplete character of the solution given in this framework. He shows that the harmony between need and reason is at this level only an abstract and dissociated solution.

Need and reason are harmonized only in law, but everyone is left a victim of the egoism of his private needs, of anarchy and of materialism. Marx aspires to the creation of a State where, as he puts it, human emancipation will be not only political but real, a State where man will find himself in a non-alienated relation to his own organization.

Now you know that, in spite of the openings that history has given to the direction pointed to by Marx, we don't seem to have produced integral man yet. On this road, Freud shows us – and it is in this sense that he doesn't go beyond Marx – that, however far the articulation of the problem has been taken by the tradition of classical philosophy, the two terms of reason and of need are insufficient to permit an understanding of the domain involved when it is a question of human self-realization. It is in the structure itself that we come up against a certain difficulty, which is nothing less than the function of desire, as I have articulated it in this seminar.

It is a curious and even paradoxical fact – but analytical experience can be registered in no other way – that reason, discourse, signifying articulation as such, is there from the beginning, *ab ovo;* it is there in an unconscious form before the birth of anything as far as human experience is concerned. It is there buried, unknown, not mastered, not available to him who is its support. And it is relative to a situation structured in this way that man at a subsequent moment has to situate his needs. Man's captivity in the field of the unconscious is primordial, fundamental in character. Now, because this field is organized logically from the beginning, it embodies a *Spaltung*, which persists in the whole subsequent development; and it is in relation to this *Spaltung* that the functioning of desire as such is to be articulated. This desire reveals certain ridges, a certain sticking point, and it is for this reason that Freudian experience has found that man's route to the integration of self is a complicated one.

The problem involved is that of *jouissance*, because *jouissance* presents itself as buried at the center of a field and has the characteristics of inaccessibility, obscurity and opacity; moreover, the field is surrounded by a barrier which makes access to it difficult for the subject to the point of inaccessibility, because *jouissance* appears not purely and simply as the satisfaction of a need but as the satisfaction of a drive – that term to be understood in the context of the complex theory I have developed on this subject in this seminar.

As you were told last time, the drive as such is something extremely complex for anyone who considers it conscientiously and tries to understand Freud's articulation of it. It isn't to be reduced to the complexity of the instinct as understood in the broadest sense, in the sense that relates it to energy. It embodies a historical dimension whose true significance needs to be appreciated by us.

This dimension is to be noted in the insistence that characterizes its appearances; it refers back to something memorable because it was remembered. Remembering, "historicizing," is coextensive with the functioning of the drive in what we call the human psyche. It is there, too, that destruction is registered, that it enters the register of experience.

This is something that I will now attempt to illustrate by leading you into the sphere, not so much of the myth of Sade (the term is inappropriate) but of the fable of Sade.

2

On page seventy-eight of Volume IV of *Juliette* in the edition that is most easily accessible to you, namely, Jean-Jacques Pauvert's, Sade expounds the *System of Pope Pius VI*, since it is to this pope that the theories in question are imputed.

Sade lays out for our benefit the theory that it is through crime that man collaborates in the new creations of nature. The idea is that the pure force of nature is obstructed by its own forms, that because the three realms present fixed forms they bind nature to a limited cycle, that is, moreover, manifestly imperfect, as is demonstrated by the chaos and abundance of conflicts as well as the fundamental disorder of their reciprocal relations. As a result, the deepest concern that can be imputed to this psychic subject that is Nature is that of wanting to wipe the slate clean, so that it may begin its task once more, set out again with a new burst of energy.

This discussion is completely literary, in the sense that it is not scientifically founded, but is rather poetic in character. In this luxuriant hodge-podge, from time to time one comes across what some people might take to be tedious digressions. But as you will see, they are entertaining to read. Thus, although reading always risks distracting one's audience's attention, I am going to read a passage from Sade's system:

> Without destruction the earth would receive no nourishment and, as a result, there would be no possibility for man to reproduce his species. It is no doubt a fateful truth, since it proves in an invincible way that the vices and virtues of our social system are nothing, and that the very vices are more necessary than the virtues, because they are creative and the virtues are merely created; or, if you prefer, the vices are causes and the virtues no more than effects. . . . A too perfect harmony would thus be a greater disadvantage than disorder; and if war, discord and crime were banished from the earth, the power of the three realms would be too violent and would destroy in its turn all the other laws of nature. The celestial bodies would all stop. Thier influences would be halted by the excessive power of one of them; there would be neither gravitation nor movement. It is thus men's crimes that introduce disorder into the sphere of the three realms and prevent this sphere from achieving a level of superiority that would disrupt all the others, by maintaining the perfect balance Horace called *rerum concordia discors*. Thus crime is necessary in the world. But the most useful crimes are no doubt those that disrupt the most, such as *the refusal of propagation* or *destruction;* all the others are worthless or rather only those two are worthy of the name of crime. Thus only the crimes mentioned are essential to the laws of the three realms and essential also to the laws of nature. A philosopher in antiquity called war *the mother of all things*. The existence of murderers is as necessary as plagues; without both of them everything in the universe would be upset. . . . such dissolution serves nature's purposes, since it

recomposes that which is destroyed. Thus every change operated by man on organized matter serves nature much more than it opposes it. What am I saying? The service of nature requires far more total destructions . . . destructions much more complete than those we are able to accomplish. Nature wants atrocities and magnitude in crimes; the more our destructions are of this type, the more they will be agreeable to it. To be of even greater service to nature, one should seek to prevent the regeneration of the body that we bury. Murder only takes the first life of the individual whom we strike down; we should also seek to take his second life, if we are to be even more useful to nature. For nature wants annihilation; it is beyond our capacity to achieve the scale of destruction it desires.

I presume that you have grasped the significance of the core of this last statement. It takes us to the heart of what was explained last time, in connection with the death drive, as the point of division between the Nirvana or annihilation principle, on the one hand, and the death drive, on the other – the former concerns a relationship to a fundamental law which might be identified with that which energetics theorizes as the tendency to return to a state, if not of absolute rest, then at least of universal equilibrium.

The death drive is to be situated in the historical domain; it is articulated at a level that can only be defined as a function of the signifying chain, that is to say, insofar as a reference point, that is a reference point of order, can be situated relative to the functioning of nature. It requires something from beyond whence it may itself be grasped in a fundamental act of memorization, as a result of which everything may be recaptured, not simply in the movement of the metamorphoses but from an initial intention.

This is to schematize what you heard last time in Mr. Kaufmann's very full and helpful summary of the work of Bernfeld and Feitelberg; it brought out the three stages at which the death drive is articulated. At the level of material systems considered to be inanimate – and, therefore, including that which involves material organization within living organisms – the operation of an irreversible tendency that proceeds in the direction of the advent of a terminal state of equilibrium is, properly speaking, something that in energetics is known as entropy. That is the first meaning that can be given to the death drive in Freud. Is that what is, in fact, involved?

Bernfeld and Feitelberg's text adds something particularly relevant to Freud's on the subject of the difference introduced by a living structure. In inanimate physical systems the dimensions of intensity and extension involved in the formula of energetics are homogeneous. According to Bernfeld living organizations as such are distinguished by the element of structure – in Goldstein's sense of the structure of an organism – that causes the two poles of the equation to become heterogeneous. That is posited at the elementary level between the nucleus and the cytoplasm as well as at the level of superior organisms between the neurological apparatus and the rest of the structure. That heterogeneity is responsible for the conflict at the level of the living structure from the beginning.

It is at this point that Bernfeld says, "I will stop here." According to him, what one finds in the drive as articulated by Freud is a general tendency of all systems to return to a state of equilibrium insofar as they are subject to the energetic equation. That may be called an instinct, as the orthodox Freudian, Bernfeld, expresses it, but it isn't what we psychoanalysts designate as the drive in our discourse.

The drive as such, insofar, as it is then a destruction drive, has to be beyond the instinct to return to the state of equilibrium of the inanimate sphere. What can it be if it is not a direct will to destruction, if I may put it like that by way of illustration?

Don't put the emphasis on the term "will" here. Whatever interest may have been aroused in Freud by an echo in Schopenhauer, it has nothing to do with the idea of a fundamental *Wille*. And it is only to make you sense the difference of register relative to the instinct to return to equilibrium that I am using the word in this way here. Will to destruction. Will to make a fresh start. Will for an Other-thing, given that everything can be challenged from the perspective of the function of the signifier.

If everything that is immanent or implicit in the chain of natural events may be considered as subject to the so-called death drive, it is only because there is a signifying chain. Freud's thought in this matter requires that what is involved be articulated as a destruction drive, given that it challenges everything that exists. But it is also a will to create from zero, a will to begin again.

This dimension is introduced as soon as the historical chain is isolated, and the history presents itself as something memorable and memorized in the Freudian sense, namely, something that is registered in the signifying chain and dependent on its existence.

That's what I am illustrating by quoting the passage from Sade. Not that Freud's notion of the death drive is not a notion that is scientifically unjustifiable, but it is of the same order as Sade's Pope Pius VI. As in Sade, the notion of the death drive is a creationist sublimation, and it is linked to that structural element which implies that, as soon as we have to deal with anything in the world appearing in the form of the signifying chain, there is somewhere – though certainly outside of the natural world – which is the beyond of that chain, the *ex nihilo* on which it is founded and is articulated as such.

I am not telling you that the notion of the death wish in Freud is not something very suspect in itself – as suspect and, I would say, almost as ridiculous as Sade's idea. Can anything be poorer or more worthless after all than the idea that human crimes might, for good or evil, contribute in some way to the cosmic maintenance of the *rerum concordia discors?*

It is even doubly suspect, since it amounts in the end to substituting a subject for Nature – and that is how I read *Beyond the Pleasure Principle.* However we construct this subject, it turns out to have as its support a subject who knows, or Freud, in effect, since he is the one who discovered the beyond of the pleasure priniple. Nevertheless, Freud is consistent with himself in also pointing, at the limit of our experience, to a field in which the subject, if he exists, is incontestably a subject who doesn't know in a point of extreme, if not absolute, ignorance. One finds there the core of Freudian exploration.

I don't even say that at this point of speculation things still have a meaning. I simply want to say that the articulation of the death drive in Freud is neither true nor false. It is suspect; that's all I affirm. But it suffices for Freud that it was necessary, that it leads him to an unfathomable spot that is problematic, since it reveals the structure of the field. It points to the site that I designate alternatively as impassable or as the site of the Thing. Freud evokes there his sublimation concerning the death instinct insofar as that sublimation is fundamentally creationist.

One also finds there the essential point of the warning whose tone and note I have given you on more than one occasion: beware of that register of thought known as evolutionism. Beware of it for two reasons. What I have to tell you now may seem dogmatic, but that's more apparent than real.

The first reason is that, however much the evolutionist movement and Freud's thought may share in terms of contemporaneity and historical affinities, there is a fundamental contradiction between the hypotheses of the one and the thought of the other. I have already indicated the necessity of the moment of creation *ex nihilo* as that which gives birth to the historical dimension of the drive. In the beginning was the Word, which is to say, the signifier. Without the signifier at the beginning, it is impossible for the drive to be articulated as historical. And this is all it takes to introduce the dimension of the *ex nihilo* into the structure of the analytical field.

The second reason may seem paradoxical to you; it is nevertheless essential: the creationist perspective is the only one that allows one to glimpse the possibility of the radical elimination of God.

It is paradoxically only from a creationist point of view that one can envisage the elimination of the always recurring notion of creative intention as supported by a person. In evolutionist thought, although God goes unnamed throughout, he is literally omnipresent. An evolution that insists on deducing from continuous process the ascending movement which reaches the summit of consciousness and thought necessarily implies that that consciousness and that thought were there at the beginning. It is only from the point of view of an absolute beginning, which marks the origin of the signifying chain as a distinct order and which isolates in their own specific dimension the memorable and the remembered, that we do not find Being *[l'être]* always implied in being *[l'étant]*, the implication that is at the core of evolutionist thought.

It isn't difficult to make what is called thought emerge from the evolution of matter, when one identifies thought with consciousness. What is difficult to make emerge from the evolution of matter is quite simply *homo faber*, production and the producer.

Production is an original domain, a domain of creation *ex nihilo*, insofar as it introduces into the natural world the organization of the signifier. It is for this reason that we only, in effect, find thought – and not in an idealist sense, but thought in its actualization in the world – in the intervals introduced by the signifier.

This field that I call the field of the Thing, this field onto which is projected something beyond, something at the point of origin of the signifying chain, this place in which doubt is cast on all that is the place of being, on the chosen place in which sublimation occurs, of which Freud gives us the most massive example – where do the view and notion of it emerge from?

It is also the place of the work that man strangely enough courts; that is why the first example I gave you was taken from courtly love. You have to admit that to place in this beyond a creature such as woman is a truly incredible idea.

Rest assured that I am in no way passing a derogatory judgment on such beings. In our cultural context, one isn't exposed to any danger by being situated as absolute object in the beyond of the pleasure principle. Let them go back to their own problems, which are homogeneous with our own, that is to say, just as difficult. That's not the issue.

If the incredible idea of situating woman in the place of being managed to surface, that has nothing to do with her as a woman, but as an object of desire. And it is that which has given rise to all the paradoxes of the famous courtly love that have caused so many headaches, because those concerned associate it with all the demands of a form of love that obviously has nothing to do with the historically specific sublimation in question.

The historians or poets who have attacked the problem cannot manage to conceive how the fever, indeed the frenzy, that is so manifestly coextensive with a lived desire, which is not at all Platonic and is indubitably manifested in the productions of courtly poetry, can be reconciled with the obvious fact that the being to whom it is addressed is nothing other than being as signifier. The inhuman character of the object of courtly love is plainly visible. This love that led some people to acts close to madness was addressed at living beings, people with names, but who were not present in their fleshly and historical reality – there's perhaps a distinction to be made there. They were there in any case in their being as reason, as signifier.

By the way this is what explains the extraordinary series of ten-line stanzas by the poet Arnaud Daniel that I read to you. One finds there the response of the shepherdess to her shepherd, for the woman responds for once from her place, and instead of playing along, at the extreme point of his invocation to the signifier, she warns the poet of the form she may take as signifier. I am, she tells him, nothing more than the emptiness to be found in my own internal cesspit, not to say anything worse. Just blow in that for a while and see if your sublimation holds up.

That's not to say there is no other solution to the perspective of the field of the Thing. Another solution that is also historically specific and, curiously enough, occurs at a period that isn't so different from the one I have just referred to, is perhaps a little more serious. It is called in Sade the Supreme-Being-in-Evil.

I say Sade because I prefer relatively close, living references to remote ones, but it is not just an invention of Sade's. It belongs to a long historical tradition, which goes at least as far back as Manicheism, if not beyond, that Manicheism which was already referred to in the time of courtly love.

In the time of courtly love there were people to whom I made a passing reference, the Cathars, and they did not doubt the fact that the Prince of this world was quite similar to this Supreme-Being-in-Evil. The *Grimmigkeit* of Boehme's God, fundamental evil as one of the dimensions of supreme life, proves that it is not simply in libertine and antireligious thought that this dimension may be evoked.

The Cathars were not Gnostics; everything indicates that they were even good Christians. The practice of their sacrament, the *consolamentum*, is sufficient proof of that. The idea they had of salvation, which is not different from the fundamental idea of Christianity, was that there is a word that saves; and the *consolamentum* was nothing more than the transmission from one subject to another of the blessing of this word. They were people who placed all of their hope in the advent of a word. In short, people who took quite seriously the message of Christianity.

The trouble is that for such a word to be not so much effective as viable, it has to be separated from discourse. Yet there is nothing more difficult than separating a word from discourse. You put your faith in a word that saves, but as soon as you begin at this level, the whole discourse comes running after you. And this is something that the Cathars didn't fail to notice in the shape of the ecclesiastical authorities, who manifested themselves briefly as the bad word and taught them that one still has to explain oneself even if one belongs to the pure. Now everybody knows that as soon as one begins to be questioned by discourse on this subject, even if it is the discourse of the

Church, then the matter can only end in one way. You are definitively silenced.

We have now arrived at a certain limit, that is to say, the field which opens on to what is involved relative to desire. How can we get any closer? How can we question this field? What happens when one doesn't project one's dreams there in a sublimated way, and that thematics emerges to which the most sober of minds are reduced, the most commonplace and the most scientific, even including a certain petty bourgeois from Vienna? What happens to us whenever the hour of desire sounds?

Well, we don't get any closer and for the best of reasons.

This will be the focus of my next lecture. One doesn't get any closer on account of the very reasons that structure the domain of the good in the most traditional sense, which is linked by a whole tradition to pleasure. It wasn't the coming of Freud that introduced a radical revolution in antiquity's point of view on the good insofar as it can be deduced from the paths of pleasure. I will try next time to show you where things stood at the time of Freud; this historical crossroads I am taking you back to is that of utility.

This time I hope to gauge for you in a definitive way and from a Freudian point of view the ethical register of utilitarianism. Freud on this occasion allows himself to go definitively beyond it; he articulates that which is basically valid in it and that which at the same time bounds it, and points to its limits.

I will try to discuss the point of view not only of the progress of thought, but also of the evolution of history, in order to demystify the Platonic and the Aristotelian view of the good, indeed of the Supreme Good, and to situate it on the level of the economy of goods.[2] It is essential to grasp the issue from the Freudian perspective of the pleasure principle and the reality principle, if one is go on to conceive the novelty of what Freud brings to the domain of ethics.

Beyond this place of restraint constituted by the concatenation and circuit of goods, a field nevertheless remains open to us that allows us to draw closer to the central field. The good is not the only, the true, or the single barrier that separates us from it.

What is this second barrier? I will tell you right away, and it will probably seem quite natural to you once I haave told you. But it isn't after all so self-evident. It is a domain in relation to which Freud always revealed a great deal of reticence; and it really is strange that he didn't identify it. The true barrier that holds the subject back in front of the unspeakable field of radical desire that is the field of absolute destruction, of destruction beyond putrefaction,

---

[2] English usage, unlike French usage, generally limits the plural of "the good," namely, "the goods" to a specific and material meaning. Here and in what follows, however, "goods" in the plural is to be read as also retaining the ethical connotations implied by the singular.

is properly speaking the aesthetic phenomenon where it is identified with experience of beauty – beauty in all its shining radiance, beauty that has been called the splendor of truth. It is obviously because truth is not pretty to look at that beauty is, if not its splendor, then at least its envelope.

In other words, I will explain next time our forward march resumes that on the scale that separates us from the central field of desire, if the good constitutes the first stopping place, the beautiful forms the second and gets closer. It stops us, but it also points in the direction of the field of destruction.

That in this sense, when one aims for the center of moral experience, the beautiful is closer to evil than to the good, shouldn't, I hope, surprise you very much. As we have long said in French: "Better is the enemy of the good."

May 4, 1960

XVII

The function of the good

SAINT AUGUSTINE AND SADE
MEMORY, FACILITATION, RITE
THE SUBJECT, ELISION OF A SIGNIFIER
THE TEXTILE FABLE
UTILITY AND *JOUISSANCE*

We have reached the barrier of desire then, and, as I indicated last time, I will speak about the good. The good has always had to situate itself on that barrier. I shall be concerned today with the way in which psychoanalysis enables one to articulate that situation.

I will speak then about the good, and perhaps what I have to say will be bad in the sense that I don't have all the goodness required to speak well of it. I won't perhaps speak too well of it because I am myself not quite well enough to speak at that high level the subject requires. But the idea of nature that I have told you about means that I will not be stopped by such an accidental contingency. I simply ask you to excuse the presentation if at the end you are not completely satisfied.

1

The question of the good is as close as possible to our sphere of action. All exchanges between men and especially interventions of the type we engage in are usually placed under the tutelage and authority of the good – the perspective is a sublime one, indeed a sublimated one. Now sublimation could be defined from a certain point of view as an opinion in the Platonic sense of the term, an opinion arranged in such a way as to reach something that might be the object of science, but that science doesn't manage to reach where it is to be found. A sublimation of any kind, even including that universal, the good itself, may be momentarily in this brief parenthesis considered to be a phony science.

Everything in your analytical experience suggests that the notion and finality of the good are problematic for you. Which good are you pursuing precisely as far as your passion is concerned? That question concerning our behavior is always on the agenda. At every moment we need to know what our effective relationship is to the desire to do good, to the desire to cure.

We have to deal with that as if it were something that is likely to lead us astray, and in many cases to do so instantly. I will even add that one might be paradoxical or trenchant and designate our desire as a non-desire to cure. Such a phrase is meaningful only insofar as it constitutes a warning against the common approaches to the good that offer themselves with a seeming naturalness, against the benevolent fraud of wanting-to-do-one's-best-for-the-subject.

But in that case what do you want to cure the subject of? There is no doubt that this is central to our experience, to our approach, to our inspiration – wanting to cure him from the illusions that keep him on the path of his desire. But how far can we go in this direction? Moreover, even if these illusions are not respectable in themselves, the subject still has to want to give them up. Is the limit of resistance here simply individual?

Here the question of different goods[1] is raised in their relation to desire. All kinds of tempting goods offer themselves to the subject; and you know how imprudent it would be for us to put ourselves in a position of promising the subject access to them all, to follow "the American way." It is nevertheless the possibility of having access to the goods of this world that determines a certain way of approaching psychoanalysis – what I have called "the American way." It also determines a certain way of arriving at the psychoanalyst's and making one's demand.

Before entering into the problem of different goods, I would like to sketch out the illusions on the path of desire. Breaking these illusions is a question of specialized knowledge – knowledge of good and evil indeed – that is located in this central field whose irreducible, ineradicable character in our experience I have attempted to show you. It is bound up with that prohibition, that reservation, that we explored specifically last year when I spoke to you about desire and its interpretation. I pointed to its essential character in the notion of "he didn't know," which is in the imperfect tense in French and which remains centrally within the field of enunciation, or in other words within the deepest relationship of the subject to signifying practice. That is to say, the subject is not the agent but the support, given that he couldn't even calculate the consequences. It is through his relationship to signifying practice that, as a consequence, he emerges as subject.

Moreover, to refer to that fantasmic experience that I chose to produce before you so as to exemplify the central field involved in desire, don't forget the moments of fantasmic creation in Sade, moments in which one finds expressed directly – in diabolically jubilatory terms that make it intolerable to read – the idea that the greatest cruelty is that the subject's fate is displayed before his eyes with his full awareness of it. The plot against the

[1] See note 2 above, p. 216.

victim is openly hatched in front of him. The value of this fantasm is that it confronts the subject with the most radical kind of interrogation, with a final "he didn't know," insofar as expressed thus in the imperfect tense, the question asked is too much for him. I just ask you to recall the ambiguity revealed by linguistic experience in connection with the French imperfect. When one says "a moment later and the bomb exploded (éclatait)," that may mean two contradictory things in French, namely, either the bomb did, in fact, explode or something happened which caused it not to explode.

We have now reached the subject of the good. The subject is in no sense new, and one has to admit that thinkers from earlier periods, whose concerns may for one reason or another seem dated to us, nonetheless sometimes formulate the issues in interesting ways. I have nothing against bringing them to your attention, however strange they may seem when presented here out of context in an apparently abstract form that doesn't seem designed to arouse our interest. Thus, when Saint Augustine writes the following in Book VII, Chapter XII, of his *Confessions*, I think it deserves far more than an indulgent smile.

> That everything that is, is good, because it is the work of God.

> I understood that all corruptible things are good, and that they wouldn't be corruptible if they were sovereignly good; no corruption would occur if they were not good. For if they were of sovereign good, they would be incorruptible, and if they had no good in them, there would be nothing in them capable of being corrupted, since corruption injures that which it corrupts, and it can only injure it if diminishes good.

And now we come to the core of the argument in the French version of the Garnier edition.

> Thus either corruption causes no damage, which cannot be upheld, or all things that are corrupted lose some good, which is undeniable. That if they had lost everything that was good, they would no longer exist at all. Or in other words, if they continued to live without being susceptible to corruption any longer, they would be in a more perfect state than they were before having lost all that was good about them, since they would remain forever in an incorruptible state.

I assume that you grasp the core and indeed the irony of this argument, and moreover that it is precisely the question that interests us. If it is unbearable to realize that everything that is good is extracted from the heart of all things, what can we say of that which remains, which is, after all, something, something different? The question goes echoing down through the centuries and down through human experience. We find it again in *The Story of Juliette*, with the difference that it is attached, as it should be, to the question of the Law, and in a no less odd way. I would like to draw your attention to this oddness because it is the oddness of a structure that is at issue. Sade writes as follows:

> Tyrants are never born out of anarchy. One only ever sees them rise up in the shadow of laws; they derive their authority from laws. The reign of law is, therefore, evil; it is inferior to anarchy. The greatest proof of this position is the obligation of any government to plunge back into anarchy whenever it wants to remake its constitution. In order to abrogate its ancient laws, it is obliged to establish a revolutionary regime in which there are no laws. Under this regime new laws are eventually born, but the second is less pure than the first since it derives from it, since the first good, anarchy, had to occur, if one wanted to achieve the second good, the State's constitution.

I give you this as a fundamental example. The same kind of argument, formulated by minds that were certainly very remote from one another in their concerns, clearly shows that some form of necessity must exist there that gives rise to this sort of logical stumbling along a certain path.

As far as we are concerned, the question of the good is articulated first of all in its relationship to the Law. On the other hand, nothing is more tempting than to evade the question of the good behind the implication of some natural law, of some harmony to be found on the way to the elucidation of desire. Yet our daily experience proves to us that beneath what we call the subject's defenses, the paths leading to the pursuit of the good only reveal themselves to us constantly, and I would add, in their original form, in the guise of some alibi on the part of the subject. The whole analytical experience is no more than an invitation to the revelation of his desire; and it changes the primitiveness of the relationship of the subject to the good compared to everything which up to that point had been articulated by the philosophers. One has undoubtedly to look closely, for it seems at first that nothing is changed, and that with Freud the compass still points toward the register of pleasure.

I have emphasized this since the beginning of the year: from the origin of moral philosophy, from the moment when the term ethics acquired the meaning of man's reflection on his condition and calculation of the proper paths to follow, all meditation on man's good has taken place as a function of the index of pleasure. And I mean all, since Plato, certainly since Aristotle, and down through the Stoics, the Epicureans, and even through Christian thought itself in Saint Thomas Aquinas. As far as the determination of different goods is concerned, things have clearly developed along the paths of an essentially hedonist problematic. It is only too evident that all that has involved the greatest of difficulties, and that these difficulties are those of experience. And in order to resolve them, all the philosophers have been led to discern not true pleasures from false, for such a distinction is impossible to make, but the true and false goods that pleasure points to.

Doesn't Freud's articulation of the pleasure principle give us an advantage, a reward in terms of knowledge and clarity?

Isn't it in a definitive way profoundly different from the meaning previously given to pleasure by anyone else?

2

Let me just draw your attention to the fact that the conception of the pleasure principle is inseparable from the reality principle, that it is in a dialectical relationship with it. But one has to begin, and I would simply like to begin by pointing out what Freud articulates exactly.

Notice how the pleasure principle is articulated from the *Entwurf*, where we began this year, right up to the end in *Beyond the Pleasure Principle*. The end illuminates the beginning, and one can already see in the *Entwurf* the nerve center to which I want to draw your attention for a moment.

Apparently there is no doubt that the pleasure principle organizes the final reactions for the human psyche, there is no doubt that pleasure is articulated in relation to the presupposition of a satisfaction, and it is driven by a lack in the order of need that the subject becomes caught up in its toils, until a perception occurs that is identical to that which first gave satisfaction. The crudest of references to the reality principle indicates that one finds satisfaction along paths that have already procured it. But look a little closer: is that all Freud has to say? Certainly not. The originality of the *Entwurf* resides in the notion of facilitations that control the distribution of libidinal investments in such a way that a certain level beyond which the degree of excitation is unbearable for the subject is never exceeded.

The introduction of the function of facilitations opens on to a theme that will become increasingly important as Freud's thought develops, in light of the fact that Freud's thought is his experience.

I have been criticized for having said that, from the point of view of ethics, our experience derives its exemplary value from the fact that it doesn't recognize the dimension of habit, in terms of which human behavior has customarily been assumed to be a process of improvement, of training. In this connection, the notion of facilitation has been used against me. I reject this opposition. The recourse to facilitation in Freud has nothing at all to do with the function of habit as it is defined when one thinks of a learning process. With Freud, it is not a question of creative imprinting but of the pleasure engendered by the functioning of the facilitations. Now the core of the pleasure principle is situated at the level of subjectivity. Facilitation is not a mechanical effect; it is invoked as the pleasure of a facility, and it will be taken up again as the pleasure of a repetition or, more precisely, as repetition compulsion. The core of Freudian thought as it is deployed by us as analysts, whether we attend this seminar or not, is that the function of memory, remembering, is at the very least a rival of the satisfactions it is charged with effecting. It has its own dimension whose reach goes beyond that of a satisfying finality. The tyranny of memory is that which is elaborated in what we call structure.

Such is the originality, the breakthrough, one cannot avoid emphasizing, if one wants to see clearly what is new in the conception of human behavior introduced by Freudian thought and experience. No doubt if someone wants to fill that fault line, he can always claim that nature involves cycles and returns. Faced with that objection, I won't affirm that he's mad; I will just suggest the terms you may use to respond.

A natural cycle is perhaps immanent in everything that exists. Moreover, it is highly diverse in its registers and levels. But I ask you to consider the break that, in the order of the manifestation of the real embodied in the cycle, is introduced by the simple fact that man is the bearer of language.

His relation to a couple of signifiers is all it takes, such as, for example, to make a traditional reference in the sketchiest of modes, *yin* and *yang*, that is to say, two signifiers, one of which is assumed to be eclipsed by the rise and return of the other – I don't care particularly for *yin* and *yang;* you can choose sine and cosine instead if you like. In other words, the structure engendered by memory must not in our experience mask the structure of memory itself insofar as it is made of a signifying articulation. If you omit it, you absolutely cannot maintain the register that is essential in the articulation of our experience, namely, the autonomy, the dominance, the agency of remembering as such, and not at the level of the real, but of the functioning of the pleasure principle.

This is not a Byzantine discussion. Thus if we create a fault line and an abyss, alternatively we fill in elsewhere something that also had the appearance of a fault line and an abyss. And it is here that one can see that the subject as such is born, a subject, moreover, whose emergence is unjustified by anything else.

As I have already pointed out, the finality of the evolution of matter toward consciousness is a mystical, elusive notion, and one that is properly speaking historically indeterminable. There is no homogeneity between the order of the apparition of phenomena, whether they be premonitory, preliminary, partial, or preparatory to consciousness, and any kind of natural order, because it is through its current state that consciousness manifests itself as a phenomenon whose activity is completely erratic and, I would even say, fragmented. It is at levels that are very different from our relationship to our own real that the mark or the touch of consciousness appears, but in the absence of any continuity or homogeneiety of consciousness. Freud came up against this fact more than once in his investigations, and he always emphasized the fact that consciousness cannot be functionalized.

With relation to the functioning of the signifying chain, on the other hand, our subject has a place in history that is quite solid and almost locatable. The function of the subject on its emergence, of the original subject, of the subject that may be traced in the chain of phenomena, we have a completely new formula for him, one that is capable of objective localization. A subject originally represents nothing more than the following fact: he can forget. Strike out that "he"; the subject is literally at his beginning the elision of a signifier as such, the missing signifier in the chain.

Such is the first place, the first person. Here the appearance of the subject is manifested as such; and it makes us directly aware of why and in what way the notion of the unconscious is central in our experience.

If you start at that point, you will see the explanation of a great many things, including that strange phenomenon that can be pinpointed in history that we call rites. I mean those rites by which man in so-called primitive civilizations believes he must accompany one of the most natural things in the world, namely, the return of natural cycles themselves. If the Emperor of China doesn't start the ploughing at a given day in spring, the rhythm of the seasons will be spoiled. If order is not preserved in the Royal House, the domain of the sea will advance upon the domain of the land. We still find echoes of this at the beginning of the sixteenth century in Shakespeare. What is this, if it isn't the essential relation, the one which binds the subject to the production of meaning and which makes him from the beginning responsible for forgetting? What relation can there be between man and the return of the sunrise, if it is not the case that as a speaking man he is sustained in a direct relation to the signifier? To refer to myth, the original position of man in relation to nature is that of Chantecler – which is a theme to be found in a minor poet, who might be approached more sympathetically, if I hadn't started another seminar by denouncing the figure of Cyrano de Bergerac by reducing him to a grotesque lucubration that had nothing to do with the monumental structure of the character.

We have now reached the point where we must raise the question of the good at this level.

3

The question of the good is situated athwart the pleasure principle and the reality principle. There's no possibility that from such a point of view we can escape conflict, given that we have regularly shifted the center.

It is impossible at this point not to bear witness to the following fact, one that is too little articulated in the Freudian conception itself, namely, that reality is not the simple dialectical correlative of the pleasure principle. Or more exactly, that reality isn't just there so that we bump our heads up against the false paths along which the functioning of the pleasure principle leads us. In truth, we make reality out of pleasure.

This is an essential notion. It is wholly summed up in the notion of praxis in the two senses that that word has acquired historically. On the one hand, in the domain of ethics, it concerns action, insofar as action has not just an ἔργον as its goal, but is also inscribed in an ἐνέργεια; on the other hand, it has to do with making, with the production *ex nihilo* I spoke to you about last time. It is no accident if these two meanings are subsumed under the same term.

We must see right away how crude it is to accept the idea that, in the ethical order itself, everything can be reduced to social constraint, as is so often the case in the theoretical writings of certain analysts – as if the fashion in which that constraint develops doesn't in itself raise a question for people who live within the realms of our experience. In the name of what is social constraint exercised? Of a collective tendency? Why in all this time hasn't such social constraint managed to focus on the most appropriate paths to the satisfaction of individuals' desires? Do I need to say anymore to an audience of analysts to make clear the distance that exists between the organization of desires and the organization of needs?

But who knows? Perhaps I need to insist after all.

Perhaps I would get a stronger reaction from an audience of school boys. They at least would realize right away that the order imposed in their school is not designed to enable them to jerk off under the best possible conditions. I nevertheless assume that the eyes of an analyst are made to interpret that which runs through a certain dream world, which we call, significantly enough, utopia. Take Fourier, for example, since reading him is by the way such fun. The farcical effect his work generates is instructive. He shows how distant what is called social progress is from whatever is done in the expectation, not so much of opening up the flood gates, as of merely thinking through a given collective order in terms of the satisfaction of desires. For the moment we just want to know if we can see a little more clearly here than others.

We are not the first to have gone along this road. As for myself, there is among those assembled here an audience of Marxists, and I assume that those who are part of it can recall the intimate, profound relationship, a relationship woven into the lines of the text, between what I am proposing here and Marx's fundamental discussions concerning the relations between man and the object of his production. To hurry things along, that brings us back to that point at which I left you in a digression of my lecture before last, namely, with Saint Martin cutting in two with his sword the large piece of cloth in which he was enveloped for his journey to Cavalla.

Let's take up the point as it stands, at the level of different goods, and let's ask ourselves the question of what that piece of cloth is.

Given that with it one can make a piece of clothing, the piece of cloth has a use value with which others before me have been concerned. You would be wrong to think that the relation of man to the object of his production at its fundamental level has been completely elucidated – even by Marx, who took things very far in this respect.

I am not going to offer here a critique of economic structures. Something very interesting did happen to me, however, one of those things I enjoy because their meaning is to be found at a level that is within our grasp but that is always more or less mystifying. It seems that in my last seminar I am supposed to have made an allusion to a given chapter of the latest book of Sartre, to his *Critique of Dialectical Reason*. I like the idea, since I am about to refer to it; the only problem is that the point in question has to do with thirty pages that I read for the first time last Sunday.

I don't know what to say about the work as a whole because I have only read these thirty pages, but I must say that they are pretty good. They concern precisely the original relations of man to the object of his needs. It seems to me that it is in this particular register that Sartre intends to take things to their final term, and if that is his purpose, if he does manage to be exhaustive, the work will certainly prove useful.

This fundamental relationship is defined starting from the notion of scarcity as that which founds man's condition, as that which makes him man in his relation to his needs. For a body of thought that aims for total dialectical transparency, such a final term is certainly rather obscure, whereas we have managed to introduce into this cloth, whether rare or not, a little breath of air which sets it floating and enables us to describe it in less opaque terms.

Psychoanalysts have given themselves plenty of room in the effort to see what this cloth symbolizes; they tell us what it both shows and hides, that the symbolism of clothes is a valid symbolism, without our knowing whether at any given moment what is being done with this cloth-phallus concerns disclosure or concealment. The profound bivalence of the whole of analytical theory on the subject of the symbolism of clothes enables us to evaluate the impasse reached with the notion of the symbol as handled up till now in psychoanalysis. If you are able to find the large volume of the *International Journal of Psychoanalysis* that was produced for Jones's fiftieth birthday, you will see an article by Flügel on the symbolism of clothes in which you will find the same impasses I pointed to, in the last issue of our journal, in Jones's own articulation of symbolism, but in an even more striking and almost caricatural form.

In any case, all the absurd things that have been said about symbolism do nevertheless lead us somewhere. There is something hidden there, and it is always, we are told, that damned phallus. We are brought back to something that one might have expected would have been thought of right off, that is to say, to the relationship of the cloth to the missing hair – but it's not missing everywhere on our body. At this point we do find a psychoanalytic writer who tells us that all the cloth we are concerned with is nothing more than the extrapolation or development of woman's fleece, the famous fleece that hides the fact that she doesn't have what it takes. These apparent revelations of the unconscious always have their comic side. But it's not completely screwy; I even think that it's a nice little fable.

Perhaps it might even contain an element of phenomenology relative to the function of nudity. Is nudity purely and simply a natural phenomenon? The whole of psychoanalytic thought is designed to prove it isn't. The thing that is particularly exalting about it and significant in its own right is that there is a beyond of nudity that nudity hides. But we don't need to engage in phenomenology; I prefer fables.

The fable on this occasion concerns Adam and Eve, with the proviso that the dimension of the signifier also be present, the signifier as introduced by the father in the benevolent directions he gives: "Adam, you must give names to everything around you." Here is Adam, then, and here is the famous hair of an Eve that we hope is worthy of the beauty that this first gesture evokes. Adam pulls out one of her hairs. Everything I am trying to show you here turns on a hair, a frog's hair.[2] Adam pulls out a hair from the woman who is given to him as his wife, who has been expected for the whole of eternity, and the next day she comes back with a mink coat over her shoulders.

Therein lies the power of the nature of cloth. It's not because man has less hair than other animals that we have to check out everything that down the ages will burst forth from his industry. If we are to believe the linguists, the problem of different goods is raised within a structure. At the beginning everything is structured as a signifier, even if only a chain of hairs is involved.

Textile is first of all a text. There is cloth, and – let me invoke the driest of minds, Marx, for example – it is impossible to posit as primary some producers' cooperative or other, unless, of course, one wants to make a psychological fable. In the beginning there is the producer's inventiveness, namely,

---

[2] The pun in the French – "poil de grenouille" – turns on the fact that as well as connoting something that does not exist, the phrase also reminds the listener of the slang meaning of "grenouille" as a pejorative term for a woman, e.g., "grenouille de bénitier."

the fact that man – and why he alone? – begins to weave something, something that isn't in the form of a covering or cocoon for his own body, but something that as cloth is going to take off on its own in the world, is going to move around. Why? Because this cloth has time value.

That's what distinguishes it from any form of natural production. One can come close to it in the creations of the animal world, but it is originated only when it is fabricated, when it is open to the world, to age and to newness; it is use value, time value; it is a reservoir of needs; it is there whether one needs it or not; and it is around this cloth that a whole dialectic of rivalry and of sharing is organized, wherein needs will be constituted.

In order to grasp this, simply set in the distance in opposition to this function, the word of the Messiah according to the Gospel when he shows men what happens to those who trust in the Father's Providence: "They weave not neither do they spin; they offer men an imitation of the robe of the lilies and the plumage of birds." This is a stupefying abolition of the text by the word. As I pointed out last time, the chief characteristic of this world is that one has to uproot it from its text if one is to have faith in it. But the history of humanity takes place in the text and it is in the text that we have the cloth.

Saint Martin's gesture means in the beginning that man as such, man with his rights, begins to be individualized as soon as one begins to make holes in this cloth through which his head and his arms can emerge, through which, in effect, he begins to organize himself as clothed, that is to say, as having needs that have been satisfied. What can there be behind this? What in spite of that can he continue to desire? – I say "in spite of that" because from that moment on we know less and less about it.

We have now reached the crossroads of utilitarianism.

Jeremy Bentham's thought is not the simple continuation of that gnoseology to which a whole tradition tirelessly devoted itself in order to reduce the transcendental or supernatural dimension of the progress of knowledge that supposedly needed elucidating. Bentham, as that work of his which has recently drawn some attention, *The Theory of Fictions*, shows, is the man who approaches the question at the level of the signifier.

With relation to institutions in their fictive or, in other words, fundamentally verbal dimension, his search has involved not attempting to reduce to nothing all the multiple, incoherent, contradictory rights of which English jurisprudence furnishes an example, but, on the contrary, observing on the basis of the symbolic artifice of these terms, which are themselves also creators of texts, what there is there that may be used to some purpose, that is to say, become, in effect, the object of a division. The long historical development of the problem of the good is in the end centered on the notion of how goods are created, insofar as they are organized not on the basis of so-called natural and predetermined needs, but insofar as they furnish the material of a distribution; and it is in relation to this that the dialectic of the good is articulated to the degree that it takes on effective meaning for man.

Man's needs find their home on the level of utility, which involves that portion of the symbolic text that may be of some use. At this stage there is no problem; the greatest utility for the greatest number – such indeed is the law in the light of which the problem of the function of goods is organized. At this level we find ourselves, in effect, prior to the moment when the subject puts his head through the holes in the cloth. The cloth is so made that the greatest number of subjects possible may put their heads and their limbs through it.

Yet all this talk wouldn't mean anything if things didn't start functioning differently. Now in this thing, whether it be rare or not, but in any case a made thing, in all this wealth finally – whatever its correlative in poverty – there is from the beginning something other than use value. There is its *jouissance* use.

As a result, the good is articulated in a wholly different way. The good is not at the level of the use of the cloth. The good is at the level where a subject may have it at his disposal.

The domain of the good is the birth of power. The notion of control of the good is essential, and if one foregrounds this, everything is revealed concerning the meaning of the claim made by man, at a certain point in his history, once he has managed to achieve control of himself.

It was Freud, not me, who took upon himself the task of unmasking what this has effectively meant historically. To exercise control over one's goods, as everyone knows, entails a certain disorder, that reveals its true nature, i.e., to exercise control over one's goods is to have the right to deprive others of them.

There is, I think, no point in making you sense the fact that historical destiny is played out around such a situation. The whole question concerns the moment when one can consider that this process has come to an end. For this function of the good engenders, of course, a dialectic. I mean that the power to deprive others is a very solid link from which will emerge the other as such.

Remember what I once told you concerning privation, which has subsequently caused a problem for some of you. You will see clearly in this connection that I don't say anything by chance.

Opposing privation to frustration and castration, I said that it was a function instituted as such in the symbolic order, to the extent that nothing is deprived of nothing – which doesn't prevent the good one is deprived of from being wholly real. The important thing is to recognize that the depriving agent is an imaginary function. It is the little other, one's fellow man, he who is given in the relationship that is half rooted in naturalness of the mirror stage, but such as he appears to us there where things are articulated at the level of the symbolic. There is a fact observed in experience that one always has to remember in analysis, namely, what is meant by defending one's goods is one and the same thing as forbidding[3] oneself from enjoying them.

The sphere of the good erects a strong wall across the path of our desire. It is, in fact, at every moment and always, the first barrier that we have to deal with.

How can we conceive crossing over it? That is a problem I will take up next time, when I point out that a radical repudiation of a certain ideal of the good is necessary, if one is to grasp the direction in which our experience is leading.

May 11, 1960.

[3] The play on words in French depends on using "défendre" both in the sense of "defend" – "défendre ses biens" – and "forbid" – "se défendre à soi-même d'en jouir."

XVIII

The function of the beautiful

THE DUPLICITY OF THE GOOD
ON THE POTLATCH
THE DISCOURSE OF SCIENCE FORGETS NOTHING
OUTRAGE AND PAIN

It seemed to me this morning that it wasn't inappropriate to begin my seminar by asking the question, Have we crossed the line?

I don't mean in what we are doing here, but in what is happening out there in the world in which we live. It isn't because what is occurring there makes such a vulgar noise that we should refuse to hear it.

At a time when I am speaking to you about the paradox of desire – in the sense that different goods obscure it – you can hear outside the awful language of power. There's no point in asking whether they are sincere or hypocritical, whether they want peace or whether they calculate the risks. The dominating impression at such a moment is that of something that may pass for a prescribed good; information addresses and captures impotent crowds to whom it is poured forth like a liquor that leaves them dazed as they move toward the slaughter house. One might even ask if one would allow the cataclysm to occur without first giving free reign to this hubbub of voices.

Is there anything more disconcerting than the transmission via those little machines that we all possess of what are known as press conferences? Or, in other words, questions that are stupidly repeated to which the leader replies with a false casualness, while he calls for more interesting questions and even on occasion engages in witticisms.

There was one somewhere yesterday, in Paris or in Brussels, that told us about our gloomy future. I swear it was absurd. Don't you think that the only way to adjust our hearing to what is proclaimed may be formulated along the lines of "What does *it* mean? What is *it* aiming at?" Yet everyone falls asleep on the soft pillow of "*It*'s not possible" – whereas, in fact, nothing is more possible, the possible is above all that. That's possible because the possible is that which can answer man's demand, and because man doesn't know what he is setting in motion with his demand.

The frightening unknown on the other side of the line is that which in man we call the unconscious, that is to say the memory of those things he forgets.

And the things he forgets – you can see in which way – are those things in connection with which everything is arranged so that he doesn't think about them, i.e., stench and corruption that always yawn like an abyss. For life after all is rottenness.

And it is even more so recently, since the anarchy of forms, that second destruction that Sade was talking about the other day in the quotation I read you – the destruction that calls for subversion even beyond the cycle of generation-corruption – are for us pressing problems. The possibility of a second destruction has suddenly become a tangible reality for us, including the threat of anarchy at the level of the chromosomes of a kind that could break the ties to given forms of life. Monsters obsessed a great deal those who up to the eighteenth century still attributed a meaning to the word "Nature." It has been a long time since we accorded any importance to calves with six feet or children with two heads. Yet we may now perhaps see them appear in the thousands.

That is why when we ask what is beyond the barrier erected by the structure of the world of the good – where is the point on which this world of the good turns, as we wait for it to drag us to our destruction – our question has a meaning that you would do well to remember has a terrifying relevance.

1

What is beyond this barrier? Don't forget that if we know there is a barrier and that there is a beyond, we know nothing about what lies beyond.

It is a false beginning to say, as on the basis of our experience some have, that it is the world of fear. To center our life, even our religion, on fear as a final term is an error. Fear with its ghosts is a localizable defense, a protection against something that is beyond, and which is precisely something unknown to us.

It is at the moment when these things are possible but wrapped in the injunction "Thinking about them is prohibited," that it is appropriate to point out the distance and the proximity that links this possible to those extraordinary texts that I have chosen this year as the fulcrum of my proof, namely, Sade's works.

One doesn't have to read very far for this collection of horrors to engender incredulity and disgust in us, and it is only fleetingly, in a brief flash, that such images may cause something strange to vibrate in us which we call perverse desire, insofar as the darker side of natural Eros enters into it.

In the end, any imaginary or indeed real relationship to the research appropriate to perverse desire only suggests the incapacity of natural desire, of the natural desire of the senses, to go very far in this direction. On this path, this desire quickly gives up, is the first to give up. It is no doubt understandable if modern man's thought seeks the beginning, the trace, the point of departure there, the path toward self-knowledge, toward the mystery of desire, but, on the other hand, all the fascination that this beginning exercises over both scientific and literary studies – witness for example the revels to be found in the works of the not untalented author of *Sexus*, *Plexus* and *Nexus*[1] – founders on a rather sterile pleasure-taking. We must be lacking in the proper method, if everything that has been elaborated on the topic by writers or scientists was outdistanced in advance some time ago, was rendered thoroughly outdated by the lucubrations of someone who was only after all a country squire, a social example of the degeneration of the nobility at a time when its privileges were about to be abolished.

It is nevertheless the case that Sade's extraordinary catalogue of horrors, which causes not only the senses and human possibilities but the imagination, too, to flinch, is nothing at all compared to what will, in effect, be seen on a collective scale, if the great and very real explosion occurs that threatens us all. The only difference between Sade's exorbitant descriptions and such a catastrophe is that no pleasure will enter into the motivation of the latter. Not perverts but bureaucrats will set things off, and we won't even know if their intentions were good or bad. Things will go off by command; they will be carried through according to regulations, mechanically, down the chain of command, with human wills bent, abolished, overcome, in a task that ceases to have any meaning. That task will be the elimination of an incalculable waste that reveals its constant and final dimension for man.

Let us not forget that that has, in effect, always been one of the dimensions in which we can recognize what a fond dreamer once charmingly referred to as "the humanization of the planet." There's never any problem in recognizing man's passage through the world, his footstep, mark, trace, touch; there where one finds a huge accumulation of oyster shells, only man can have manifestly been. The geological ages have left their waste, too, waste that allows us to recognize order. But the pile of garbage is one of the sides of the human dimension that it would be wrong to mistake.

Having sketched the outlines of this sepulchral mound at the limit of the politics of the good, of the general good, of the good of the community, we will pick up again where we left off last time.

What is the sphere of the search for the good composed of, once it has been undeceived of the error of judgment that I cited by way of example in Saint Augustine?

His reasoning is as follows: it is by the mental process of the subtraction of the good from the good that one ends up refuting the existence of anything else but the good in being, given that that which remains, since it is more

---

[1] The author referred to is, of course, Henry Miller.

perfect than that which previously was, can in no way be evil. Saint Augustine's reasoning here is calculated to surprise us, and we cannot help wondering what the historical emergence of such a form of thought signifies. It's a question I will leave open.

Last time we defined the good in symbolic creation as the *initium* that is the point of departure of the human subject's destiny in his coming to terms with the signifier. The true nature of the good, its profound duplicity, has to do with the fact that it isn't purely and simply a natural good, the response to a need, but possible power, the power to satisfy. As a result, the whole relation of man to the real of goods is organized relative to the power of the other, the imaginary other, to deprive him of it.

Let us recall the terms around which, in the first year of my seminar devoted to Freud's *Technical Writings*, I organized the ideal ego and the ego ideal, terms that I represented in my graph. The big I designates the identification of omnipotence with the signifier, with the ego ideal. On the other hand, as image of the other, it is the *Urbild* of the ego, the original form on the basis of which the ego models itself, sets itself up, and operates under the auspices of pseudomastery. We will now define the ego ideal of the subject as representing the power to do good, which then opens up within itself the beyond that concerns us today. How is it that as soon as everything is organized around the power to do good, something completely enigmatic appears and returns to us again and again from our own action – like the ever-growing threat within us of a powerful demand whose consequences are unknown? As for the ideal ego, which is the imaginary other who faces us at the same level, it represents by itself the one who deprives us.

At these two poles of the structuralization of the world of goods, what is it we see outlined?

On the one hand, starting with the unveiling with which the revelation of classical philosophy terminates, that is to say, starting with the point at which Hegel is said to have been stood on his feet, the social conflict proves to be the thread which gives meaning to the enlightened segment of history in the classical sense of the term.

On the other hand, at the other end, there appears something that looks to us like a question offering hope.

2

Scientific research conducted in what is problematically referred to as the "human sciences" has revealed that for a very long time, outside the domain of classical history, man in non-historical societies has, it is believed, invented a practice conceived to have a salutary function in the maintenance of intersubjective relations. In my eyes this is like the little stone that was miraculously made to inform us that not everything is caught up in the necessary dialectic of the competition for goods, of the conflict between goods, and of the necessary catastrophe that it gives rise to, and that, moreover, in the world we are exploring, there have existed signs that positively show how men have thought that the destruction of goods as such might be a function expressive of value.

I assume you are all well enough informed so that I don't have to remind you what a potlatch is. Let me just note briefly that it concerns ritual ceremonies involving the extensive destruction of a variety of goods, consumer goods as well as luxury goods and goods for display. The practice is found in societies that are now no more than relics, vestiges of a form of human social existence that our expansion has tended to wipe out. The potlatch bears witness to man's retreat from goods, a retreat which enabled him to link the maintenance and discipline of his desire, so to speak – insofar as this is what concerns him in his destiny – to the open destruction of goods, that were both personal and collective property. The problem and the drama of the economy of the good, its ricochets and rebounds, all turn on this point.

Furthermore, as soon as that key is given us, we clearly see that it is not simply the privilege of primitive societies. I couldn't find today the piece of paper on which I noted that at the beginning of the twelfth century – that through courtly love marked the rise to the surface in European culture of a problematic of desire as such – we see appear in a feudal rite the manifestation of something wholly analogous. The rite in question occurred at a festival, a meeting of barons somewhere in the region of Narbonne, and it involved huge destruction, not only of the goods that were consumed directly as part of the festivities, but also of animals and harnesses. Everything occurred as if the foregrounding of the problematic of desire required as its necessary correlative the need for ostentatious forms of destruction, insofar as they are gratuitous. Those who in the community claim to be privileged subjects, feudal Lords, those who set themselves up as such in this ceremony, throw down challenges to each other, rival each other in attempting to destroy the most.

This is at the other extreme the only example we have of the order of destruction that is carried out consciously and in a controlled way, that is to say, in a very different way from that massive destruction which we have all witnessed, given that we belong to generations that are relatively close to it. This latter destruction seems to us to be an inexplicable accident, a resurgence of savagery, whereas it is rather necessarily linked to the leading edge of our discourse.

A new problem arises for us, one that even Hegel found obscure. For a long time in *The Phenomenology of Mind*, Hegel tried to articulate the problem of human history in terms of conflicts between discourses. The tragedy of Antigone especially appealed to him because he saw the clear opposition there between the discourse of the family and that of the state. But in my opinion things are much less clear.

As far as we are concerned, we find in the discourse of the community, of the general good, the effects of a scientific discourse in which we see revealed for the first time the power of the signifier as such. That question is our very own. As far as we are concerned, the question raised is subsumed beneath the order of thought that I am trying to present to you here.

The sudden, prodigious development of the power of the signifier, of the discourse that emerged from the little letters of mathematics and that is distinct from all previously existing discourses, becomes an additional alienation. In what way? Insofar as it is a discourse that by reason of its structure forgets nothing. That is why it is different from the discourse of primary memorization, which carries on inside us without our knowledge, different from the memorizing discourse of the unconscious whose center is absent, whose place is identified through the phrase "he didn't know," that is precisely the sign of that fundamental omission in which the subject is situated. At a certain moment in time, man learned to emit and place the discourse of mathematics in circulation, in the real as well as in the world, and that discourse cannot function unless nothing is forgotten. It only takes a little signifying chain to begin to function based on this principle, for things to move forward as if they were functioning by themselves. So much so that we even wonder if the discourse of physics, as engendered by the omnipotence of the signifier, will reach the point of the integration of nature or its disintegration.

This fact strangely complicates the problem of our desire, even if it is doubtless no more than one of its phases. Let us just say that, as far as the man who is talking to you is concerned, it is there that one finds the revelation of the decisive and original character of the place where human desire is situated in the relationship of man to the signifier. Should this relationship be destroyed?

I take it that you might have heard in the report we had on the contribution of one of Freud's disciples – an open-minded and cultured man, but not exactly a genius – that it is in that direction that the question of the meaning of the death drive lies. It is insofar as this question is tied to history that the problem is raised. It is a question of the here and now, and not *ad aeternum*. It is because the movement of desire is in the process of crossing the line of a kind of unveiling that the advent of the Freudian notion of the death drive is meaningful for us. The question is raised at the level of the relationship of the human being to the signifier as such, to the extent that at the level of the signifier every cycle of being may be called into question, including life in its movement of loss and return.

And it is this that gives a no less tragic meaning to something that we analysts are the bearers of. In its own cycle the unconscious now appears to us as the field of a non-knowledge, even though it is locatable as such. Yet in this field where we have to function everyday, we cannot fail to recognize the following fact that every child could understand.

The desire of the man of good will is to do good, to do the right thing, and he who comes to seek you out, does so in order to feel good, to be in agreement with himself, to identify with or be in conformity with some norm. Now you all know what we nevertheless find in the margin, but also perhaps at the limit of that which occurs on the level of the dialectic and progress of the knowledge of the unconscious. In the irreducible margin as well as at the limit of his own good, the subject reveals himself to the never entirely resolved mystery of the nature of his desire.

The reference the subject makes to some other seems quite absurd, when we see him continually refer to the other – and we certainly see more than a few of these others – as if he were someone who lives harmoniously and who in any case is happier than the analysand, doesn't ask any questions, and sleeps soundly in his bed. We don't need to see this other come and lie down on our couch, however solid and together he may be, to know that this mirage, this reference of the dialectic of the good to a beyond that, by way of illustration, I will call "the good that musn't be touched," is the very text of our experience.

I would even add that this register of a *jouissance* as that which is only accessible to the other is the only dimension in which we can locate the strange malaise that, if I'm not mistaken, only the German language has managed to point to – along with other psychological nuances concerning the gap in man – with the word *Lebensneid*.

Lebensneid is not an ordinary jealousy, it is the jealousy born in a subject in his relation to an other, insofar as this other is held to enjoy a certain form of *jouissance* or superabundant vitality, that the subject perceives as something that he cannot apprehend by means of even the most elementary of affective movements. Isn't it strange, very odd, that a being admits to being jealous of something in the other to the point of hatred and the need to destroy, jealous of something that he is incapable of apprehending in any way, by any intuitive path? The identification of this other virtually in the form of a concept may in itself suffice to provoke the movement of malaise concerned; and I don't think one has to be an analyst to see such disturbing undulations passing through subjects' behaviors.

Now we have reached the frontier. What will enable us to cross it?

3

One finds at this frontier another crossing point, which enables us to locate precisely an element of the field of the beyond-the-good principle. That element, as I have said, is the beautiful.

I just want to introduce you to the problematic today. I will limit myself to two articulations.

Freud was extremely prudent in this connection. On the nature of the creation that is manifested in the beautiful, the analyst has by his own admission nothing to say. In the sphere that calculates the value of the work of art, we find ourselves reduced to a position that isn't even that of schoolchildren, but of pickers up of crumbs. Moreover, that's not all, and Freud's text is very weak on the topic. The definition he gives of sublimation at work in artistic creation only manages to show us the reaction or repercussions of the effects of what happens at the level of the sublimation of the drive, when the result or the work of the creator of the beautiful reenters the field of goods, that is to say, when they have become commodities. One must recognize that the summary Freud gives of the artist's career is practically grotesque. The artist, he says, gives a beautiful form to the forbidden object in order that everyone, by buying his little artistic product, rewards and sanctions his daring. That is a way of shortcircuiting the problem. And Freud is perfectly aware of the limits he imposes on himself in a way that is perfectly obvious when the problem of creation – which he leaves aside as outside the range of our experience – is added to it.

We are thus brought back again to all the pedantic thoughts that in the course of centuries have been expressed about the beautiful.

Everyone knows that in every field those who have something to say – that is in this case the creators of beauty – are understandably the most dissatisfied by pedantic formulas. Yet something that has been expressed by almost all of them, especially by the best but also at the level of common experience, does make the rounds, namely, that there is a certain relationship between beauty and desire.

This relationship is strange and ambiguous. On the one hand, it seems that the horizon of desire may be eliminated from the register of the beautiful. Yet, on the other hand, it has been no less apparent – from the thought of antiquity down to Saint Thomas who has some valuable things to say on the question – that the beautiful has the effect, I would say, of suspending, lowering, disarming desire. The appearance of beauty intimidates and stops desire.

That is not to say that on certain occasions beauty cannot be joined to desire, but in a mysterious way, and in a form that I can do no better than refer to by the term that bears within it the structure of the crossing of some invisible line, i.e., outrage. Moreover, it seems that it is in the nature of the beautiful to remain, as they say, insensitive to outrage, and that is by no means one of the least significant elements of its structure.

I will show it to you then in the detail of analytical experience, show it to you with pointers that will enable you to be alert to it when it occurs in an analytical session. With the precision of a Geiger counter, you can pick it up by means of references to the aesthetic register that the subject will give you in his associations, in his broken, disconnected monologue, either in the form of quotations or of memories from his schooldays. You don't, of course, always deal with creators, but you do deal with people who have had a relationship to the conventional sphere of beauty. You can be sure that the more these references become strangely sporadic and peremptory with relation to the text of the discourse, the more they are correlative of something that makes its presence felt at that moment, and that belongs to the register of a destructive drive. It is at the very moment when a thought is clearly about to appear in a subject, as in the narration of a dream for example, a thought that one recognizes as aggressive relative to one of the fundamental terms of his subjective constellation, that, depending on his nationality, he will make some reference to a passage from the Bible, to an author, whether a classic or not, or to some piece of music. I mention this today to show that we are not far from the very text of our experience.

The beautiful in its strange function with relation to desire doesn't take us in, as opposed to the function of the good. It keeps us awake and perhaps helps us adjust to desire insofar as it is itself linked to the structure of the lure.

You can see this place illustrated by the fantasm. If there is "a good that mustn't be touched," as I was saying earlier, the fantasm is "a beauty that mustn't be touched," in the structure of this enigmatic field.

The first side of this field is known to us, it is the side that along with the pleasure principle prevents us from entering it, the side of pain.

We must ask ourselves what it is that constitutes that field. The death drive, says Freud, primary masochism. But isn't that to take too big a leap? Is the pain that denies access to the side the whole content of the field? Are all those who express demands for this field masochists after all? And I can tell you right off, I don't think so.

Masochism is a marginal phenomenon and it possesses something almost caricatural that moral inquiry at the end of the nineteenth century has pretty much laid bare. The economy of masochistic pain ends up looking like the economy of goods. One wants to share pain as one shares heaps of other things that are left over; and one even comes close to fighting over it.

But isn't there something there that involves a panicky return to the dialectic of goods? In truth, the whole behavior of the masochist – and I mean by that the perverse masochist – points to the fact that it is a question of a structural feature in his behavior. Read Mr. Sacher-Masoch. He's an enlightening writer, although he doesn't have the stature of Sade, and you will see that in the end the point aimed at by the position of the perverse masochist is the desire to reduce himself to this nothing that is the good, to this thing that is treated like an object, to this slave whom one trades back and forth and whom one shares.

But one shouldn't after all proceed too quickly to break inventive homonymy, and the fact the masochism has been called by this name for so long by psychoanalysis is not without reason. The unity that emerges from all the fields which analytical thought has labeled masochism has to do with the fact that in all these fields pain shares the character of a good.

We will continue our inquiry next time with relation to a document.

It's not exactly a new document. Down through the centuries longwinded commentators have cut their teeth and sharpened their nails on it. This text appeared in the field where the morality of happiness was theorized and it gives us its underlying structure. It is there that its underlying structure is the most visible, there where it appears on the surface. That which over the centuries has caused the greatest problems, from Aristotle down to Hegel and Goethe, is a tragedy, one that Hegel considered the most perfect, but for the wrong reason, namely, *Antigone*.

Antigone's position relates to a criminal good. One would have to have a character that was deeply out of touch with the cruelties of our time to attack the subject, if I may say so, by focusing on the tyrant.

We will, therefore, take up the text of *Antigone* together, since it will enable us to point to a fundamental moment, to reach an essential reference point in our investigation of what it is man wants and what he defends himself against. We will see what an absolute choice means, a choice that is motivated by no good.

May 18, 1960

THE ESSENCE OF TRAGEDY
A commentary on Sophocles's *Antigone*

XIX

The splendor of Antigone

THE MEANING OF CATHARSIS
HEGEL'S WEAKNESS
THE FUNCTION OF THE CHORUS
GOETHE'S WISH

I told you that I would talk about *Antigone* today.

I am not the one who has decreed that *Antigone* is to be a turning point in the field that interests us, namely, ethics. People have been aware of that for a long time. And even those who haven't realized this are not unaware of the fact that there are scholarly debates on the topic. Is there anyone who doesn't evoke *Antigone* whenever there is a question of a law that causes conflict in us even though it is acknowledged by the community to be a just law?

And what is one to think of the scholars' contribution to the discussion of *Antigone?* What is one to think of it when one has, like me, gone over the ground for one's own interest and for the interest of those one is speaking to?

Well now, while I have tried to omit nothing that seemed important in all that has been said on the question, so as not to deprive either you or me of the help that I might derive from this lengthy historical survey, I have nevertheless often had the impression that I was lost in quite extraordinary byways. One learns that the opinions formulated by the pens of our great thinkers over the centuries are strange indeed.

1

Antigone is a tragedy, and tragedy is in the forefront of our experiences as analysts – something that is confirmed by the references Freud found in *Oedipus Rex* as well as in other tragedies. He was attracted by his need of the material he found in their mythical content. And if he himself didn't expressly discuss *Antigone* as tragedy, that doesn't mean to say it cannot be done at this crossroads to which I have brought you. It seems to me to be what it was for Hegel, although in a different way, namely, the Sophoclean tragedy that is of special significance.

In an even more fundamental way than through the connection to the

Oedipus complex, tragedy is at the root of our experience, as the key word "catharsis" implies.

For you the word is no doubt more or less closely associated with the term "abreaction," which presupposes that the problem outlined by Freud in his first work with Breuer, namely, that of discharge, has already been broached – discharge in an act, indeed motor discharge, of something that is not so simple to define, and that we still have to say remains a problem for us, the discharge of an emotion that remains unresolved. For that is what is involved here: an emotion or a traumatic experience may, as far as the subject is concerned, leave something unresolved, and this may continue as long as a resolution is not found. The notion of unfulfillment suffices to fill the role of comprehensibility which is required here.

Read over Freud and Breuer's opening pages and, in the light of what I have attempted to focus on for your benefit in our experience, you will see how difficult it now is to be content with the word "fulfillment" that is employed in this context, and to state simply, as Freud does, that the action may be discharged in the words that articulate it.

That catharsis which in this text is linked to the problem of abreaction, and which is already specifically invoked in the background, has its origins in the thought of classical antiquity. It is centered on Aristotle's formula at the beginning of Chapter VI of his *Poetics:* Aristotle there explains at length, in a classification of the genres, what must be present for a work to be defined as a tragedy.

The passage is a long one and we will return to it later. One finds there a description of the distinguishing characteristics of tragedy, of its composition, and of what, for example, distinguishes it from epic discourse. I simply put on the blackboard the end point or final words of this passage, what in logical causality is known as its τέλος. It is formulated by Aristotle as δί ἐλέου καὶ φόβου περαίνουσα τὴν τῶν τοιούτων παθημάτων κάθαρσιν. That is to say, a means of accomplishing the purgation of the emotions by a pity and fear similar to this.

These words which seem so simple have over the centuries produced a flood – indeed a whole world – of commentaries, whose history I can't even begin to trace here.

The references I will make to this history are highly selective and to the point. We usually translate the word "catharsis" by something like "purgation." And thus, all of us here, especially if we are doctors, are, from the school desks of our so-called secondary schools on, more or less familiar with the term "purgation," which has a certain Moliéresque meaning. And this is the case because the Moliéresque element here merely echoes an ancient medical concept, namely, in Molière's own words, the one which involves the elimination of "peccant humors."

Moreover, that is not very far from what the term still, in fact, evokes. But it also has a different resonance. And to make you sense it right away, I can simply point out what in the course of our work here I recently expounded for you with reference to the name of the Cathars.

What are the Cathars? They are the pure. Καθαρός is a pure person. And the word in its original sense doesn't mean illumination or discharge, but purification.

Doubtless in classical antiquity, too, the term "catharsis" was already used in a medical context, in Hippocrates, for example, with a specifically medical meaning; it is linked to forms of elimination, to discharge, to a return to normality. But, on the other hand, in other contexts it is linked to purification and especially to ritual purification. Hence the ambiguity which we, as you might suspect, are far from the first to discover.

So as to refer to a specific individual, I will mention the name of Denis Lambin, who reinterprets Aristotle in order to emphasize the ritual function of tragedy and the ceremonial sense of purification. It's not a matter of affirming that he is more or less right than someone else, but of simply identifying the sphere in which the question is raised.

We shouldn't, in fact, forget that the term catharsis is strangely isolated in the context of the *Poetics*. It's not that it isn't developed and commented on there, but we will learn very little about it until some new papyrus is discovered. I assume you know that what we have of the *Poetics* is only a part, roughly half, in fact. And in the half that we have there is only the passage referred to which discusses catharsis. We know that there was more because at the beginning of Book VIII, in the numbering of Didot's classic edition of the *Politics*, Aristotle speaks of "that catharsis which I discussed elsewhere in the *Poetics*." In Book VIII his subject is catharsis in connection with music, and as things turned out, it is there that we learn much more about catharsis.

In this text catharsis has to do with the calming effect associated with a certain kind of music, from which Aristotle doesn't expect a given ethical effect, nor even a practical effect, but one that is related to excitement. The music concerned is the most disturbing kind, the kind that turned their stomachs over, that made them forget themselves, in the same way that hot jazz (*le hot*) or rock 'n' roll does for us; it was the kind of music that in classical antiquity gave rise to the question of whether or not it should be prohibited.

Well now, says Aristotle, once they have experienced the state of exaltation, the Dionysian frenzy stimulated by such music, they become calm. That's what catharsis means as it is evoked in Book VIII of the *Politics*.

Yet not everyone enters into such states of excitement, even if everyone is in the position of being at least slightly susceptible. There are the παθητικοί as opposed to the ἐνθουσιαστικοί. The former are in the position of being prey to other passions, namely, fear and pity. Well, it turns out that a form of catharsis or calming effect will be granted them by a certain music also, by the music, one may assume, that has a role in tragedy. And this comes about through pleasure, Aristotle tells us, leaving us once again to reflect on what might be meant by pleasure and at what level and why it is invoked on this occasion. What is this pleasure to which one returns after a crisis that occurs in another dimension, a crisis that sometimes threatens pleasure, for we all know to what extremes a certain kind of ecstatic music may lead? It is at this point that the topology we have defined – the topology of pleasure as the law of that which functions previous to that apparatus where desire's formidable center sucks us in – perhaps allows us to understand Aristotle's intuition better than has been the case heretofore.

In any case, before I go on to define the beyond of the apparatus referred to as the central point of that gravitational pull, I want to emphasize that element in modern literature which has given rise to the use of the term catharsis in its medical sense.

The medical notion of Aristotelian catharsis is, in effect, more or less current in a sphere that goes far beyond the realm of our colleagues, the writers, critics, and literary theoreticians. But if one seeks to determine the culminating moment of this conception of catharsis, one reaches a point of origin beyond which the concept is much broader and where it is far from obvious that the word catharsis has only the medical connotation.

The triumph of the latter conception of its meaning has a source to which it is worth making an erudite reference here. The paper in question is by Jakob Bernays and it appeared in a review in Breslau. I couldn't tell you why Breslau is involved, since I wasn't able to consult enough biographical material on this Jakob Bernays. If I am to believe Jones's book on Freud, the latter, as you will probably have realized, belongs to the same family from which Freud took his wife, namely, a distinguished Jewish bourgeois family, that had long since acquired a form of nobility in the sphere of German culture. Jones refers to Michael Bernays as a professor in Munich, who was condemned by his family as a political apostate, as someone who changed his political allegiance for the sake of his career. As for Jakob Bernays, if I am to believe the person who looked into this for me, he is simply mentioned as someone who had a distinguished career as a Latinist and a Hellenist. Nothing further is said except that he didn't achieve his academic success at the same cost as Michael.

What I have here is an 1880 version of two papers by Jakob Bernays, reprinted in Berlin, on the subject of Aristotle's theory of drama. They are excellent. It is rare to find such a satisfying work by an academic in general, and even more so by a German academic. It is as clear as crystal. And it is no accident if the virtual universal adoption of the medical notion of catharsis occurs at that time.

It is a pity that Jones, who was himself so knowledgeable, didn't believe it appropriate to place a greater emphasis on the personality and the work of Jakob Bernays; little attention has been paid to him. It is nevertheless difficult to imagine that Freud, who was by no means indifferent to the reputation of the Bernays' family, wasn't aware of him. It would have been a way of referring Freud's original use of the word catharsis to its best source.

Having said that, I will now return to what most concerns us in this commentary on *Antigone*, namely, the essence of tragedy.

2

Tragedy – we are told in a definition that we can hardly avoid paying attention to, since it appeared scarcely a century after the time of the birth of tragedy – has as its aim catharsis, the purgation of the τιαθήματα, of the emotions of fear and pity.

How is one to understand that formula? We will approach the problem from the perspective imposed on us by what we have articulated on the subject of the proper place of desire in the economy of the Freudian Thing. Will this allow us to take the additional step required by this historical revelation?

If the Aristotelian formulation appears at first sight to be so closed, it is due to the loss of a part of Aristotle's work as well as to a certain conditioning within the very possibilities of thought. Yet is it so closed to us after all as a consequence of the progress made in our discussions of ethics here over the past two years? What in particular has been said about desire enables us to bring a new element to the understanding of the meaning of tragedy, above all by means of the exemplary approach suggested by the function of catharsis – there are no doubt more direct approaches.

In effect, *Antigone* reveals to us the line of sight that defines desire.

This line of sight focuses on an image that possesses a mystery which up till now has never been articulated, since it forces you to close your eyes at the very moment you look at it. Yet that image is at the center of tragedy, since it is the fascinating image of Antigone herself. We know very well that over and beyond the dialogue, over and beyond the question of family and country, over and beyond the moralizing arguments, it is Antigone herself who fascinates us, Antigone in her unbearable splendor. She has a quality that both attracts us and startles us, in the sense of intimidates us; this terrible, self-willed victim disturbs us.

It is in connection with this power of attraction that we should look for the true sense, the true mystery, the true significance of tragedy – in connection with the excitement involved, in connection with the emotions and, in particular, with the singular emotions that are fear and pity, since it is through their intervention, δι' ἐλέου καὶ φόβου, through the intervention of pity and

...at we are purged, purified of everything of that order. And that order, ...now immediately recognize, is properly speaking the order of the ...ary. And we are purged of it through the intervention of one image among others.

And it is here that a question arises. How do we explain the dissipatory power of this central image relative to all the others that suddenly seem to descend upon it and disappear? The articulation of the tragic action is illuminating on the subject. It has to do with Antigone's beauty. And this is not something I invented; I will show you the passage in the song of the Chorus where that beauty is evoked, and I will prove that it is the pivotal passage. It has to do with Antigone's beauty and with the place it occupies as intermediary between two fields that are symbolically differentiated. It is doubtless from this place that her splendor derives, a splendor that all those who have spoken worthily of beauty have never omitted from its definition.

Moreover, as you know, this is the place that I am attempting to define. I have already come close to it in previous lectures, and I attempted to grasp it the first time by means of the second death imagined by Sade's heroes – death insofar as it is regarded as the point at which the very cycles of the transformations of nature are annihilated. This is the point where the false metaphors of being (*l'étant*) can be distinguished from the position of Being (*l'être*) itself, and we find its place articulated as such, as a limit, throughout the text of *Antigone*, in the mouths of all the characters and of Tiresias. But how can one also not fail to see this position in the action itself? Given that the middle of the play is constituted of a time of lamentation, commentary, discussions, and appeals relative to an Antigone condemned to a cruel punishment. Which punishment? That of being buried alive in a tomb.

The central third of the text is composed of a detailed series of vowel gradations, which informs us about the meaning of the situation or fate of a life that is about to turn into certain death, a death lived by anticipation, a death that crosses over into the sphere of life, a life that moves into the realm of death.

It is surprising that dialecticians or indeed aestheticians as eminent as Hegel and Goethe haven't felt obliged to take account of this whole field in their evaluation of the effect of the play.

The dimension involved here is not unique to *Antigone*. I could suggest that you look in a number of places and you will find something analogous without having to search too hard. The zone defined in that way has a strange function in tragedy.

It is when passing through that zone that the beam of desire is both reflected and refracted till it ends up giving us that most strange and most profound of effects, which is the effect of beauty on desire.

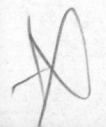

It seems to split desire strangely as it continues on its way, for one cannot say that it is completely extinguished by the apprehension of beauty. It continues on its way, but now more than elsewhere, it has a sense of being taken in, and this is manifested by the splendor and magnificence of the zone that draws it on. On the other hand, since its excitement is not refracted but reflected, rejected, it knows it to be most real. But there is no longer any object.

Hence these two sides of the issue. The extinction or the tempering of desire through the effect of beauty that some thinkers, including Saint Thomas, whom I quoted last time, insist on. On the other hand, the disruption of any object, on which Kant insists in *The Critique of Judgment*.

I was talking to you just now of excitement. And I will take a moment to have you reflect on the inappropriate use that is made of this word in the usual translation into French of *Triebregung*, namely, "émoi pulsionnel," "instinctual excitement."[1] Why was this word so badly chosen? "Emoi" (excitement) has nothing to do with emotion nor with being moved. "Emoi" is a French word that is linked to a very old verb, namely, "émoyer" or "esmayer," which, to be precise, means "faire perdre à quelqu'un ses moyens," as I almost said, although it is a play on words in French, "to make someone lose" not "his head," but something closer to the middle of the body, "his means." In any case a question of power is involved. "Esmayer" is related to the old gothic word "magnan" or "mögen" in modern German. As everybody knows, a state of excitement is something that is involved in the sphere of your power relations; it is notably something that makes you lose them.

We are now in a position to be able to discuss the text of *Antigone* with a view to finding something other than a lesson in morality.

A thoroughly irresponsible individual wrote a short time ago that I am powerless to resist the seductions of the Hegelian dialectic. The reproach was formulated at a time when I was beginning to articulate for you the dialectic of desire in terms that I have continued to employ since. And I don't know if the reproach was deserved at the time, but no one could claim that the individual involved is especially sensitive to these things. It is in any case true that Hegel nowhere appears to me to be weaker than he is in the sphere of poetics, and this is especially true of what he has to say about *Antigone*.

According to Hegel, there is a conflict of discourses, it being assumed that the discourses of the spoken dialogues embody the fundamental concerns of the play, and that they, moreover, move toward some form of reconciliation. I just wonder what the reconciliation of the end of *Antigone* might be. Fur-

---

[1] There is an additional problem in English, since the equivalent for the German "Triebe" and the French "pulsion," i.e., "drive," has no adjectival form.

ther, it is not without some astonishment that one learns that, in addition, this reconciliation is said to be subjective.

Let us not forget that in Sophocles's last play, *Oedipus at Colonus*, Oedipus's final malediction is addressed to his sons; it is the malediction that gives rise to the catastrophic series of dramas to which *Antigone* belongs. *Oedipus at Colonus* ends with Oedipus's last curse, "Never to have been born were best . . ." How can one talk of reconciliation in connection with a tone like that?

I am not tempted to regard my own indignation as particularly worthy; others have had a similar reaction before me. Goethe notably seems to have been somewhat suspicious of such a view, and so was Erwin Rohde. When I went and looked up his *Psyche* recently, a work that I made use of to bring together classical antiquity's different conceptions of the immortality of the soul, and that is an admirable work, which I strongly recommend, I was pleased to come across an expression of the author's astonishment at the traditional interpretation of *Oedipus at Colonus*.

Let us now attempt to wash our brains clean of all we have heard about *Antigone* and look in detail at what goes on there.

3

What does one find in *Antigone?* First of all, one finds Antigone.

Have you noticed that she is only ever referred to throughout the play with the Greek word ἡ παῖς, which means "the child"? I say that as a way of coming to the point and of enabling you to focus your eye on the style of the thing. And, of course, there is the action of the play.

The question of the action in tragedy is very important. I don't know why someone whom I'm not very fond of, probably because he is always being shoved under my nose, someone called La Bruyère, said that we have arrived too late in a world that is too old in which everything has already been said. It's not something I've noticed. As far as the action of tragedy is concerned, there's still a lot to be said. It's far from being resolved.

To return to Erwin Rohde, whom I complimented just now, I was astonished to find that in another chapter he explains a curious conflict between the tragic author and his subject, a conflict that is caused by the following: the laws of the genre oblige the author to choose as frame a noble action in preference to a mythic action. I suppose that is so that everyone already knows what it's all about, what's going on. The action has to be emphasized in relation to the ethos, the personalities, the characters, the problems, and so forth, of the time. If that's true, then Mr. Anouilh was right to give us his little fascist Antigone. The conflict that results from the dialogue between the poet and his subject is, according to Erwin Rohde, capable of generating conflicts between action and thought, and in this connection, echoing a great many things that have already been said before, he refers with some relevance to the figure of Hamlet.

It's entertaining, but it must be difficult for you to accept, if what I explained last year about *Hamlet* meant anything to you. *Hamlet* is by no means a drama of the importance of thought in the face of action. Why on the threshold of the modern period would *Hamlet* bear witness to the special weakness of future man as far as action is concerned? I am not so gloomy, and nothing apart from a cliché of decadent thought requires that we should be, although it is a cliché Freud himself falls into when he compares the different attitudes of Hamlet and Oedipus toward desire.

I don't believe that the drama of Hamlet is to be found in such a divergence between action and thought nor in the problem of the extinction of his desire. I tried to show that Hamlet's strange apathy belongs to the sphere of action itself, that it is in the myth chosen by Shakespeare that we should look for its motives; we will find its origin in a relationship to the mother's desire and to the father's knowledge of his own death. And to take a step further, I will mention here the moment at which our analysis of *Hamlet* is confirmed by the analysis I am leading up to on the subject of the second death.

Don't forget one of the effects in which the topology I refer to may be recognized. If Hamlet stops when he is on the point of killing Claudius, it is because he is worried about that precise point I am trying to define here: simply to kill him is not enough, he wants him to suffer hell's eternal torture. Under the pretext that we have already busied ourselves a great deal with this hell, should we see it as beneath our dignity to make a little use of it in the analysis of a text? Even if he doesn't believe in hell anymore than we do, even if he's not at all sure about it, since he does after all question the notion – "To sleep, perchance to dream . . ." – it is nevertheless true that Hamlet stops in the middle of his act because he wants Claudius to go to hell.

The reason why we are always missing the opportunity of pointing to the limits and the crossing-points of the paths we follow is because we are unwilling to come to grips with the texts, preferring to remain within the realm of what is considered acceptable or, in other words, the realm of prejudices. If I were not to have taught you anything more than an implacable method for the analysis of signifiers, then it would not have been in vain – at least I hope so. I even hope that that is all you will retain. If it is true that what I teach represents a body of thought, I will not leave behind me any of those handles which will enable you to append a suffix in the form of an "-ism." In other words, none of the terms that I have made use of here one after the other – none of which, I am glad to see from your confusion, has yet managed to impress itself on you as the essential term, whether it be the symbolic, the signifier or desire – none of the terms will in the end enable anyone of you to turn into an intellectual cricket on my account.

Next then in a tragedy, there is a Chorus. And what is a Chorus? You will be told that it's you yourselves. Or perhaps that it isn't you. But that's not the point. Means are involved here, emotional means. In my view, the Chorus is people who are moved.

Therefore, look closely before telling yourself that emotions are engaged in this purification. They are engaged, along with others, when at the end they have to be pacified by some artifice or other. But that doesn't mean to say that they are directly engaged. On the one hand, they no doubt are, and you are there in the form of a material to be made use of; on the other hand, that material is also completely indifferent. When you go to the theater in the evening, you are preoccupied by the affairs of the day, by the pen that you lost, by the check that you will have to sign the next day. You shouldn't give yourselves too much credit. Your emotions are taken charge of by the healthy order displayed on the stage. The Chorus takes care of them. The emotional commentary is done for you, The greatest chance for the survival of classical tragedy depends on that. The emotional commentary is done for you. It is just sufficiently silly; it is also not without firmness; it is more or less human.

Therefore, you don't have to worry; even if you don't feel anything, the Chorus will feel in your stead. Why after all can one not imagine that the effect on you may be achieved, at least a small dose of it, even if you didn't tremble that much? To be honest, I'm not sure if the spectator ever trembles that much. I am, however, sure that he is fascinated by the image of Antigone.

In this he is a spectator, but the question we need to ask is, What is he a spectator of? What is the image represented by Antigone? That is the question.

Let us not confuse this relationship to a special image with the spectacle as a whole. The term spectacle, which is usually used to discuss the effect of tragedy, strikes me as highly problematic if we don't delimit the field to which it refers.

On the level of what occurs in reality, an auditor rather than a spectator is involved. And I can hardly be more pleased with myself since Aristotle agrees with me; for him the whole development of the arts of theater takes place at the level of what is heard, the spectacle itself being no more than something arranged on the margin. Technique is not without significance, but it is not essential; it plays the same role as elocution in rhetoric. The spectacle here is a secondary medium. It is a point of view that puts in its place the modern concerns with *mise en scène* or stagecraft. The importance of *mise en scène* should not be underrated, and I always appreciate it both in the theater and in the cinema. But we shouldn't forget that it is only important – and I hope you will forgive the expression – if our third eye doesn't get a hard-on; it is, so to speak, jerked off a little with the *mise en scène*.

In this connection I have no intention of giving myself up to the morose pleasure I was denouncing earlier by affirming a supposed decline in the spectator. I don't believe in that at all. From a certain point of view, the audience must always have been at the same level. *Sub specie aeternitatis* everything is equal, everything is always there, although it isn't always in the same place.

But I would just mention in passing that you really have to be a student in my seminar – by which I mean someone especially alert – to find something in the spectacle of Fellini's *La Dolce Vita*.

I am amazed at the murmur of pleasure that that name seems to have aroused among a significant number of you here today. I am ready to believe that this effect is only due to the moment of illusion produced by the fact that the things I say are calculated to emphasize a certain mirage, which is, in effect, the only one aimed at in the series of cinematographic images referred to. But it isn't reached anywhere except at one single moment. That is to say at the moment when early in the morning among the pines on the edge of the beach, the jet-setters suddenly begin to move again after having remained motionless and almost disappearing from the vibration of the light; they begin to move toward some goal that pleased a great many of you, since you associated it with my famous Thing, which in this instance is some disgusting object that has been caught by a net in the sea. Thank goodness, that hadn't yet been seen at the moment I am referring to. Only the jet-setters start to walk, and they remain almost always as invisible, just like statues moving among trees painted by Uccello. It is a rare and unique moment. Those of you who haven't been should go and observe what I've been teaching you here. It happens right at the end, so that you can take your seats at the right moment, if there are any seats left.

Now we are ready for *Antigone*.

Our Antigone is on the point of entering the action of the play, and we will follow her.

4

What else can I tell you today? I am hesitating because it is late. What I want to do is lead you from one end to the other to make you appreciate its scope.

There is nevertheless one thing that you could do between now and next time, and that is read the play. I don't suppose that alerting you last time by telling you that I would be talking about *Antigone* was even enough to make you glance at it, given the average level of zeal you display. It would, however, not be without interest if you did so before next time.

There are a thousand ways of doing so. First of all, there's Mr. Robert Pignarre's critical edition. For those who know Greek, I recommend the interlinear translation, since a word by word rendering is amazingly instructive, and I will be able to make you see the extent to which my points of reference are perfectly articulated in the text by the signifiers, so that I don't have to search for them all over the place. If I find a word now and then which echoes what I have to say, that would be a by no means arbitrary mode of confirmation. On the contrary, I will show you that the words I use are the words that are to be found running like a single thread from one end of the play to the other, and that these words give it its structure.

There is one other thing I would like to point out.

One day Goethe in a conversation with Eckermann was in a speculative mood. A few days previously he had invented the Suez canal and the Panama canal. I must say that you have to be quite brilliant to have extremely clear views on the subject of the historical function of these two pieces of equipment in 1827. Then one day he comes across a book that had just come out and has been completely forgotten since by a certain Irish, which is a nice little commentary on Antigone, and that I know through Goethe.

I don't see how it is so different from Hegel's commentary; it's a little more simpleminded, but there are some amusing things in it. Those who sometimes criticize Hegel for the extraordinary difficulty of his statements will find their taunts ratified by Goethe's authority. Goethe certainly rectifies the Hegelian view that Creon is opposed to Antigone as one principle of the law, of discourse, to another. The conflict is thus said to be linked to structures. Goethe, on the other hand, shows that Creon is driven by his desire and manifestly deviates from the straight path; he seeks to break through a barrier in striking at his enemy Polynices beyond limits within which he has the right to strike him. He, in fact, wants to inflict on him that second death that he has no right to inflict on him. All of Creon's speeches are developed with that end in view, and he thus rushes by himself toward his own destruction.

If it's not exactly stated in those terms, it is implied, intuited, by Goethe. It is not for him a question of a right opposed to a right, but of a wrong opposed to – what? To something else that is represented by Antigone. Let me tell you that it isn't simply the defense of the sacred rights of the dead and of the family, nor is it all that we have been told about Antigone's saintliness. Antigone is borne along by a passion, and I will try to tell you which one it is.

But one thing is strange, and that is that Goethe tells us he was shocked, rattled, by one point in her speeches. When every move has been made, her capture, her defiance, her condemnation, and even her lamentations, and she stands on the edge of the celebrated tomb with the martyrdom that we have witnessed already behind her, Antigone stops to justify herself. When she has already seemed to have been moved to a kind of "Father, why hast thou forsaken me?", she steps back and says, "Understand this: I would not have defied the law of the city for a husband or a child to whom a tomb had been denied, because after all," she says, "if I had lost a husband in this way, I could have taken another, and even if I had lost a child with my husband, I could have made another child with another husband. But it concerned my brother αὐτάδελφος, born of the same father and the same mother." The Greek term that expresses the joining of oneself to a brother or sister recurs throughout the play, and it appears right away in the first line when Antigone is speaking to Ismene. Now that Antigone's mother and father are hidden away in Hades, there is no possibility of another brother ever being born:

μητρὸς δ'ἐν Ἅιδου καὶ πατρὸς κεκευθότοιν
οὐκ ἔστ' ἀδελφὸς ὅστις ἄν βλάστοι ποτέ

The sage from Weimar finds that all that is a bit strange. He's not the only one. Over the centuries the reasoning found in that extraordinary justification has always left people uncertain. It's important that some madness always strike the wisest of discourses, and Goethe cannot help emitting a wish. "I wish," he says, "that one day some scholar will reveal to us that this passage is a later addition."

This is the truth of a prudent man, one who knows the value of a text, one who always takes care not to formulate ideas prematurely – for isn't that how one exposes oneself to all kinds of risks? – and naturally when one makes such a wish, one can always hope that it will be realized. But there were at least four or five nineteenth-century scholars who said that such a position is untenable.

A story just like it is said to be in Herodotus, in the third book. In truth, there isn't too great a relationship apart from the fact that it is a question of life and death and of a brother, father, husband and child. It concerns a woman who as a result of her lamentations is offered the possibility of choosing one person in her family to be pardoned, the whole family having been condemned, as was possible at the Persian court. The woman explains why she chooses her brother over her husband.

On the other hand, just because two passages resemble each other doesn't mean to say that one is copied from the other. Why, in any case, would the copied lines have been inserted there? In other words, this passage is so little apocryphal that these two lines are quoted roughly ninety years later by Aristotle in the third book of his *Rhetoric* in a passage that explains how one should explain one's acts. It is difficult to believe the someone who was living ninety years after Sophocles would have quoted these lines as a literary example, if they carried with them the odor of a scandal. That seems to render the thesis of a latter addition highly doubtful.

In the end, precisely because it carries with it the suggestion of a scandal, this passage is of interest to us. You can already see why; it is only there so as to furnish additional evidence to something that next time I will try to define as the aim of *Antigone*.

May 25, 1960

XX

The articulations of the play

I would like to try today to talk about *Antigone*, the play written by Sophocles in 441 B.C., and in particular about the economy of the play.

With the category of the beautiful, Kant says that only the example – which doesn't mean the object – is capable of assuring its transmission insofar as this is both possible and demanded. Now, from every point of view, this text deserves to play such a role for us.

As you in any case know, I am reopening the question of the function of the beautiful in relation to that which we have been considering as the aim of desire. In a word, it may be that something new on the subject of the function of desire may come to light here. That is the point we have reached.

It is only a single point on our path. Don't be astonished at how long that path is, Plato says somewhere in the *Phaedrus*, which is itself a dialogue on the beautiful: Don't be astonished if the detour is such a long one, for it is a necessary detour.

Today we need to make progress in our commentary on *Antigone*.

Read this truly admirable text. It is an unimaginable highpoint, a work of overwhelming rigor, whose only equivalent in Sophocles's work is his final work, *Oedipus at Colonus*, which was written in 401.

I will now attempt to analyze this text with you so as to make you appreciate its extraordinary stature.

1

As I said last time then, we have Antigone, we have something going on, we have the Chorus.

On the other hand, as far as the nature of tragedy is concerned, I quoted the end of Aristotle's sentence on pity and fear effecting the catharsis of the emotions, that famous catharsis the true meaning of which we will try to grasp at the end. Strangely enough, Goethe saw the function of this fear and pity in the action itself. That is, the action would provide us with a model of the balance between fear and pity. That is certainly not what Aristotle says; what he says is as inaccessible to us as a closed road on account of the curious fate that has left us with so little material to confirm what he says in his text, because so much of it has been lost down through the centuries.

I will tell you one thing right away. Please note, and this is my first point, that at first glance, of the two protagonists, Creon and Antigone, neither one seems to feel fear or pity. If you doubt that, it is because you haven't read *Antigone*, and since we are going to read the play together, I hope to point it out to you in the text.

My second point is that it is not "seems," but it is "certain" that at least one of the protagonists right through to the end feels neither fear nor pity, and that is Antigone. That is why, among other things, she is the real hero. Creon, on the other hand, is moved by fear toward the end, and if it isn't the cause of his ruin, it is certainly the sign of it.

Let us now take up the question from the beginning.

It's not even that Creon says the play's opening words. As composed by Sophocles, the play begins by introducing us to Antigone in her dialogue with Ismene; and she affirms her position and her reasons from the opening lines. Creon isn't even there as a foil. He only appears later. He is nevertheless essential for our demonstration.

Creon exists to illustrate a function that we have shown is inherent in the structure of the ethic of tragedy, which is also that of psychoanalysis; he seeks the good. Something that after all is his role. The leader is he who leads the community. He exists to promote the good of all.

What does his fault consist of? Aristotle tells us, using a term that he affirms falls directly within the province of tragic action, ἁμαρτία. We have some trouble translating that word. "Error," we say, and in order to relate it to ethics, we interpret it as "error of judgment." But perhaps it isn't as simple as that.

As I told you last time, almost a century separates the period of the creation of great tragedies from their interpretation by philosophical thought. Minerva, as Hegel has already said, takes flight at twilight. I'm not too sure, but I think we should remember this formula, which has been so often evoked, to recall that there is after all some distance between the teachings embodied in tragic rites as such and their subsequent interpretation in the form of an ethics, which with Aristotle is a science of happiness.

Nevertheless, it is true that we do note the following. And I would not have any difficulty finding ἁμαρτία in others of Sophocles's tragedies: it exists, it is affirmed. The terms ἁμαρτάνειν and ἁμαρτήματα are to be found in Creon's own speeches, when at the end he succumbs to the blows of fate. But ἁμαρτία does not appear at the level of the true hero, but at the level of Creon.

His error of judgment (and we come closer to it here than that thought which is fond of wisdom ever has) is to want to promote the good of all – and I don't mean the Supreme Good, for let us not forget that 441 B.C. is very early, and our friend Plato hadn't yet created the mirage of that Supreme Good – to promote the good of all as the law without limits, the sovereign law, the law that goes beyond or crosses the limit. He doesn't even notice that he has crossed that famous limit about which one assumes enough has been said when one says that Antigone defends it and that it takes the form of the unwritten laws of the Δίκη. One thinks one has said enough when one interprets it as the Justice or the Doctrine of the gods, but one hasn't, in fact, said very much. And there is no doubt that Creon in his innocence crosses over into another sphere.

Note that his language is in perfect conformity with that which Kant calls the *Begriff* or concept of the good. It is the language of practical reason. His refusal to allow a sepulcre for Polynices, who is an enemy and a traitor to his country, is founded on the fact that one cannot at the same time honor those who have defended their country and those who have attacked it. From a Kantian point of view, it is a maxim that can be given as a rule of reason with a universal validity. Thus, before the ethical progression that from Aristotle to Kant leads us to make clear the identity of law and reason, doesn't the spectacle of tragedy reveal to us in anticipation the first objection? The good cannot reign over all without an excess emerging whose fatal consequences are revealed to us in tragedy.

What then is this famous sphere that we must not cross into? We are told that it is the place where the unwritten laws, the will or, better yet, the Δίκη of the gods rules. But we no longer have any idea what the gods are. Let us not forget that we have lived for a long time under Christian law, and in order to recall what the gods are, we have to engage in a little ethnography. If you read the *Phaedrus* I was talking about just now, which is a reflection on the nature of love, you will see that we have changed the very axis of the words that designate it.

What is this love? Is it that which, as a result of the fluctuations of the whole Christian adventure, we have come to call sublime love? Is it, in effect, very close, although it was reached by other paths? Is it desire? Is it that which some people believe I identify with a certain central sphere, namely, some natural evil in man? Is it that which Creon somewhere calls anarchy? In any case, you will see that the way in which the lovers in the *Phaedrus* act in relation to love varies according to the "epopteia" in which they have participated. "Epopteia" here means initiation in the sense that the term has in antiquity; it designates very detailed ceremonies in the course of which certain phenomena occur. One comes upon these down through the centuries – and down to the present time, if one is willing to go to other regions of the globe – in the form of trances or phenomena of possession in which a divine being manifests itself through the mouth of someone who is, so to speak, willing to cooperate.

Thus Plato tells us that those who have undergone an initiation to Zeus do not react in love in the same way as those who were initiated to Ares. Just replace those names with those who in a given province of Brazil stand for a spirit of the earth or war or of a sovereign being. It is not our intention to engage in exoticism here, but that is what is involved.

In other words, this whole sphere is only really accessible to us from the outside, from the point of view of science and of objectification. For us Christians, who have been educated by Christianity, it doesn't belong to the text in which the question is raised. We Christians have erased the whole sphere of the gods. And we are, in fact, interested here in that which we have replaced it with as illuminated by psychoanalysis. In this sphere, where is the limit? A limit that has no doubt been there from the beginning, but which doubtless remains isolated and leaves its skeleton in this sphere that we Christians have abandoned. That is the question I am asking here.

The limit involved, the limit that it is essential to situate if a certain phenomenon is to emerge through reflection, is something I have called the phenomenon of the beautiful, it is something I have begun to define as the limit of the second death.

I first brought this to your attention in connection with Sade as something that sought to pursue nature to the very principle of its creative power, which regulates the alternation of corruption and generation. Beyond that order, which it is no longer easy for us to think of and assume in the form of knowledge – and that is taken to be a reference point in the development of Christian thought – Sade tells us that there is something else, that a form of transgression is possible, and he calls it "crime."

As I indicated, the form of the crime may only be a ridiculous fantasm, but what is in question is that which the thought points to. The crime is said to be that which doesn't respect the natural order. And Sade's thought goes as far as forging the strangely extravagant notion that through crime man is given the power to liberate nature from its own laws. For its own laws are chains. What one has to sweep aside in order to force nature to start again from zero, so to speak, is the reproduction of forms against which nature's both harmonious and contradictory possibilities are stifled in an impasse of conflicting forces. That is the aim of Sadean crime. It isn't for nothing that crime is one boundary of our exploration of desire or that it is on the basis of a crime that Freud attempted to reconstruct the genealogy of the law. The frontiers represented by "starting from zero," *ex nihilo*, is, as I indicated at the beginning of my comments this year, the place where a strictly atheist thought necessarily situates itself. A strictly atheist thought adopts no other perspective than that of "creationism."

Moreover, nothing demonstrates better that Sadean thought is situated at that limit than the fundamental fantasm one finds in Sade, a fantasm that is illustrated in a thousand or more exhausting images that he gives us of the manifestations of human desire. The fantasm involved is that of eternal suffering.

In the typical Sadean scenario, suffering doesn't lead the victim to the point where he is dismembered and destroyed. It seems rather that the object of all the torture is to retain the capacity of being an indestructible support. Analysis shows clearly that the subject separates out a double of himself who is made inaccessible to destruction, so as to make it support what, borrowing a term from the realm of aesthetics, one cannot help calling the play of pain. For the space in question is the same as that in which aesthetic phenomena disport themselves, a space of freedom. And the conjunction between the play of pain and the phenomena of beauty is to be found there, though it is never emphasized, for it is as if some taboo or other prevented it, as if some prohibition were there, which is related to the difficulty we are familiar with in our patients of admitting something that properly speaking belongs to the realm of fantasm.

I will point it out to you in Sade's texts, where it is so obvious that one fails to see it. The victims are always adorned not only with all kinds of beauty, but also with grace, which is beauty's finest flower. How does one explain this necessity, if not by the fact that we need to find it hidden, though imminent, however we approach the phenomenon, in the moving presentation of the victim or also in every form of beauty that is too obvious, too present, so that it leaves man speechless at the prospect of the image that is silhouetted behind it and threatens it. But what precisely is the threat, since it isn't the threat of destruction?

The whole question is so crucial that I intend to have you go over the passages of Kant's *Critique of Judgment* that are concerned with the nature of beauty; they are extraordinarily precise. I will leave them aside for the moment except to note the following: the forms that are at work in knowledge, Kant tells us, are interested in the phenomenon of beauty, though the object itself is not involved. I take it you see the analogy with the Sadean fantasm, since the object there is no more than the power to support a form of suffering, which is in itself nothing else but the signifier of a limit. Suffering is conceived of as a stasis which affirms that that which is cannot return to the void from which it emerged.

Here one encounters the limit that Christianity has erected in the place of all the other gods, a limit that takes the form of the exemplary image which attracts to itself all the threads of our desire, the image of the crucifixion. If we dare, not so much look it in the face – given that mystics have been staring at it for centuries, we can only hope that it has been observed closely – but speak about it directly, which is much more difficult, shall we say that what is involved there is something that we might call the apotheosis of sadism? And by that I mean the divinization of everything that remains in this sphere, namely, of the limit in which a being remains in a state of suffering, otherwise he can only do so by means of a concept that moreover represents the disqualification of all concepts, that is, the concept of *ex nihilo*.

Suffice it for me to remind you of what you as analysts encounter directly, in other words the extent to which the fantasm that guides feminine desire – from the reveries of pure young virgins to the couplings fantasized by middle-aged matrons—may be literally poisoned by the favored image of Christ on the cross. Need I go further and add that in connection with that image Christianity has been crucifying man in holiness for centuries? In holiness.

For some time now we have discovered that administrators are saints. Can't one turn that around and say that saints are administrators, administrators of the access to desire, for Christianity's influence over man takes place at the level of the collectivity? Those gods who are dead in Christian hearts are pursued throughout the world by Christian missionaries. The central image of Christian divinity absorbs all other images of desire in man with significant consequences. From an historical point of view, we have perhaps reached the edge of this. It is what in the language of administration is referred to as the cultural problems of underdeveloped countries.

I am not as a result going to promise you a surprise here, whether it be a good one or a bad one. You will come upon it, as *Antigone* says, soon enough.

Let us go back to *Antigone*.

2

Antigone is the heroine. She's the one who shows the way of the gods. She's the one, according to the Greek, who is made for love rather than for hate. In short, she is a really tender and charming little thing, if one is to believe the bidet-water commentary that is typical of the style used by those virtuous writers who write about her.

By way of introduction, I would just like to make a few remarks. And I will come right to the point in stating the term that is at the center of Antigone's whole drama, a term that is repeated twenty times, and that given the shortness of the text, sounds like forty – which, of course, does not prevent its not being read – ἄτη.

It is an irreplaceable word. It designates the limit that human life can only briefly cross. The text of the Chorus is significant and insistent – ἐκτὸς ἄτας. Beyond this *Atè*, one can only spend a brief period of time, and that's where Antigone wants to go. It's not a moving little journey at all. One learns from Antigone's own mouth testimony on the point she has reached: she literally cannot stand it anymore. Her life is not worth living. She lives with the memory of the intolerable drama of the one whose descendence has just been destroyed in the figures of her two brothers. She lives in the house of Creon; she is subject to his law; and that is something she cannot bear.

She cannot bear, you tell yourselves, to live with someone whom she abhors. But why not after all? She is fed and housed, and in Sophocles, she isn't married off like Giraudoux's Electra. Don't imagine by the way that Giraudoux invented that. It was Euripides, but in his play she isn't married off to the gardener. So that's the situation: Antigone cannot bear it, and it weighs down on her in such a way as to explain the resolution, which is affirmed from the beginning in her dialogue with Ismene.

This dialogue is of an exceptional harshness. Ismene points out that "Really, given our situation, we don't have much room to maneuver, so let's not make things worse." Antigone jumps on her right away, saying, "Especially now, don't ever say that again, for even if you wanted to, I won't have anything to do with you." And the term ἔχθρα, emnity, is used in connection with her relationship with her sister and what she will find in the other life when she finds her dead brother again. She who later on will say, "I am made for love rather than hate," is immediately introduced with the word emnity.

In the course of events, when her sister comes back to her to share her fate, and even though she hasn't committed the forbidden deed, Antigone will reject her also with a cruelty and a scorn that are consciously calculated. She says to Ismene, "Go back to your Creon, since you love him so."

This then is how the enigma of Antigone is presented to us: she is inhuman. But we shouldn't situate her at the level of the monstrous, for what would that mean from our point of view? That's all right for the Chorus, which is present throughout the whole story, and which at a certain moment after one of those breath-taking lines that are typical of Antigone, cries out, "She is ὠμός." We translate that as best we can by "inflexible." It literally means something uncivilized, something raw. And the word "raw" comes closest, when it refers to eaters of raw flesh. That's the Chorus's point of view. It doesn't understand anything. She is as ὠμός as her father – that's what the Chorus says.

What does it mean to us if Antigone goes beyond the limits of the human? What does it mean if not that her desire aims at the following – the beyond of *Atè?*

That same word *Atè* is to be found in "atrocious." That's what is involved here, and that's what the Chorus repeats at a given moment in its speech with an emphasis that is technical. One does or does not approach *Atè*, and when one approaches it, it is because of something that is linked to a beginning and a chain of events, namely, that of the misfortune of the Labdacides family. As one starts to come close to it, things come together in a great hurry, and what one finds at the bottom of everything that goes on at every level in this family, the text tells us, is a μέριμνα, which is almost the same word as μνήμη, with an emphasis on "resentment." But it is very wrong to translate it thus, for "resentment" is a psychological notion, whereas μέριμνα is one of those ambiguous words that are between the subjective and the objective, and that properly speaking give us the terms of signifying speech. The μέριμνα of the Labdacides is that which drives Antigone to the border of *Atè*.

One can no doubt translate *Atè* by "misfortune," but it doesn't have anything to do with misfortune. It is this meaning that is assigned by doubtless implacable gods, as she might say, which renders her pitiless and fearless. It is also this that, so as to have her appear in the course of carrying out her act, causes the poet to create the following fascinating image, namely, that first occasion when during the night she goes and covers her brother's body with a fine layer of dust, so that it is disguised enough to be hidden from view. One cannot, of course, expose to the eyes of the world that carrion flesh visited by dogs and birds, who come to tear off strips and carry them away, as the text says, only to leave them on the altars in town centers where they promote horror and pestilence.

Thus Antigone carries out the deed the first time. But what goes beyond a given limit must not be seen. The messenger goes and tells Creon what has happened, assuring him that no trace has been found, that there is no way of knowing who did it. The order is given to scatter the dust once again. But this time Antigone is caught in the act. Upon his return the messenger describes what happened in the following terms: first, they removed the dust that was covering the body, and then, they placed themselves up-wind so as to avoid the awful smells, because it stank. But a strong wind began to blow, and the dust started to fill the air and even, the text tells us, the heavens themselves. And at the very moment when everyone tries to escape, to cover their heads with their arms, and to go to earth at the spectacle of the change in nature, little Antigone appears at the height of the total darkness, of the cataclysmic moment. She appears once more beside the corpse, emitting moans, the text says, like a bird that has just lost its young.

It's a very strange image. And it is even stranger that it should be taken up and repeated by other authors. I found in Euripides' *Phoenissae* four lines where she is also compared to the lonely mother of a lost brood, who emits pathetic cries. That proves what the image of a bird always symbolizes in classical poetry. Let us not forget how close pagan myth is to ideas of metamorphosis – remember the transformation of Philomen and Baucis. It is the nightingale that appears in Euripides as the image of that which a human being is transformed into through his plaintive cries. The limit we have reached here is the one where the possibility of metamorphosis is located – metamorphosis that has come down through the centuries hidden in the works of Ovid and that regains its former vitality, its energy, during that turning point of European sensibility, the renaissance, and bursts forth in the theater of Shakespeare. That's what Antigone is.

The movement of the play toward its climax will from now on be obvious to you.

I must clear the ground further, but it's impossible not to point in passing to a few lines spoken by Antigone. Lines 48, 70, and 73, where Antigone expresses a kind of idiocy that is apparent at the end of a sentence in the word μετά.

Μετά means "with" or "after." Prepositions don't have the same function in Greek as they do in French, in the same way that particles play a different role in English from what we know in French. Μετά is, properly speaking, that which implies a break. In response to Creon's edict, she says, "But it has nothing to do *with* my concerns." At another moment, she says to her sister, "If you wanted to come *with* me now and to carry out the sacred task, I would no longer accept you." She says to her brother, "I will lie down, my loving friend, my almost lover, here *with* you." Μετά is placed each time at the end of the line in an inverse position, for normally this preposition like the word "with" is placed in front of the noun. This feature implies in a signifying form the kind of fierce presence Antigone represents.

I will skip the details of her dialogue with Ismene. The commentary could go on and on; it could take at least a year. I am sorry that I cannot contain the extraordinary substance of the style and metre involved in the framework of a seminar. I will pass on. After this opening, which demonstrates that the die is already cast, we have the Chorus. This alternation between action and the Chorus is something that, I believe, recurs five times.

But be careful. It is said that tragedy is an action. Is it ἄγειν? Is it πράττειν? The signifier introduces two orders in the world, that of truth and that of the event. But if one wants to retain it at the level of man's relations to the dimension of truth, one cannot also at the same time make it serve to punctuate the event. In tragedy in general there is no kind of true event. The hero and that which is around him are situated with relation to the goal of desire. What occurs concerns subsidence, the piling up of different layers of the presence of the hero in time. That's what remains undetermined: in the collapse of the house of cards represented by tragedy, one thing may subside before another, and what one finds at the end when one turns the whole thing around may appear in different ways.

An illustration of that is the following: after having broadcast the fact that he will never yield an inch in his responsibilities as ruler, Creon starts to lose his nerve once old Tiresias has finished giving him a piece of his mind. He then says to the Chorus, "Shouldn't I perhaps, after all . . . perhaps yield?" He says it in terms that, from the point of view of what I am arguing here, are extraordinarily precise, for *Atè* is used there again with a special appositeness. At that moment it is clear that if he had been to the grave before finally and belatedly granting the corpse its funeral honors, something that does after all take a little time, the worst might have been avoided.

Only there it is, it is probably not for nothing that he begins with the corpse; he wants, as they say, to come to terms with his conscience. Believe me, that is always the element that leads everyone astray whenever reparations are to be made. I have only given you a little illustration, for at every moment in the unfolding of the drama the question of temporality, of the way in which the threads in place are joined together, remains decisive, essential. But it is no more comparable to an action than what I referred to earlier as subsidence, as a collapse back onto its premises.

Thus, after the first dialogue between Antigone and Ismene, the music, the Chorus, the song of liberation, Thebes is beyond the power of those whom one might well call the barbarians. The style of the poem, which is that of the Chorus, represents Polynices's soldiers and his shadow strangely enough as a huge bird hovering above the houses. The image of our modern wars as something that glides overhead was already made concrete in 441 B.C.

Once this first musical entrance is finished – and one cannot help feeling that there is some irony involved on the part of the author – it's over or, in other words, things are about to begin.

3

Creon arrives and makes a long speech justifying his actions. But in reality there is only a docile Chorus there to hear him, a collection of yes-men. There follows a dialogue between Creon and the Chorus. The Chorus itself hasn't altogether given up the idea that there is something excessive in Creon's statements, but at the very moment when it is about to express the thought, that is when the messenger arrives and narrates what has happened, it gets told off in no uncertain terms.

The character of the messenger in this tragedy is a formidable one. He turns up shuffling and mumbling, and he says, "You can't imagine how much I have been thinking things over on my way here, and how many times I came close to taking off in a hurry. That's how a short trip turns into a long one." He's an impressive talker. He even goes so far as to say, "I am sorry to see that you are of the opinion that it is your opinion that you believe in lies."

In short, I am suspected of being suspicious. That style of δοκεῖ ψευδῆ δοκεῖν resonates with the discourse of the Sophists, since Creon answers him right away, "You are in the process of making points on the subject of the δόξα." In brief, throughout a whole ridiculous scene the messenger engages in idle speculations about what has happened, and in particular speculations about their safety, in the course of which the guards are in a state of panic, in which they nearly come to blows before they draw lots in order to decide which one of them will be chosen to go as messenger. After having got it all out, he is the object of a stream of threats from Creon, who is the person in power and who on this occasion is excessively limited; Creon lets him know that they can all expect the worst if the guilty person is not found in a hurry. "I've come out of this in quite good shape," the messenger comments, "since I haven't been strung up right away to the end of a branch. They won't see me again in a hurry."

This scene is a bit like the entrance of the clowns. But the messenger is quite subtle; he is very clever when he says to Creon, "What is offended just now? Is it your heart or your ears?" He makes Creon turn around in circles; Creon is forced to face the situation in spite of himself. The messenger then explains, "If it is your heart, then it is the one who did the deed that offends it; I only offend your ears." We have already reached the height of cruelty but we're having fun.

And what happens immediately afterwards? A hymn of praise to mankind. The Chorus sets out to praise mankind. I am constrained by the time, so I can't go on, but I will take up this praise of mankind next time.

Then right after the extraordinary tall tale that is this hymn of praise to man, we see Antigone's guard turn up without any concern for verisimilitude, temporal verisimilitude at least. The guard is delighted. He's had a rare piece of luck; his responsibility in the case has been absolved once he has laid hands on the guilty party. Then the Chorus sings its song on mankind's relation to *Atè*. I'll come back to that, too, another time.

Next comes Hemon, who is Creon's son and Antigone's fiancé. He begins a dialogue with his father. The only confrontation between the father and son causes the dimension to appear that I began to discuss concerning the relations of man to his good; there is a moment of doubt, a hesitation. This point is extremely important if we want to be clear about Creon's stature. We will see later what he is, that is, like all executioners and tyrants at bottom, a human character. Only the martyrs know neither pity nor fear. Believe me, the day when the martyrs are victorious will be the day of universal conflagration. The play is calculated to demonstrate that fact.

Creon doesn't lose his nerve, far from it; his son leaves to the sound of the most terrible threats. And what bursts forth again at that very moment? The Chorus once more, and what does it have to say? Ἔρως ἀνίκατε μάχαν,

"Invincible love of combat." I suppose that even those who do not know Greek have heard at one time or other those three words that have come down through the centuries with a number of melodies in their wake.

That song bursts forth at the very moment when Creon decrees the punishment Antigone will be made to undergo: she will be placed alive in a tomb – something that doesn't suggest too tender an imagination. Let me remind you that in Sade it is number seven or eight on the list of ordeals to which the hero is submitted – the reference is a useful one for you to realize the significance of what is involved here. It is precisely at this moment that the Chorus says in so many words: "This story is driving us mad; we are losing our grip; we are going out of our minds; as far as this child is concerned we are moved to . . . ," what the text, using a term whose appositeness I ask you to remember, calls ἵμερος ἐναργής.

Ἵμερος is the same term that in the *Phaedrus* points to what I am trying to grasp here as the reflection of desire of the kind by which even the gods are bound. It is the term used by Jupiter to designate his relations with Ganymede. Ἵμερος ἐναργής is literally desire made visible. This is what appears at the moment when the long scene that leads up to the punishment takes place.

After Antigone's speech, in which is to be found the passage discussed by Goethe that I talked about the other day, the Chorus starts up again with a mythological song in which at three different moments it evokes three especially dramatic destinies that are all on the boundary between life and death, the boundary of the still living corpse. Antigone herself even refers to the image of Niobe, who is imprisoned in the narrow cavity of a rock and will be exposed forever to the assault of rain and weather. It is around this image of the limit that the whole play turns.

At the moment when it is moving more and more toward a kind of explosive climax of divine delirium, the blind Tiresias appears. He doesn't simply announce the future, however, because the revelation of his prophecy has a role to play in the preparation of that future. In his dialogue with Creon he withholds what he has to say until the latter – in whose rigid mind everything is political or, in other words, a question of interest – is foolish enough to say a sufficient number of insulting things for Tiresias to come out with his prophecy. The value attributed to the words of a seer is, as in all circumstances where tradition counts, decisive enough for Creon to give in and resign himself to countermanding his own orders, which, of course, proves catastrophic.

The situation is heightened even further. In its penultimate appearance the Chorus breaks out in a hymn to the most hidden and supreme god, Dionysos. The spectators imagine that this is once again a hymn of liberation, that everyone is comforted, everything will work out all right. Those, on the other hand, who knew what Dionysos and his savage followers represent realize that the hymn breaks out because the limits of the field of the conflagration have been breached.

After that there is hardly room for the final twist of the action, the one in which the deluded Creon goes and knocks in desperation at the doors of the tomb within which Antigone has hanged herself. Hemon kisses her and emits a few final groans, but we do not know what happened in the sepulcre any more than we know what goes on when Hamlet goes down into the sepulcre. Antigone was after all walled in at the limit of *Atè*, and one is justified in wondering at which moment Hemon entered the tomb. As when the actors turn their faces away from the spot where Oedipus disappears, we don't know what happened in Antigone's tomb.

In any case, when Hemon emerges, he is possessed by divine μανία. He shows all the signs of someone who has lost his reason. He attacks his father, misses him, and kills himself. And when Creon returns to the palace where a messenger has already preceded him, he discovers his wife is dead.

At that point the text shows us, in terms that are calculated to remind us where the limit is situated, a Creon who is out of his mind demanding that he be carried off – "Drag me out by my feet." And the Coryphaeus manages to find the strength to engage in a play of words in saying, "You're right to say that: the pain that one feels in one's feet is the best kind of pain; unlike other kinds, it doesn't last long."

Sophocles is no pedantic schoolmaster, but unfortunately he has been translated by pedants. In any case, that's how the corrida ends. Have the arena raked over, the bull removed, and cut off his you-know-what, if there is any left. That's the style in which he has been rendered. May he go off to the bright sound of little bells.

It is more or less in these terms that the play of Antigone has been translated. Next time I will take a little time to point out a few essential points that will enable you to link my interpretation directly to the very terms used by Sophocles.

I hope that that will take no more than half of my time, and that I will be able to speak afterwards about what Kant has to say on the subject of the beautiful.

June 1, 1960

XXI

Antigone between two deaths

THE-RACE-IS-RUN
SOPHOCLES'S ANTI-HUMANISM
THE LAW OF *EX NIHILO*
THE DEATH DRIVE ILLUSTRATED
COMPLEMENT

I did recommend an interlinear edition of *Antigone* to those of you who know enough Greek to get by, but it's not available. Use the Garnier translation instead, since it's not bad at all.[1]

The following lines of the Greek text are the ones that concern us: 4–7, 323–325, 332–333, 360–375, 450–470, 559–560, 581–584, 611–614, 620–625, 648–650, 780–805, 839–841, 852–862, 875, 916–924, 1259–1260.

Lines 559–560 give us Antigone's attitude toward life. She tells us that her soul died long ago and that she is destined to give help, ὠφελεῖν, to the dead – we spoke about the same word in connection with Ophelia.

Lines 611–614 and 620–625 have to do with the Chorus's statements on the limit that is *Atè*, and it is around this that what Antigone wants is played out.

I already pointed out last time the importance of the term that ends both of these passages, ἐκτὸς ἄτας. Ἐκτός signifies an outside or what happens once the limit of *Atè* has been crossed. When, for example, the guard comes and tells of the event that challenges Creon's authority, he says at the end that he is ἐκτὸς ἐλπίδος, outside or beyond all hope; he no longer hopes to be saved. Ἐκτὸς ἄτας has the meaning of going beyond a limit in the text. And it is around this notion that the Chorus's song is developed at that moment, in the same way that it says that man goes toward πρὸς ἄταν, that is, toward *Atè*. In this business the whole prepositional system of the Greeks is so vital and suggestive. It is because man mistakes evil for the good, because something beyond the limits of *Atè* has become Antigone's good, namely, a good that is different from everyone else's, that she goes toward, πρὸς ἄταν.

So as to take up the problem in a way that allows me to bring my comments together, I must return to a simple, clean, unencumbered view of the tragic hero, and in particular of the one who concerns us, Antigone.

---

[1] The best equivalent in English is, of course, the Loeb bilingual edition.

1

One thing has struck a commentator on Sophocles – commentator in the singular, for I have been surprised to find that it is only in a relatively recent book on Sophocles by Karl Reinhardt that something important has been brought out, namely, the special solitude of Sophoclean heroes, μονούμενοι, which is a nice term used by Sophocles, along with ἄφιλοι and φρενὸς οἰοβῶται, that is to say, those who lead their thoughts to graze far off. But it is nevertheless certain that it is not this that is involved here, for in the end tragic heroes are always isolated, they are always beyond established limits, always in an exposed position and, as a result, separated in one way or another from the structure.

It is strange that something very obvious has been overlooked. Let us examine the seven plays of Sophocles that are extant of the twenty-five which he is said to have produced during a life of ninety years, sixty of which he devoted to tragedy. They are *Ajax, Antigone, Electra, Oedipus Rex, The Trachiniae, Philoctetes,* and *Oedipus at Colonus.*

A certain number of these plays remain familiar to us, but you are not perhaps aware that *Ajax* is a very odd piece of work. It begins with the massacre of the Greeks' flock by Ajax. Because Athena doesn't wish him well, he goes crazy. He imagines he is massacring the Greek army, but it is their flock instead. Afterwards he awakens from his craziness, is overcome with shame, and goes and kills himself in a corner. There is absolutely nothing else in the play but that, which is, after all, rather peculiar. As I was saying the other day, there isn't even the suggestion of a perepetia. Everything is there from the beginning; the trajectories that are set in motion have only to come crashing down one on top of the other as best they can.

We will leave *Antigone* aside for one moment, since we are discussing it.

Electra, too, is an odd play of Sophocles. In Aeschylus we find the *Choephoroe* and the *Eumenides,* where the death of Agamemnon gives rise to all kinds of things. And once his murder has been avenged, Orestes then has to deal with the avenging divinities who protect the maternal blood. There is nothing comparable in Sophocles. Electra is in certain ways the very double of Antigone – "Dead in life," she says, "I am already dead to everything." Moreover, at that climactic moment when Orestes is making Aegisthus jump for it, he says to him, "Do you realize you are talking to people who are just like the dead? You are not talking to the living." It is an extremely odd note and the whole thing ends abruptly just like that. There isn't the least trace of anything superfluous. Everything ends abruptly. The end of *Electra* involves an execution in the proper sense of the word.

We can leave aside *Oedipus Rex,* given the perspective I am adopting here.

In any case, I am not claiming to promulgate a general law, since we know nothing of the greater part of Sophocles's work.

The Trachiniae has to do with the end of Hercules. Hercules has come to the end of his labors, and he knows it. He is told he will be able to go and rest, that his work is over. Unfortunately, he mixed up the last of his labors with the desire for a female captive, and because she loves him, his wife sends him the delightful tunic that she has been keeping since the beginning in case of need, as a kind of weapon to be reserved for the right moment. She sends it to him and you know what happens. The whole end of the play is taken up with Hercules's groans and roars of pain as he is consumed by the burning cloth.

Then there is *Philoctetes*. Philoctetes is a character who has been exiled on an island. He has been rotting away there for ten years, and then he is asked to render the community a service. All kinds of things happen, including the moving struggle with his conscience of the young Neoptolemes, who is dispatched to serve as bait in an attempt to deceive the hero.

Finally, there is *Oedipus at Colonus*.

You have no doubt noted the following. If there is a distinguishing characteristic to everything we ascribe to Sophocles, with the exception of *Oedipus Rex*, it is that for all his heroes the race is run. They are at a limit that is not accounted for by their solitude relative to others. There is something more; they are characters who find themselves right away in a limit zone, find themselves between life and death. The theme of between-life-and-death is moreover formulated as such in the text, but it is also manifest in the situations themselves.

One could even fit *Oedipus Rex* into this context. The hero has a characteristic that is both unique to him and paradoxical in relation to others. At the beginning of the drama he has attained the height of happiness. Yet Sophocles represents him as driven to bring about his own ruin through his obstinacy in wanting to solve an enigma, to know the truth. Everyone tries to prevent him, including especially Jocasta, who is always saying, "That's enough; we already know enough." Still he wants to know and in the end he does know. Yet I do grant that *Oedipus Rex* is an exception; it doesn't fit the general formula of the Sophoclean hero, who is marked by a stance of the-race-is-run.

Let us now return to Antigone, whose race is run in the most obvious of ways.

On one occasion I showed you an anamorphosis; it was the finest I could find for our purpose, and it is indeed exemplary, far beyond anything one could have hoped for. Do you remember the cylinder from which this strange phenomenon rises up? It cannot properly speaking be said that from an optical point of view there is an image as such. Without going into the optical definition of the phenomenon, one can say that it is because an infinitesimal fragment of image is produced on each surface of the cylinder that we see a series of screens superimposed; and it is as a result of these that a marvelous illusion in the form of a beautiful image of the passion appears beyond the mirror, whereas something decomposed and disgusting spreads out around it.

That's the kind of thing that is involved here. What is the surface that allows the image of Antigone to rise up as an image of passion? The other day I evoked in connection with her the phrase, "Father, why hast thou abandoned me?" which is literally expressed in one line. Tragedy is that which spreads itself out in front so that that image may be produced. When analyzing it, we follow an inverse procedure; we study how the image had to be constructed in order to produce the desired effect. So let's begin.

I have already emphasized the implacable side of Antigone; the side that shows neither fear nor pity is apparent at every point. Somewhere in order to deplore this, the Chorus calls her, line 875, αὐτόγνωτος. That should be heard alongside the γνῶθι σεαυτόν of the Delphic oracle. One cannot ignore the meaning of the kind of self-knowledge attributed to her.

I have already indicated her extreme harshness when she tells Ismene of her purpose at the beginning. "Do you realize what is happening?" she asks. Creon has just promulgated what is called a κήρυγμα – a term that plays an important role in modern protestant theology as a dimension of the revelation. Her manner is as follows: "Here's the situation then. This is what he has proclaimed for you and me." Then she adds in the lively style of the text: "I speak for me." And she goes on to affirm that she will bury her brother.

We will see what that means.

2

From then on things move fast. The guard comes and announces that the brother has been buried. At this point I am going to draw your attention to something that reveals the importance of Sophocles's work for us.

Some people have said, and I seem to remember that it is the name of one of the many works that I consulted, that Sophocles is a humanist. He is found to be human since he gives the idea of a properly human measure between a rootedness in archaic ideals represented by Aeschylus and a move toward bathos, sentimentality, criticism, and sophistry that Aristotle had already reproached Euripides with.

I don't disagree with the notion that Sophocles is in that median position, but as far as finding in him some relationship to humanism is concerned, that would be to give a wholly new meaning to the word. As for us, we consider ourselves to be at the end of the vein of humanist thought. From our point of view man is in the process of splitting apart, as if as a result of a spectral analysis, an example of which I have engaged in here in moving along the joint between the imaginary and the symbolic in which we seek out the relationship of man to the signifier, and the "splitting" it gives rise to in him. Claude Lévi-Strauss is looking for something similar when he attempts to formalize the move from nature to culture or more exactly the gap between nature and culture.

It is curious to note that on the edge of humanism it is also in this analysis, in this gap of analysis, of limits, in this attitude that the race is run, that the images rise up that turn out to be the most fascinating of that whole period of history which can be dubbed humanist.

I find for example the point in the text that you have in your hands, lines 360–375, very striking; it concerns the moment when the Chorus bursts forth just after the departure of the messenger whose comic responses and shuffling movements, when he comes to announce the news that may cost him dearly, I referred to earlier. It is really terrible, the Chorus says, to see someone so obstinate about believing he believes. Believing he believes what? Something that no one for the moment has the right to imagine, that is the play of δοκεῖ δοκεῖν. That's the element I sought to emphasize in that line along with the other response: "You're playing the fool with your stories about the δόξα." That's an obvious allusion to the philosophical games of the time that focused on a theme. The scene itself is quite ridiculous, for we are not really interested in whether the guard will be skinned alive or not on account of the bad news he bears, and he in any case gets out of it with a flourish.

Immediately afterwards in line 332 the Chorus breaks out in the chant that I said the other day was a celebration of mankind. It begins as follows:

πολλὰ τὰ δεινὰ κ' οὐδὲν ἀν-
θρώπου δεινότερον πέλει·

The lines mean literally: "There are a lot of wonders in the world, but there is nothing more wonderful than man."

As far as Lévi-Strauss is concerned, what the Chorus says about man here is really the definition of culture as opposed to nature: man cultivates speech and the sublime sciences; he knows how to protect his dwelling place from winter frosts and from the blasts of a storm; he knows how to avoid getting wet. Yet there is a slippage here; there is, it seems to me, an undeniable irony in what follows, in the famous phrase παντοπόρος ἄπορος, which has given rise to a debate on the subject of its punctuation. The accepted punctuation seems to be the following: παντοπόρος, ἄπορος ἐπ' οὐδὲν ἔρχεται τὸ μέλλον.

Παντοπόρος means "he who knows all kinds of tricks" – man knows a lot of tricks. Ἄπορος is the opposite; it means when one has no resources or defenses against something. You are, I suppose, familiar with the term aporia. Ἄπορος means one that is "screwed." As the proverb from the Vaud region has it, "Nothing is impossible for man; what he can't do, he ignores." That's the tone of the text.

Next we have – ἐπ' οὐδὲν ἔρχεται τὸ μέλλον.

Ἔρχεται means "he advances." Ἐπ' οὐδὲν means "toward nothing." Τὸ μέλλον can be translated quite innocently as "the future"; it also means "that which must happen," but at other moments it signifies μέλλειν, "to delay." As a result, τὸ μέλλον opens up a semantic field that isn't easy to identify precisely with a corresponding French term. The problem is usually solved by saying, "Since he is highly resourceful, he will never be without resources whatever he has to face." The thought strikes me as a little petty bourgeois. It's not clear that it was the poet's intention to emit such a platitude.

In the first place, it is difficult to disconnect the two terms that are joined at the beginning of the sentence, παντοπόρος ἄπορος. I also note that later on in line 370 we find another conjunction, ὑψίπολις ἄπολις, that is to say "he who is both above and outside the city." And this is the definition of a character generally identified, as I will explain later, with Creon, with his deformation. At the same time I am not sure that ἄπορος ἐπ' οὐδὲν ἔρχεται can be translated as "because he doesn't approach anything without resources." It isn't at all in conformity with the genius of the Greek language in this case. Ἔρχεται requires that ἐπ'οὐδὲν be attached to it. Ἐπ' agrees with ἔρχεται, not with ἄπορος. We are the ones who find there someone who is ready for everything, whereas it is literally a question of the following: "He advances toward nothing that is likely to happen, he advances and he is παντοπόρος, "artful," but he is ἄπορος, always "screwed." He knows what he's doing. He always manages to cause things to come crashing down on his head.

You should respond to this turning point as to something in the style of Prévert. And I will confirm that such is the case. Just afterwards one finds the line Ἅιδα μόνου ψεῦξιν οὐκ ἐπάξεται, which means that there is only one thing he can't come to terms with and that has to do with Hades. Dying is something he doesn't know how to come to terms with. The important point occurs in what follows, – νότων δ'ἀμηχάνων φυγὰς. Having said that there is one thing that man hasn't managed to come to terms with, and that is death, the Chorus says that he has come up with an absolutely marvelous gimmick, namely, translated literally, "an escape *into* impossible sicknesses." There is no way of ascribing another meaning to that phrase than the one I ascribe. The translations usually attempt to say that man even manages to come to deal with sickness, but that's not what it means at all. He hasn't managed to come to terms with death but he invents marvelous gimmicks in the form of sicknesses he himself fabricates. There is something extraordinary about finding that notion expressed in 441 B.C. as one of mankind's essential dimensions. It wouldn't make any sense to translate that as "an escape *from* sicknesses." Sickness is involved here μηχανόεν. That's quite a gimmick he has invented; make of it what you will.

In any case, the text repeats that man has failed relative to Hades, and we enter immediately afterwards into μηχανόεν. There is something related to σοφόν in that, a term that isn't so simple. I would just remind you of the analysis of the Heraclitean sense of σοφόν, "wise," and ὁμολογεῖν, "to say the same thing," that is to be found in the Heidegger text I translated for the first issue of *La Psychanalyse*. That σοφόν still has all of its primitive vigor. There is something of *sophos* in the mechanism, μηχανόεν. There is something ὑπὲρ ἐλπίδ'ἔχων, which transcends all hope and which ἔρπει. It's this that directs him sometimes toward evil and sometimes toward the good. That is to say that this power or *mandate*, as I translated the word *sophos* in the article I was talking about, which is laid upon him by this good, is an eminently ambiguous one.

Right afterwards we find the passage beginning νόμους παρείρων, etc., upon which the whole of the play is going to turn. For παρείρων means undeniably "to arrange the laws wrongly, to weave them together wrongly, to get them all mixed up." Χθονός is "the earth," and Θεῶν τ'ἔνορκον δίκαν is "that which is formulated or told in the law." That's the thing we appeal to in the silence of the analysand. We don't say "Speak." We don't say "Enunciate" or "Recount," but "Tell." But that's exactly what we shouldn't do. That Δίκη is essential and constitutes the dimension of enunciation or ἔνορκον, confirmed by an oath of the gods.

There are two obvious dimensions that may be distinguished without difficulty: on the one hand, the laws of the earth and, on the other, the commandments of the gods. But they may be confused. They don't belong to the same order, and if one mixes them up, there will be trouble. There will be so much trouble that the Chorus, which in spite of its vacillations does cleave to a fixed line, affirms, "In any case, we don't want to be associated with so and so." The point is to proceed in that direction is properly speaking τὸ μὴ καλόν or something that isn't "beautiful," and not, as it is translated, because of the very audacity of the idea, something that isn't "good." Thus the Chorus doesn't want the character in question as its πάρεδρος, that is as its companion or immediate neighbor. The Chorus doesn't want to be with him in the same central point we are talking about. It doesn't want to have close relations with him, nor does it want to ἴσον φρονῶν, to have the same desire. It separates its own desire from the desire of the other. And I don't think I am forcing the issue when I find here an echo of certain formulas that I have given you.

Does Creon confuse νόμους χθονός with the Δίκη of the gods? The classical interpretation is clear: Creon represents the laws of the city and identifies them with the decrees of the gods. But it's not as obvious as that, for it cannot be denied that Antigone is after all concerned with the chthonic laws, the laws of the earth. I haven't stopped emphasizing the fact that it is for the sake of her brother who has descended into the subterranean world that she opposes κήρυγμα, that she resists Creon's order; it is in the name of the most radically chthonian of relations that are blood relations. In brief, she is in a position to place the Δίκη of the gods on her side. In any case the ambiguity is obvious. And this is something that we will shortly see confirmed.

I have already pointed out how, after the condemnation of Antigone, the Chorus emphasizes the fact that she went in search of her *Atè*. In a similar vein, Electra says, "Why do you always plunge yourself into the *Atè* of your house, why do you persist in referring to the fatal murder in front of Aegisthus and your mother? Aren't you the one who brings down all kinds of evil on your head as a result?" To which the other responds, "I agree but I can't help it."

It is because she goes toward *Atè* here, because it is even a question of going ἐκτὸς ἄτας, of going beyond the limit of *Atè*, that Antigone interests the Chorus. It says that she's the one who violates the limits of *Atè* through her desire. The lines I referred to above concern this and especially those that end with the formula ἐκτὸς ἄτας, to go beyond the limit of *Atè*. *Atè* is not ἁμαρτία, that is to say a mistake or error; it's got nothing to do with doing something stupid.

When at the end Creon returns bearing something in his arms, lines 1259–1260, and, as the Chorus tells us, it seems to be nothing other than the body of his son who has committed suicide, the Chorus then says, "If we may say so, it is not a misfortune that is external to him; it is αὐτὸς ἁμαρτών, his own mistake. He's the one who made the mistake of getting himself into the mess." Ἁμαρτία is the word used, that is "mistake" or "blunder."

That's the meaning Aristotle insists on, and to my mind he's wrong, for that is not the quality which leads the tragic hero to his death. It's only true for Creon the counter- or secondary hero, who is indeed ἁμαρτών. At the moment when Eurydice commits suicide, the messenger uses the word ἁμαρτάνειν. He hopes, we are told, that she isn't going to do something stupid. And naturally he and the Coryphaeus stiffen in anticipation because no noise is heard. The Coryphaeus says, "That's a bad sign." The mortal fruit that Creon harvests through his obstinacy and his insane orders is the dead son he carries in his arms. He has been ἁμαρτών; he has made a mistake. It's not a question here of ἀλλοτρία ἄτη. *Atè* concerns the Other, the field of the Other, and it doesn't belong to Creon. It is, on the other hand, the place where Antigone is situated.

3

And it is to Antigone that we must now turn.

Is she, as the classic interpretation would have it, the servant of a sacred order, of respect for living matter? Is hers the image of charity? Perhaps, but only if we confer on the word charity a savage dimension. Yet the path from Antigone's passion to her elevation is a long one.

When she explains to Creon what she has done, Antigone affirms the advent of the absolute individual with the phrase "That's how it is because that's how it is." But in the name of what? And to begin with on the basis of what? I must quote the text.

She says clearly, "You made the laws." But once again the sense is missed. Translated word for word, it means, "For Zeus is by no means the one who proclaimed those things to me." Naturally, she is understood to have said – and I have always told you that it is important not to understand for the sake of understanding – "It's not Zeus who gives you the right to say that." But she doesn't, in fact, say that. She denies that it is Zeus who ordered her to do it. Nor is it $\Delta i\kappa\eta$, which is the companion or collaborator of the gods below. She pointedly distinguishes herself from $\Delta i\kappa\eta$. "You have got that all mixed up," she, in effect, says. "It may even be that you are wrong in the way you avoid the $\Delta i\kappa\eta$. But I'm not going to get mixed up in it; I'm not concerned with all these gods below who have imposed laws on men." $\H{\omega}\rho\iota\sigma\alpha\nu$, $\hat{o}\rho i\xi\omega$, $\H{o}\rho o\varsigma$ means precisely the image of an horizon, of a limit. Moreover, the limit in question is one on which she establishes herself, a place where she feels herself to be unassailable, a place where it is impossible for a mortal being to $\hat{v}\pi\epsilon\rho\delta\rho\alpha\mu\epsilon\hat{\iota}\nu$, to go beyond $\nu\acute{o}\mu\iota\mu\alpha$, the laws. These are no longer laws, $\nu\acute{o}\mu o\varsigma$, but a certain legality which is a consequence of the laws of the gods that are said to be $\check{\alpha}\gamma\rho\alpha\pi\tau\alpha$, which is translated as "unwritten," because that is in effect what it means. Involved here is an invocation of something that is, in effect, of the order of law, but which is not developed in any signifying chain or in anything else.

Involved is an horizon determined by a structural relation; it only exists on the basis of the language of words, but it reveals their unsurpassable consequence. The point is from the moment when words and language and the signifier enter into play, something may be said, and it is said in the following way: "My brother may be whatever you say he is, a criminal. He wanted to destroy the walls of his city, lead his compatriots away in slavery. He led our enemies on to the territory of our city, but he is nevertheless what he is, and he must be granted his funeral rites. He doubtless doesn't have the same rights as the other. You can, in fact, tell me whatever you want, tell me that one is a hero and a friend, that the other is an enemy. But I answer that it is of no significance that the latter doesn't have the same value below. As far as I am concerned, the order that you dare refer me to doesn't mean anything, for from my point of view, my brother is my brother."

That's the paradox encountered by Goethe's thought and he vacillates. My brother is what he is, and it's because he is what he is and only he can be what he is, that I move forward toward the fatal limit. If it were anyone else with whom I might enter into a human relationship, my husband or my children for example, they are replaceable; I have relations with them. But this brother who is ἄθαπτος, who has in common with me the fact of having been born in the same womb – the etymology of the word ἀδελφός embodies an allusion to the womb – and having been related to the same father – that criminal father the consequences of whose crimes Antigone is still suffering from – this brother is something unique. And it is this alone which motivates me to oppose your edicts.

Antigone invokes no other right than that one, a right that emerges in the language of the ineffaceable character of what is – ineffaceable, that is, from the moment when the emergent signifier freezes it like a fixed object in spite of the flood of possible transformations. What is, is, and it is to this, to this surface, that the unshakeable, unyielding position of Antigone is fixed.

She rejects everything else. The stance of the-race-is-run is nowhere better illustrated than here. And whatever else one relates it to, is only a way of causing uncertainty or disguising the absolutely radical character of the position of the problem in the text.

The fact that it is man who invented the sepulchre is evoked discretely. One cannot finish off someone who is a man as if he were a dog. One cannot be finished with his remains simply by forgetting that the register of being of someone who was identified by a name has to be preserved by funeral rites.

No doubt all kinds of things may be added to that. All the clouds of the imaginary come to be accumulated around it as well as the influences that are released by the ghosts who multiply in the vicinity of death. But at bottom the affair concerns the refusal to grant Polynices a funeral. Because he is abandoned to the dogs and the birds and will end his appearance on earth in impurity, with his scattered limbs an offense to heaven and earth, it can be seen that Antigone's position represents the radical limit that affirms the unique value of his being without reference to any content, to whatever good or evil Polynices may have done, or to whatever he may be subjected to.

The unique value involved is essentially that of language. Outside of language it is inconceivable, and the being of him who has lived cannot be detached from all he bears with him in the nature of good and evil, of destiny, of consequences for others, or of feelings for himself. That purity, that separation of being from the characteristics of the historical drama he has lived through, is precisely the limit or the *ex nihilo* to which Antigone is attached. It is nothing more than the break that the very presence of language inaugurates in the life of man.

That break is manifested at every moment in the fact that language punctuates everything that occurs in the movement of life. Αὐτόνομος is the word the Chorus uses to situate Antigone; it tells her, "You are going off toward death without knowing your own law." Antigone knows what she is condemned to, that is, to take part, so to speak, in a game whose outcome is known in advance. It is, in effect, posited as a game by Creon. She is condemned to the sealed chamber of the tomb in which she will be put to the test, namely, that of knowing if the gods below will come to her aid. It is at this point in her ordeal that Creon pronounces his condemnation, when he says, "We'll see how useful your loyalty to the gods below will be. You will have the food that is always placed next to the dead by way of an offering, and we'll see just how long you last with that."

It is at that moment that the tragedy is illuminated with a new light, in the form of Antigone's κομμός, her complaint or lamentation. And it is significant that certain commentators have been scandalized by it.

4

When does this complaint begin? From the moment when she crosses the entrance to the zone between life and death, that is to say, when what she has already affirmed herself to be takes on an outward form. She has been telling us for a long time that she is in the kingdom of the dead, but at this point the idea is consecrated. Her punishment will consist in her being shut up or suspended in the zone between life and death. Although she is not yet dead, she is eliminated from the world of the living. And it is from that moment on that her complaint begins, her lamentation on life.

Antigone will lament that she is departing ἄταφος, without a tomb, even though she is to be shut up in a tomb, without a dwelling place, mourned by no friend. Thus her separation is lived as a regret or lamentation for everything in life that is refused her. She even evokes the fact that she will never know a conjugal bed, the bond of marriage, that she will never have any children. The speech is a long one.

It has occurred to some commentators to cast doubt on this side of the tragedy in the name of the so-called unity of the character represented as the cold and inflexible Antigone. The term ψυχρόν is that of coldness and frigidity. Creon calls her "a cold object to caress," line 650, in a dialogue with his son, so as to let him know that he's not losing very much. Antigone's character is contrasted with her complaint so as to bring out the lack of verisimilitude in an outburst that, it is held, should not be attributed to the poet.

It's an absurd misinterpretation, for from Antigone's point of view life can only be approached, can only be lived or thought about, from the place of that limit where her life is already lost, where she is already on the other side. But from that place she can see it and live it in the form of something already lost.

And it is from the same place that the image of Antigone appears before us as something that causes the Chorus to lose its head, as it tells us itself, makes the just appear unjust, and makes the Chorus transgress all limits, including casting aside any respect it might have for the edicts of the city. Nothing is more moving than that ἵμερος ἐναργής, than the desire that visibly emanates from the eyelids of this admirable girl.

The violent illumination, the glow of beauty, coincides with the moment of transgression or of realization of Antigone's *Atè*, which is the characteristic that I have chiefly insisted on and which introduced us to the exemplary function of Antigone's problem in allowing us to determine the function of certain effects. It is in that direction that a certain relationship to a beyond of the central field is established for us, but it is also that which prevents us from seeing its true nature, that which dazzles us and separates us from its true function. The moving side of beauty causes all critical judgment to vacillate, stops analysis, and plunges the different forms involved into a certain confusion or, rather, an essential blindness.

The beauty effect is a blindness effect. Something else is going on on the other side that cannot be observed. In effect, Antigone herself has been declaring from the beginning: "I am dead and I desire death." When Antigone depicts herself as Niobe becoming petrified, what is she identifying herself with, if it isn't that inanimate condition in which Freud taught us to recognize the form in which the death instinct is manifested? An illustration of the death instinct is what we find here.

It is at the moment when Antigone evokes Niobe that the Coryphaeus sings her praise, line 840: "You then are half-goddess." Then Antigone's response bursts forth, and she is far from being a half-goddess: "This is absurd; you are making fun of me." And the word she uses means "outrage," which, as I have already indicated, is manifestly correlated to the moment of crossing over. The Greek word is used here in its proper sense, which is directly related to the term meaning to cross over – "outrage" is to go "out" or beyond (*c'est aller outre*), go beyond the right one has to make light of what happens at the greatest of costs. Ὑβρίζεις is the term Antigone confronts the Chorus with: "You do not realize what you are saying. You outrage me." But her stature is far from diminished as a result, and her complaint, the κομμός, her long complaint, follows immediately.

The Chorus then goes on to make an enigmatic reference to three quite disparate episodes from the history of mythology. The first concerns Danae, who was shut up in a bronze chamber. The second is to Lycurgus, the son of Dryas, King of the Edonians, who was mad enough to persecute the servants of Dionysos, to pursue and terrify them, and even to rape their women and to make divine Dionysos jump into the sea. This is the first mention we have of the Dionysiac. In Book II of the *Iliad* we find Dionysos in a death-like state, and he goes on to revenge himself by transforming Lycurgus into a madman. There are a number of different forms of the myth – perhaps he was imprisoned; blinded by Dionysos's madness he even killed his own sons whom he mistook for vine shoots, and he hacked off his own limbs. But that's not important because the text only refers to the vengeance of Dionysos the God. The third example, which is even more obscure, concerns the hero Phineas, who is at the center of a whole bundle of legends that are full of contradictions and extremely difficult to reconcile. He is found on a cup as the object of a conflict between the Harpies, who torment him, and the Boreads, the two sons of Boreas who protect him, and on the horizon there passes, strangely enough, the wedding procession of Dionysos and Ariadne.

There is certainly a lot to be gained in the interpretation of these myths, if it turns out to be possible. Their disparate character and the apparent lack of relevance to the issues at hand is certainly one of the burdens that the tragic texts impose on their commentators. I don't pretend to be able to solve the problem, but it was by bringing to the attention of my friend Lévi-Strauss the difficulty of this passage, that I recently managed to interest him in Antigone.

There is nevertheless something that one can point to in this rash of tragic episodes evoked by the Chorus at the moment when Antigone is at the limit. They all concern the relationship of mortals to the gods. Danae is entombed because of the love of a god; Lycurgus is punished because he attempted to commit violence on a god, and it is also because she is of divine descent that Cleopatra the Boread and rejected companion of Phineas is implicated in the story – she is referred to as $ἄμιππος$, that is to say, as swift as a horse, and it is said that she also moves faster across solid ice than any steed; she's a skater. Now the striking thing about Antigone is that she undergoes a misfortune that is equal to that of all those who are caught up in the cruel sport of the gods. Seen from the outside by us as $ατραγωδόι$, she appears as the victim at the center of the anamorphic cylinder of the tragedy. She is there in spite of herself as victim and holocaust.

Antigone appears as $αὐτόνομος$, as a pure and simple relationship of the human being to that of which he miraculously happens to be the bearer, namely, the signifying cut that confers on him the indomitable power of being what he is in the face of everything that may oppose him.

Anything at all may be invoked in connection with this, and that's what the Chorus does in the fifth act when it evokes the god that saves.

Dionysos is this god; otherwise why would he appear there? There is nothing Dionysiac about the act and the countenance of Antigone. Yet she pushes to the limit the realization of something that might be called the pure and simple desire of death as such. She incarnates that desire.

Think about it. What happens to her desire? Shouldn't it be the desire of the Other and be linked to the desire of the mother? The text alludes to the fact that the desire of the mother is the origin of everything. The desire of the mother is the founding desire of the whole structure, the one that brought into the world the unique offspring that are Eteocles, Polynices, Antigone and Ismene; but it is also a criminal desire. Thus at the origin of tragedy and of humanism we find once again an impasse that is the same as Hamlet's, except strangely enough it is even more radical.

No mediation is possible here except that of this desire with its radically destructive character. The fruit of the incestuous union has split into two brothers, one of whom represents power and the other crime. There is no one to assume the crime and the validity of crime apart from Antigone.

Between the two of them, Antigone chooses to be purely and simply the guardian of the being of the criminal as such. No doubt things could have been resolved if the social body had been willing to pardon, to forget and cover over everything with the same funeral rites. It is because the community refuses this that Antigone is required to sacrifice her own being in order to maintain that essential being which is the family *Atè*, and that is the theme or true axis on which the whole tragedy turns.

Antigone perpetuates, eternalizes, immortalizes that *Atè*.

June 8, 1960

SUPPLEMENTARY NOTE

I would like now to focus on the meaning I give to such an exploration of the tragedy of *Antigone*.

It may have seemed demanding to some of you. For some time now I have used the metaphor of the rabbit and the hat in connection with a certain way of making something appear from analytical discourse that isn't there. I might almost say that on this occasion I have put you to the test of eating raw rabbits. You can relax now. Take a lesson from the boa constrictor. Have a little nap and the whole thing will pass through. You will even notice on waking that you have digested something after all.

It is on account of the procedure I have adopted – and it's no doubt quite a demanding one obviously, quite a tough one – of requiring you to accompany me in breaking the stones along the road of the text that it will enter your body. You will see in retrospect that even if you are not aware of it, the latent, fundamental image of Antigone forms part of your morality, whether you like it or not. That's why it is important to analyze its meaning, and it's not the watered-down meaning in the light of which its lesson is usually transmitted.

Involved here is nothing more nor less than the reinterpretation of the Sophoclean message. You can certainly resist this resharpening of the text's high points, but if you decide to reread Sophocles, you will perceive the distance we have traveled. Even if I am challenged on a given point – for I don't exclude the possibility that I, too, on occasion may misinterpret something – I believe I have dissipated the all-encompassing nonsense in which Sophocles is carefully preserved by a certain tradition.

While I was discussing that with some of you who were countering my views with memories they had of reading *Oedipus at Colonus* – memories that were obviously influenced by the scholarly interpretation – I remembered a little footnote. There are people here who like footnotes. So I will read one that is to be found in a work that psychoanalysts ought to have read at least once, namely, Erwin Rohde's *Psyche*, of which there exists an excellent French translation.

On the whole, you will find more there, and more that is certain, concerning that which Greek civilization has handed down to us than in any work originally written in French. The most brilliant people on earth don't have all the arrows in their quiver. As it is, we are unfortunate enough to have a romantic movement that didn't rise much above the level of a certain idiocy, and we by no means possess all the advantages when it comes to erudition.

On page 463 of the French translation of Erwin Rohde's book, you will find a little footnote on *Oedipus at Colonus*, which I have already discussed with you in terms that are directly related to what I am concerned with today. Rohde writes: "One only has to read the play with an open mind to realize that this savage, angry, pitiless old man who calls down horrible curses on his sons" – Rohde is perfectly correct, for twenty minutes before the end of the play, Oedipus is still crushing Polynices beneath the weight of his curses – "and who as a man thirsty for revenge looks forward passionately to the misfortunes that are about to descend on his native town, has none of that profound peace of the gods, of that transfiguration associated with the penitent, which traditional exegesis is pleased to observe in him. The poet does not make a habit of disguising life's realities, and here he shows himself to be fully aware that destitution and misfortune do not usually have the effect of transfiguring man; they depress him rather and strip him of his nobility. His Oedipus is pious. He was from the beginning in *Oedipus Rex*, but in his distress he turns savage."

That is the testimony of a reader who is not especially concerned with the problems of tragedy, since his work is an historical account of the different concepts that the Greeks had of the soul.

As far as we are concerned, I have tried to show you that at a time that preceded the ethical formulations of Socrates, Plato and Aristotle, Sophocles presents us with man and questions him along the paths of his solitude; he situates the hero in a sphere where death encroaches on life, in his relationship, that is, to what I have been calling the second death here. This relationship to being suspends everything that has to do with transformation, with the cycle of generation and decay or with history itself, and it places us on a level that is more extreme than any other insofar as it is directly attached to language as such.

To put it in the terms of Lévi-Strauss – and I am certain that I am not mistaken in invoking him here, since I was instrumental in having had him reread *Antigone* and he expressed himself to me in such terms – Antigone with relation to Creon finds herself in the place of synchrony in opposition to diachrony.

I have stopped half-way in what I might have said about the text. We are not in a position to exhaust its significance this year, if only for reasons of time, but it is clear that the question raised at the end concerns what I shall call the divine use of Antigone.

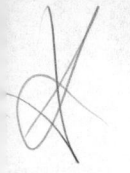

In this connection one might make a number of comparisons. Antigone hanging in her tomb evokes something very different from an act of suicide, since there are all kinds of myths of hanged heroines, including girls, such as that of Erigone, who is linked to the advent of the cult of Dionysos. Dionysos has given wine to her father, but because he doesn't know its properties, he violates her and dies. She then hangs herself on his tomb. It is an explanatory myth of a whole rite in which we see more or less simplified and symbolic images of girls hanging from trees. In short, one finds there a whole ritual and mythical background, which may be brought back to resituate in its religious harmony all that is produced on the stage. It is nevertheless true that from a Sophoclean perspective the hero has nothing to do with that kind of use. Antigone is someone who has already set her sights on death. The invocation that is wrapped around this stem is something else; it doesn't have to do with human defiance here.

That's as far as I will go today. Involved in what I had to say to you about catharsis is the beauty effect. The beauty effect derives from the relationship of the hero to the limit, which is defined on this occasion by a certain *Atè*. And on that subject I will now, so to speak, pass the word to someone else (*passer la parole*), conscious of the fact that I am using the very definitions of the structure of the seminar.

In effect, I don't want to be the one who, like some jack-of-all trades, takes upon himself alone the task of poking about in all those more-or-less heterogeneous fields that offer the traditional formulations of these things.

At a certain level within you, I mean all of you individually at a certain point in your thinking, there is a form of resistance to the things I am trying to express, and it consists of making sympathetic comments that are more-or-less ambiguous in kind on what has come to be known as my learning or, as is also said, my cultural background. It's something I don't like. It also has a negative side; one wonders where I find the time to assemble all that. But you will recognize that my existence began a little before yours. I may not have had two hundred years of mowing like an English lawn, but I am getting there. In any case, I am closer than you are, and I've had time to forget several times over the things I discuss with you.

I would, therefore, like today to ask someone to speak about the beautiful who seems to me to be particularly well-equipped to discuss it in relation to something that I take to be essential for the continuation of my argument; that something is the definition of the beautiful and the sublime as articulated by Kant.

Involved there is a form of category analysis that is of the highest significance in any effort to connect up with the topological structuration that I am pursuing with you here. It seems to me essential to take the time to recall Kant's insights, if you have already read *The Critique of Judgment*, or to hear what they are, if you haven't yet had the opportunity to read that work. That is why I have asked Mr. Kaufmann to speak to us now.

You will see afterwards the use that we might make of the work he will be presenting for your benefit today. [Mr. Kaufmann's presentation followed.]

You were certainly right to state that infinitesimal calculus is evoked behind the experience of the sublime. One should note that in Kant's time infinitesimal calculus still harbored a kind of mystery of the signifier that has totally disappeared since that time.

The 1764 passage you quoted from Kant should really be communicated to Claude Lévi-Strauss, as the inaugural speech he gave on being appointed to his Chair at the *Collège de France* is already implied there. I don't mean by that antedated, but anticipated precisely in a way that is not emphasized at all in Rousseau. Kant already founds the ethics of ethnography there.

The work you presented today suggested to the audience here, which is heterogeneous in its educational background, the idea of structures around which Kant both regroups and dissociates the idea of the beautiful. We might have placed in the background the idea of pleasure in Aristotle and have quoted the nice little definition he gives of it in the *Rhetoric*.

We will use that as a fulcrum – something that is in traditional philosophy – when we take up again where we left off the question of the effect of tragedy. Although we think we always have to defer to Aristotle, that effect concerned cannot be fully explained in terms of moral catharsis.

June 15, 1960

THE TRAGIC DIMENSION OF PSYCHOANALYTIC EXPERIENCE

XXII

The demand for happiness and the promise of analysis

DESIRE AND THE LAST JUDGMENT
THE SECOND DEATH
THE FABLE OF THE CLODHOPPERS
HADES AND DIONYSOS
THE ANALYST'S DESIRE

The report I gave two years ago at Royaumont on "The Direction of the Cure" is to appear in the next issue of our review. The text is somewhat thrown together because I wrote it between two seminars I was giving here. I shall keep its improvised form, although I will try to fill out and rectify certain things to be found there.

1

I said somewhere that an analyst has to pay something if he is to play his role.

He pays in words, in his interpretations. He pays with his person to the extent that through the transference he is literally dispossessed. The whole current development of analysis involves the misrecognition of the analyst, but whatever he thinks of that and whatever panic reaction the analyst engages in through "the countertransference," he has no choice but to go through it. He's not the only one there with the person to whom he has made a commitment.

Finally, he has to pay with a judgment on his action. That's the minimum demanded. Analysis is a judgment. It's required everywhere else, but if it seems scandalous to affirm it here, there is probably a reason. It is because, from a certain point of view, the analyst is fully aware that he cannot know what he is doing in psychoanalysis. Part of this action remains hidden even to him.

And it is this that justifies the direction I have been taking you in this year, the point to which I have suggested you follow me, namely, there where the question of exploring the general ethical consequences involved in Freud's opening up of the relationship to the unconscious is raised.

I grant that there was the appearance of a detour, but it was necessary so as to bring you closer to our ethics as analysts. A few reminders were necessary before I could bring you closer to the practice of analysis and its technical problems. In the present state of affairs, they can hardly be resolved through such reminders.

In the first place, is it the end of analysis that is demanded of us? What is demanded can be expressed in a simple word, *bonheur* or "happiness," as they say in English. I'm not saying anything new in that; a demand for happiness is doubtless involved here.

In the report I referred to earlier – which, now that I see it in print, seems a little too aphoristic, which explains why I will attempt here to lubricate its hinges a little – I allude to the question without explaining it further. The business is not helped by the fact that happiness has become a political matter. I won't go any further into this, but it is the reason why I ended the lecture called "Dialectical Psychoanalysis" – a lecture in which I brought to an end a certain period of activity in a group that we have broken with since – with the words, "There is no satisfaction for the individual outside of the satisfaction of all."

To refocus analysis on the dialectic makes evident the fact that the goal is indefinitely postponed. It's not the fault of analysis if the question of happiness cannot be articulated in any other way at the present time. I would say that it is because, as Saint-Just says, happiness has become a political matter. It is because happiness has entered the political realm that the question of happiness is not susceptible to an Aristotelian solution, that the prerequisite is situated at the level of the needs of all men. Whereas Aristotle chooses between the different forms of the good that he offers the master, and tells him that only certain of these are worthy of his devotion – namely, contemplation – the dialectic of the master has, I insist, been discredited in our eyes for historical reasons that have to do with the period of history in which we find ourselves. Those reasons are expressed in politics by the following formula: "There is no satisfaction for the individual outside of the satisfaction of all."

It is in such a context that analysis appears to be – without our being able to explain why precisely it is the case in this context – and the analyst sets himself up to receive, a demand for happiness.

I have set out to show you this year the distance traveled since Aristotle, say, by choosing among some of the most crucial concepts. I wanted to make you feel the extent to which we approach these things differently, how far we are from any formulation of a discipline of happiness.

There is in Aristotle a discipline of happiness. He shows the paths along which he intends to lead anyone who is willing to follow him in his problematic, paths which in different spheres of potential human activity lead to the realization of one of the functions of virtue. Such virtue is achieved through μεσότης, something that is far from being a simple golden mean or a process linked to the avoidance of excess; instead it is supposed to enable man to choose that which might reasonably allow him to realize himself in his own good.

Please note that one finds nothing similar in psychoanalysis. Along paths that would appear surprising to someone straight out of high school, we claim to allow the subject to put himself in a position such that things mysteriously and almost miraculously work themselves out right, provided he grasp them at the right end. Goodness only knows how obscure such a pretension as the achievement of genital objecthood (*l'objectalité genitale*) remains, along with what is so imprudently linked to it, namely, adjustment to reality.

One thing only alludes to the possibility of the happy satisfaction of the instinct, and that is the notion of sublimation. But it is clear that if one looks at the most esoteric formulation of the concept in Freud, in the context of his representing it as realized preeminently in the activity of the artist, it literally means that man has the possibility of making his desires tradeable or salable in the form of products. The frankness and even cynicism of such a formulation has in my eyes a great merit, although it is far from exhausting the fundamental question, and that is, How is it possible?

The other formulation consists of informing us that sublimation is the satisfaction of the drive with a change of object, that is, without repression. This definition is a profounder one, but it would also open up an even knottier problematic, if it weren't for the fact that my teaching allows you to spot where the rabbit is hidden.

In effect, the rabbit to be conjured from the hat is already to be found in the instinct. This rabbit is not a new object; it is a change of object in itself. If the drive allows the change of object, it is because it is already deeply marked by the articulation of the signifier. In the graph of desire that I gave you, the instinct is situated at the level of the unconscious articulation of a signifying series and is for this reason constituted as fundamental alienation. That is why, on the other hand, each of the signifiers composing this series is joined by a common element.

In the definition of sublimation as satisfaction without repression, whether implicitly or explicitly, there is a passage from not-knowing to knowing, a recognition of the fact that desire is nothing more than the metonymy of the discourse of demand. It is change as such. I emphasize the following: the properly metonymic relation between one signifier and another that we call desire is not a new object or a previous object, but the change of object in itself.

Let me cite as an example something that occurred to me when I was preparing these comments for you, so that I could give an image of what I mean by sublimation. Think of the shift from a verb to what in grammar is called its complement or, in a more philosophical grammar, its determinative. Think of the most radical of verbs in the development of the phases of the drive, the verb "to eat." There is "eating." That is how the verb, the action, appears head-first in many languages, before there is any determination as to who is involved. Thus one sees here the secondary character of the subject, since we don't even have the subject, the something that is there to be eaten.

There is eating – the eating of what? Of the book.

When in the *Apocalypse* we read this powerful image, "eat the book," what does it mean? – if it isn't that the book itself acquires the value of an incorporation, the incorporation of the signifier itself, the support of the properly apocalyptic creation. The signifier in this instance becomes God, the object of the incorporation itself.

In daring to formulate a satisfaction that isn't rewarded with a repression, the theme that is central or preeminent is, What is desire? And in this connection I can only remind you of what I have articulated in the past: realizing one's desire is necessarily always raised from the point of view of an absolute condition. It is precisely to the extent that the demand always under- or overshoots itself that, because it articulates itself through the signifier, it always demands something else; that in every satisfaction of a need, it insists on something else; that the satisfaction formulated spreads out and conforms to this gap; that desire is formed as something supporting this metonymy, namely, as something the demand means beyond whatever it is able to formulate. And that is why the question of the realization of desire is necessarily formulated from the point of view of a Last Judgment.

Try to imagine what "to have realized one's desire" might mean, if it is not to have realized it, so to speak, in the end. It is this trespassing of death on life that gives its dynamism to any question that attempts to find a formulation for the subject of the realization of desire. To illustrate what I am saying, if we pose directly the question of desire on the basis of that Parminedean absolutism, which eliminates everything that is not being, then we will say, nothing is from that which is not born, and all that exists lives only in the lack of being.

2

Does life have anything to do with death? Can one say that the relationship to death supports or subtends, as the string does the bow, the curve of the rise and fall of life? It is enough for us to take up again the question that Freud himself thought he could raise on the basis of his experience – everything points to the fact that it is effectively raised by our experience.

In what I was saying a moment ago, I wasn't talking about that death. I am interested in the second death, the one that you can still set your sights on once death has occurred, as I showed you with concrete examples in Sade's texts.

After all, the human tradition has never ceased to keep this second death in mind by locating the end of our sufferings there; in the same way it has never ceased to imagine a second form of suffering, a suffering beyond death that is indefinitely sustained by the impossibility of crossing the limit of the second death. And that is why the tradition of hell in different forms has always remained alive, and it is still present in Sade in the idea he has of making the sufferings inflicted on a victim go on indefinitely. This refinement is attributed to one of the heroes of his novels, a Sadist who tries to assure himself of the damnation of the person he sends out of life into death.

Whatever the significance of the metapsychological imagining of Freud's that is the death instinct, whether or not he was justified in forging it, the question it raises is articulated in the following form by virtue of the mere fact that it has been raised: How can man, that is to say a living being, have access to knowledge of the death instinct, to his own relationship to death?

The answer is, by virtue of the signifier in its most radical form. It is in the signifier and insofar as the subject articulates a signifying chain that he comes up against the fact that he may disappear from the chain of what he is.

In truth, it's as dumb as can be. Not to recognize it, not to promote it as the essential articulation of non-knowledge as a dynamic value, not to recognize that the discovery of the unconscious is literally there in the form of this last word, simply means that they don't know what they are doing. Not remembering this fundamental principle causes the proliferation that one can observe in analytical theory, a whole jungle, a veritable downpour of references – "It's coming down in handfuls," as they say in Charente – and one cannot help noticing the note of disorientation with which it resonates.

I read no doubt a little hastily the translation of Bergler's last work. He always has something scathing and interesting to say, except that one has the impression of a wild stream of unmastered notions.

I wanted to show you how the function of the signifier in permitting the subject's access to his relationship to death might be made more concrete than is possible through a connotation. That is why I have tried to have you recognize it in our recent meetings in an aesthetic form, namely, that of the beautiful – it being precisely the function of the beautiful to reveal to us the site of man's relationship to his own death, and to reveal it to us only in a blinding flash.

Since I asked Mr. Kaufmann to remind you last time of the terms according to which, right at the beginning of the period of man's relation to happiness that we are still living in, Kant thought it necessary to define the relation to the beautiful, I have subsequently heard the complaint that the thing wasn't made vivid enough for you by means of an example. Well, let me try to give you one.

Remember the four moments of the beautiful as they were articulated for you. I will try by means of a graduated process to illustrate that for you. For the first step I will draw on an element of my daily experience.

My experience is not that vast, and I have often said to myself that I haven't had sufficient taste for it – things don't always seem to me to be that much fun. Nevertheless, something always turns up to enable one to find an image for that path of the in-between where I am attempting to lead you.

Let us just say that, unlike Mr. Teste, if stupidity is not my strong point, I'm not particularly proud of the fact.[1]

I'm just going to tell you a little incident.

I was in London once in what they call a kind of "Home," where I was being welcomed as a guest of an institution which disseminates French culture. It was in one of those charming little areas of London at some distance from the center, toward the end of October when the weather is often delightful. I was the recipient of a form of hospitality that was marked by a kind of Victorian monasticism in a charming little building. The style of the establishment was marked by the delicious smell of toast and the menace of those inedible gelatine desserts that they are in the habit of consuming over there.

I wasn't alone but was with someone who has agreed to accompany me through life, one of whose characteristics is an extreme sense of uniqueness. In the morning this person, that is to say my wife, suddenly says out of the blue: "Professor D . . . is here." He is or was one of my mentors at the *Ecole des Langues Orientales*. It was very early in the morning. "How do you know?" I asked her, since I assure you Professor D . . . is not a close friend of mine. I was told: "I've seen his shoes."

I must say that I couldn't help feeling startled by that answer; I was also skeptical. To read the highly personal traits of an individuality into a pair of clodhoppers sitting outside a door didn't seem to me to be sufficiently convincing evidence, and there was nothing else that allowed me to believe that Professor D . . . might be in London. I found the thing quite funny and didn't attach any importance to it.

I made my way at that early hour along the corridors without thinking anything more about it. And it was then that to my astonishment I saw Professor D . . . in person slipping out of his bedroom in his dressing gown, exposing as he went a pair of long and highly academic drawers.

I find that experience highly instructive, and it is on that basis that I intend to suggest to you the notion of the beautiful.

Nothing less was required than an experience in which the universality

---

[1] The reference is to Paul Valéry's short work of fiction, *Monsieur Teste*.

belonging to the shoes of an academic was intimately joined to whatever it was that was absolutely specific to Professor D . . . , for me to invite you quite simply to think of Van Gogh's old shoes – on the basis of which Heidegger has given us a dazzling image of what a work of beauty is.

You must imagine Professor D . . .'s clodhoppers *ohne Begriff*, with no thought of the academic, without any connection to his endearing personality, if you are to begin to see Van Gogh's own clodhoppers come alive with their own incommensurable quality of beauty.

They are simply there; they communicate a sign of understanding that is situated precisely at equal distance from the power of the imagination and that of the signifier. This signifier is not even a signifier of walking, of fatigue, or of anything else, such as passion or human warmth. It is just a signifier of that which is signified by a pair of abandoned clodhoppers, namely, both a presence and a pure absence – something that is, if one likes, inert, available to everyone, but something that seen from certain sides, in spite of its dumbness, speaks. It is an impression that appears as a function of the organic or, in a word, of waste, since it evokes the beginning of spontaneous generation.

That factor which magically transforms these clodhoppers into a kind of reverse side and analogue of two buds proves that it is not a question of imitation – something that has always taken in those who have written on the topic – but of the capture, by virtue of their situation in a certain temporal relationship, of that quality through which they are themselves the visible manifestation of beauty.

If you don't find this example convincing, find others. What I am, in effect, attempting to show here is that the beautiful has nothing to do with what is called ideal beauty. It is only on the basis of the apprehension of the beautiful at the very point of the transition between life and death that we can try to reinstate ideal beauty or, in other words, the function of that which sometimes reveals itself to us as the ideal form of beauty, and in the first place the famous human form.

If you read that work of Lessing's which is so rich in all kinds of insights, the *Laocoon*, you will find that he is absorbed from the beginning in the conception of the dignity of the object. Not that it is as the result of historical progress that the dignity of the object has finally been abandoned, thank God, since everything seems to indicate that it always was. Greek artists didn't restrict themselves to producing images of the gods; as we learn from Aristophanes's writings, paintings of onions cost a lot of money. It is thus not just with the Dutch painters that people began to realize that any object may be the signifier by means of which that reflection, mirage, or more or less unbearable brilliance we call the beautiful starts to vibrate.

But since I have just referred to the Dutch, take the example of the still life. You will find there moving in the opposite direction from that of the clodhoppers discussed above, as they began to bud, the same crossing of the line. As Claudel showed so admirably in his study of Dutch painting, it is to the extent that the still life both reveals and hides that within it which constitutes a threat, denouement, unfolding, or decomposition, that it manifests the beautiful for us as a function of a temporal relation.

Moreover, insofar as it engages the ideal, the question of the beautiful can only be found at this level as operating at the limit. Even in Kant's time it is the form of the human body that is presented to us as the limit of the possibilities of the beautiful, as ideal *Erscheinen*. It once was, though it no longer is, a divine form. It is the cloak of all possible fantasms of human desire. The flowers of desire are contained in this vase whose contours we attempt to define.

And it is this that leads me to posit the form of the body, and especially its image, as I have previously articulated it in the function of narcissism, as that which from a certain point of view represents the relationship of man to his second death, the signifier of his desire, his visible desire.

The central mirage is to be found in Ἵμερος ἐναργής, which both indicates the site of desire insofar as it is desire of nothing, the relationship of man to his lack of being, and prevents that site from being seen.

3

Here we can take the question even further. Is it the same shadow that is represented by the human body; is it this same image that constitutes a barrier to the Other-thing that lies beyond?

That which lies beyond is not simply the relationship to the second death or, in other words, to man to the extent that language demands of him that he realize the following, namely, that he is not. There is also the libido, that is to say, that which at fleeting moments carries us beyond the encounter that makes us forget it. And Freud was the first to articulate boldly and powerfully the idea that the only moment of *jouissance* that man knows occurs at the site where fantasms are produced, fantasms that represent for us the same barrier as far as access to *jouissance* is concerned, the barrier where everything is forgotten.

I should like to introduce here, as a parallel to the function of the beautiful, another function. I have named it on a number of occasions without emphasizing it particularly, but it seems to me essential to refer to it here. It is with your permission what I shall call Αἰδώς or, in other words, a sense of shame. The omission of this barrier, which prevents the direct experience of that which is to be found at the center of sexual union, seems to me to be at the origin of all kinds of questions that cannot be answered, including notably the matter of feminine sexuality, which is a subject that is on the agenda of our research activities – though I am not responsible for that.

The end of *Antigone* offers us the substitution of some bloody image of sacrifice that is realized in the mystical suicide. Clearly, beyond a certain point we do not know what goes on in Antigone's tomb. Everything points to the fact that what occurs there takes place as a crisis of μανία – Antigone attains the same level as that at which both Ajax and Hercules perish. I won't take up the question of Oedipus's end.

In this connection I have found no better a source than the Heraclitean aphorisms that we owe to the denunciatory references of Saint Clement of Alexandria – he found in them the sign of pagan abominations. I have retained a small fragment that says, εἰ μὴ γὰρ Διονύσωι Πομπὴν ἐποιοῦντο καὶ ὕμνεον αἶσμα, "clearly, if they did not organize processions and feasts to Dionysos accompanied by the singing of hymns" – and it is here that the ambiguity begins—αἰδοίοισιν ἀναιδέστατα Εἰργασίάν – what would they perform? the most disrespectful of homages to something shameful." That is in a sense one way of reading it. And, Heraclites goes on, Hades and Dionysos are the same thing to the extent that both of them μαίνονται, they enter a state of delirium and start to perform like hyenas. The reference is to bacchic processions that are linked to the appearance of all manner of forms of trance.

You should realize that Heraclites didn't at all like extreme religious ceremonies and had no sympathy for ecstacy – a lack of sympathy that is very different from that of a Christian or a rationalist. And he leads us up to the point where he says that if it weren't a reference to Hades or a ceremony of ecstacy, it would be nothing more than an odious phallic ceremony, an object of disgust.

Yet it isn't clear that one should rely on this translation. There is an obvious play on words between αἰδοίοισιν ἀναιδέστατα and Ἅιδης, which means invisible. Αἰδοῖα means the shameful parts, but it can also mean something respectable and venerable. The term song isn't missing. In the end, in singing their praises with great pomp to Dionysos, the members of his sect do not really know what they are doing. Aren't Hades and Dionysos one and the same thing?

It's a question that is also raised for us. Do the fantasm of the phallus and the beauty of the human image find their legitimate place at the same level? Or is there, on the contrary, an imperceptible distinction, an irreducible difference, between them? The whole Freudian enterprise has come up against that issue. At the end of one of his final papers, "Analysis Terminable and Interminable," Freud tells us that in the end the aspiration of the patient collapses into an ineradicable nostalgia for the fact that there is no way he can be the phallus, and that since he cannot be it, he can only have it in the condition of the *Penisneid* in a woman or of castration in a man.

That's something to remember whenever the analyst finds himself in the position of responding to anyone who asks him for happiness. The question of the Sovereign Good is one that man has asked himself since time immemorial, but the analyst knows that it is a question that is closed. Not only doesn't he have that Sovereign Good that is asked of him, but he also knows there isn't any. To have carried an analysis through to its end is no more nor less than to have encountered that limit in which the problematic of desire is raised.

That this problematic is central for access to any realization of oneself whatsoever constitutes the novelty of the analysis. There is no doubt that in the course of this process the subject will encounter much that is good for him, all the good he can do for himself, in fact, but let us not forget what we know so well because we say it everyday of our lives in the clearest of terms: he will only encounter that good if at every moment he eliminates from his wishes the false goods, if he exhausts not only the vanity of his demands, given that they are all no more than regressive demands, but also the vanity of his gifts.

Psychoanalysis makes the whole achievement of happiness turn on the genital act. It is, therefore, necessary to draw the proper consequences from this. It is doubtless possible to achieve for a single moment in this act something which enables one human being to be for another in the place that is both living and dead of the Thing. In this act and only at this moment, he may simulate with his flesh the consummation of what he is not under any circumstances. But even if the possibility of this consummation is polarizing and central, it cannot be considered timely.

What the subject achieves in analysis is not just that access, even if it is repeated and always available, but something else that through the transference gives everything living its form – the subject, so to speak, counts the vote relative to his own law. This law is in the first place always the acceptance of something that began to be articulated before him in previous generations, and which is strictly speaking *Atè*. Although this *Atè* does not always reach the tragic level of Antigone's *Atè*, it is nevertheless closely related to misfortune.

What the analyst has to give, unlike the partner in the act of love, is something that even the most beautiful bride in the world cannot outmatch, that is to say, what he has. And what he has is nothing other than his desire, like that of the analysand, with the difference that it is an experienced desire.

What can a desire of this kind, the desire of the analyst, be? We can say right away what it cannot be. It cannot desire the impossible.

I will give you an example of that in a compact definition, which an author managed to come up with before he disappeared, of a function that seemed to him to be essential in the dual relationship with the analyst, a relationship that exists to the extent that we respond to the demand of happiness, but that does not exhaust the analysis. This function, which is namely that of distance, is defined in the following terms: the gap between the way in which the subject expresses his instinctual "drives"[2] and the way in which he would be able to express them if the process of arranging and organizing them weren't available.

In the light of my teaching, the truly aberrant and contradictory character of such a formulation is apparent. If the instinct is the effect of the mark of the signifier on needs, their transformation as an effect of the signifier into something fragmented and panic-stricken that we call the drive, what can such a definition of distance mean?

In the same way, if the analyst's desire is an experienced desire, it is impossible for the analyst to agree to remain in the trap that is the desire to reduce such a distance to nothing. The function of the analyst would essentially be that of a "joiner" (*un rappocher*), as the same theoretician expresses it. The same fantasm is involved here, namely, that of the incorporation or ingestion of the phallic image to the extent that it is actualized in a relationship that is entirely governed by the imaginary. In that direction the subject can achieve nothing but some form of psychosis or perversion, however mild its character, for the term "joiner" that is placed by the author concerned at the center of the analytical dialectic does no more than reflect a desire of the analyst, whose nature the latter misperceives as a result of an inadequate theory of his position; it is the desire to draw closer to the point of being joined to the one who is in his charge.

One can only say of such an aspiration that it is pathetic in its naiveté. And one is only surprised that it could have been formulated other than as a dead-end to be dismissed.

That, then, is what I wanted to remind you of today, so as to indicate to you the direction taken by our research on the subject of the beautiful and, I would add, the sublime. We haven't yet extracted from the Kantian definitions of the sublime all the substance we might. The conjunction of this term with that of sublimation is probably not simply an accident nor simply homonymic.

We will take up the question of this satisfaction next time for our profit; the promise of analysis grants no other.

June 22, 1960

2. In English in text.

XXIII

The moral goals of psychoanalysis

THE BOURGEOIS DREAM
OEDIPUS, LEAR, AND THE SERVICE OF GOODS
THE INCORPORATION OF THE SUPEREGO
THE THREE FATHERS
UNRECONCILED OEDIPUS

At the point where I am about to bring to an end the risky topic that I chose to explore with you this year, I believe I cannot do enough to articulate the limit of the progress I wanted you to make.

I will spend next year outlining the ends and the means of analysis in relation to each other. Though that's not necessarily the title I will give the Seminar. It seems to me to be indispensable that we stop for a moment to consider something that remains obscure in what might be called the moral goals of psychoanalysis.

1

To promote in the practice of analysis a form of psychological normalization implies what might be called rationalizing moralization. Furthermore, to aim for the fulfillment of what is known as the genital stage, that is, a maturation of the drive and object, which would set the standard for a right relationship to reality, definitely embodies a certain moral implication.

Should the theoretical and practical purpose of our action be limited to the ideal of psychological harmonization? In the hope of allowing our patients to achieve the possibility of an untroubled happiness should we assume that the reduction of the antimony that Freud himself so powerfully articulated may be complete? I am referring to what he expresses in *Civilization and Its Discontents* when he affirms that the form in which the moral agency is concretely inscribed in man – and that is nothing less than rational according to him – the form he called the superego, operates according to an economy such that the more one sacrifices to it, the more it demands.

Are we entitled to forget that threat, that cleavage in the moral being of man, in the doctrine and practice of psychoanalysis? In truth, that is what happens; we are only too inclined to forget it, both in the promises that we believe we can make, and in those that we believe we can make to ourselves in the matter of a given outcome of our therapy. It's serious, and it's even more serious when we are in a position to give to an analysis its full significance; I mean when we are faced by the conceivable end of an analysis in its training function in the fullest sense of the term.

If we are to consider an analysis completed for someone who is subsequently to find himself in a responsible position relative to an analysis, in the sense that he becomes an analyst himself, should it ideally or by right end with the position of comfort that I categorized just now as a moralizing rationalization of the kind in which it often tends to express itself?

When in conformity with Freudian experience one has articulated the dialectic of demand, need and desire, is it fitting to reduce the success of an analysis to a situation of individual comfort linked to that well-founded and legitimate function we might call the service of goods? Private goods, family goods, domestic goods, other goods that solicit us, the goods of our trade or our profession, the goods of the city, etc.

Can we, in fact, close off that city so easily nowadays? It doesn't matter. However we regulate the situation of those who have recourse to us in our society, it is only too obvious that their aspiration to happiness will always imply a place where miracles happen, a promise, a mirage of original genius or an opening up of freedom, or if we caricature it, the possession of all women for a man and of an ideal man for a woman. To make oneself the guarantor of the possibility that a subject will in some way be able to find happiness even in analysis is a form of fraud.

There's absolutely no reason why we should make ourselves the guarantors of the bourgeois dream. A little more rigor and firmness are required in our confrontation with the human condition. That is why I reminded you last time that the service of goods or the shift of the demand for happiness onto the political stage has its consequences. The movement that the world we live in is caught up in, of wanting to establish the universal spread of the service of goods as far as conceivably possible, implies an amputation, sacrifices, indeed a kind of puritanism in the relationship to desire that has occurred historically. The establishment of the service of goods at a universal level does not in itself resolve the problem of the present relationship of each individual man to his desire in the short period of time between his birth and his death. The happiness of future generations is not at issue here.

As I believe I have shown here in the sphere I have outlined for you this year, the function of desire must remain in a fundamental relationship to death. The question I ask is this: shouldn't the true termination of an analysis – and by that I mean the kind that prepares you to become an analyst – in the end confront the one who undergoes it with the reality of the human condition? It is precisely this, that in connection with anguish, Freud designated as the level at which its signal is produced, namely, *Hilflosigkeit* or distress, the state in which man is in that relationship to himself which is his own death – in the sense I have taught you to isolate it this year – and can expect help from no one.

At the end of a training analysis the subject should reach and should know the domain and the level of the experience of absolute disarray. It is a level at which anguish is already a protection, not so much *Abwarten* as *Erwartung*. Anguish develops by letting a danger appear, whereas there is no danger at the level of the final experience of *Hilflosigkeit*.

I have already told you how the limit of this region is expressed for man; it touches the end of what he is and what he is not. That is why the myth of Oedipus acquires its full significance here.

2

Today I will once again bring you back to the passage through that intermediary region, and I remind you that in the Oedipus story one must not overlook the time that passes between the moment when Oedipus is blinded and the moment when he dies. And it is, moreover, a special, unique death that, as I have already said, constitutes a genuine enigma in Sophocles.

One shouldn't forget that in a sense Oedipus did not suffer from the Oedipus complex, and he punished himself for a sin he did not commit. He simply killed a man whom he didn't know was his father, a man whom, according to the realistically motivated form in which the myth is presented, he met on the road along which he was fleeing because he had got wind of something quite unpleasant concerning him with relation to his father. He flees those whom he thinks are his parents, and commits a crime in trying to avoid it.

He doesn't know that in achieving happiness, both conjugal happiness and that of his job as king, of being the guide to the happiness of the state, he is sleeping with his mother. One might therefore ask what the treatment he inflicts on himself means. Which treatment? He gives up the very thing that captivated him. In fact, he has been duped, tricked by reason of the fact that he achieved happiness. Beyond the sphere of the service of goods and in spite of the complete success of this service, he enters into the zone in which he pursues his desire.

Note carefully the dispositions he makes; at the moment of death, he remains unmoved. The irony of the French expression for hale and hearty, *bon pied bon oeil*,[1] should not mean too much in his case, since the man whose feet are swollen has also lost the sight of his eyes. But that doesn't prevent him from demanding everything or, in other words, all the honors due his rank. The

---

[1] It means literally "good foot good eye."

memory of the legend allows us to perceive something that is emphasized by modern ethnography, because after the sacrifice he was sent the victim's thigh instead of its shoulder – it might be the other way round – and he sees in this lapse an intolerable insult and breaks with his sons to whom he had handed over power. Then in the end his curse on his sons bursts forth, and it is absolute.

It is important to explore what is contained in that moment when, although he has renounced the service of goods, nothing of the preeminence of his dignity in relation to these same goods is ever abandoned; it is the same moment when in his tragic liberty he has to deal with the consequence of that desire that led him to go beyond the limit, namely, the desire to know. He has learned and still wants to learn something more.

In order to make myself understood, I should perhaps evoke another tragic figure, one who is no doubt closer to us – King Lear.

I cannot give a detailed analysis of the significance of the play here. I just wanted to make you understand what Oedipus's crossing over means on the basis of *King Lear*, where we find that crossing over in a derisory form.

King Lear, too, gives up the service of goods, gives up his royal duties; the old fool believes he is lovable and, therefore, hands over the service of goods to his daughters. But you must not assume that he gives up anything. It's supposed to be the beginning of freedom, a life of festivities with his fifty knights, lots of fun, during which time he stays in turn with each of those two shrews whom he thought he could entrust with the duties of power.

In the meantime, there he is with no other warrant than that of loyalty, of an agreement founded on honor, since he conceded the power he had of his own free will. Shakespeare's formidable irony mobilizes a whole swarm of destinies that devour each other, for it isn't just Lear but all the good people in the play whom we see condemned to suffering without remission for having trusted to simple loyalty and to agreements founded on honor. I don't have to emphasize the fact; just read the play again.

Lear as well as Oedipus shows us that he who enters that space, whether it be by the derisory path of Lear or the tragic one of Oedipus, finds himself alone and betrayed.

Oedipus's last word is, as you know, that phrase μὴ φύναι which I have repeated here any number of times, since it embodies a whole exegesis on negation. I indicated to you how the French language raises it in that little pleonastic "ne" which no one knows what to do with, since it dangles there in an expression such as "je crains qu'il ne vienne" ("I'm afraid he is coming"), which would be just as pleased if it weren't there like a particle oscillating between a coming and fear of it.[2] It has no *raison d'être* except for that

---

[2] See note 2 on p. 64 on the pleonastic "ne."

of the subject itself. In French it is the remains of that which means μή in Greek, a word that does not signify a negation. I could show it to you in any text.

Other texts give expression to it, such as *Antigone,* for example, in the passage where the guard, in speaking about the person whom he does not yet know to be Antigone, says: "He left without leaving a trace." And the guard adds in the lesson chosen by the editor: "ἔφευγε μὴ εἰδέναι." In principle that means he avoided its being known that it was him – τό μὴ εἰδέναι – as a variant suggests. But if one took the first version with its two negations literally, one would have to say he avoided its not being known that it was him. The μή is there to indicate the *Spaltung* between the enunciation and the enunciated that I have already explained. Μή φύναι means "rather not to be."

That's the choice with which a human existence such as Oedipus's has to end. It ends so perfectly that he doesn't die like everybody else, that is to say accidentally; he dies from a true death in which he erases his own being. The malediction is freely accepted on the basis of the true subsistence of a human being, the subsistence of the subtraction of himself from the order of the world. It's a beautiful attitude, and as the madrigal says, it's twice as beautiful on account of its beauty.

Oedipus shows us where the inner limit zone in the relationship to desire ends. In every human experience that zone is always relegated to a point beyond death, since the ordinary human being conducts himself in the light of what needs to be done so as not to risk the other death, the death that simply involves kicking the bucket. *Primum vivere* – questions relating to being are always postponed to later, which does not, of course, mean that they aren't there on the horizon.

Here then are the topological notions without which it is our experience that it is impossible to find one's way or to say anything that is not simply confusing and a going round in circles – and that's true of even the most eminent of authors. Take, for example, the article by Jones that is remarkable in all kinds of ways, "Hatred, Culpability and Fear," in which he shows the circularity of these terms, though it's not an absolute one. I beg you to study it pen in hand, for we will be dealing with it next year. You will see how many things would be illuminated if the principles we are articulating were applied.

Let us take up those principles again in connection with the common man who concerns us here; let us try to see what they imply. Jones, for example, has perhaps expressed better than others the moral alibi that he called *moralisches Entgegenkommen,* that is, a kind of consent to the moral demand. In effect, he shows that very often there is nothing more in the duties man imposes on himself than the fear of the risks involved in failing to impose those duties. One should call things by their name, and it's not because one hangs up a triple analytical veil that it doesn't mean what it says: psychoanalysis teaches that in the end it is easier to accept interdiction than to run the risk of castration.

Let's try to practice a little brain-washing on ourselves. Before going into the question further, which is often a way of avoiding it, what does it mean to say, as Freud does, that the superego appears at the moment of the decline of the Oedipus complex? Of course, we have in the meantime made a little progress by demonstrating that one was born before, in reaction to sadistic drives, according to Melanie Klein, although no one has been able to prove that the same superego is involved. But let's limit ourselves to the Oedipal superego. The fact that it is born at the moment of the decline of the Oedipus complex means that the subject incorporates its authority into himself.

That ought to put you on the right track. In a famous article called "Mourning and Melancholia," Freud also says that the work of mourning is applied to an incorporated object, to an object which for one reason or another one is not particularly fond of. As far as the loved object that we make such a fuss about in our mourning is concerned, we do not, in fact, simply sing its praises, if only because of the lousy trick it played on us by leaving us. Thus, if we are sufficiently cruel to ourselves to incorporate the father, it is perhaps because we have a lot to reproach this father with.

It is here that the distinctions I presented to you last year may prove useful. Castration, frustration, and privation are not the same thing. If frustration properly belongs to the symbolic mother, he who is responsible for castration, according to Freud, is the real father, and as far as privation is concerned, it's the imaginary father. Let us try to understand the function of each of these elements at the moment of decline of the Oedipus complex and of the formation of the superego. Perhaps that will shed a little light, and we won't have the impression of reading two different lines at the same time when we take account of the castrating father, on the one hand, and the father as origin of the superego, on the other. This distinction is basic to everything Freud articulated, and in particular to the question of castration once he began to spell it out – the phenomenon is indeed a stupefying one since it is a notion that had never even been broached before him.

The real father, Freud tells us, is a castrating father. In what way? Through his presence as real father who effectively occupies that person with whom the child is in a state of rivalry, namely, the mother. Whether or not that is the case in experience, in theory there is no doubt about it: the real father is elevated to the rank of Great Fucker – though not, believe me, in the face of the Eternal, which isn't even around to count the number of times. Yet doesn't this real and mythical father fade at the moment of the decline of the Oedipus complex into the one whom the child may easily have already discovered at the relatively advanced age of five years old, namely, the imaginary father, the father who has fucked the kid up.

Isn't that what the theoreticians of analytical experience say as they mumble away? And doesn't one find the point of difference there? Isn't it in connection with the experience of privation the small child undergoes – not because he is small but because he is human – in connection with what the child experiences as privation, that the mourning for the imaginary father is forged? – that is a mourning for someone who would really be someone. The perpetual reproach that is born at that moment, in a way that is more or less definitive and well-formed depending on the individual case, remains fundamental in the structure of the subject. It is this imaginary father and not the real one which is the basis of the providential image of God. And the function of the superego in the end, from its final point of view, is hatred for God, the reproach that God has handled things so badly.

I believe that that is the true structure of the articulation of the Oedipus complex. If you break it down in that way, you will find that the detours, hesitations, and gropings of different authors in their attempts to explain various difficulties and details will be much clearer. In particular, you will also be able to see, in a way that is otherwise impossible, what Jones really means when he speaks of the relationship between hate, fear, and guilt in connection with the genesis of the superego.

3

To pick up the thread, let us say, would to God that the drama took place at the bloody level of castration and that the poor little man flooded the whole world with his blood like Kronos Uranus!

Everyone knows that castration is there on the horizon and that it never, of course, occurs. What does happen relates to the fact that the little man is rather a paltry support for that organ, for that signifier, and that he seems rather to be deprived of it. And here one can see that his fate is common to that of the little girl, who also can be explained much more clearly from this angle of vision.

What is in question is the moment when the subject quite simply perceives that his father is an idiot or a thief, as the case may be, or quite simply a weakling or, routinely, an old fogey, as in Freud's case. He was if you like an agreeable and kind old fogey, but he must, like all fathers, have communicated in spite of himself the series of shocks we call the contradictions of capitalism; he left Freiberg where there was nothing to do anymore in order to move to Vienna, and it is the kind of thing that doesn't go unnoticed in the mind of a child, even if he is only three years old. And it was because Freud loved his father that he felt obliged to restore his stature to the point of attributing to him the gigantic proportions of the father of the primitive horde.

But that's not what resolves the fundamental questions; that's not the essential question, as the story of Oedipus tells us. If Oedipus is a whole man, if Oedipus doesn't have an Oedipus complex, it is because in his case there is no father at all. The person who served as father was his adoptive father. And, my good friends, that's the case with all of us, because as the Latin has it, *pater is est quem justae nuptiae demonstrant*, that is to say, the father is he who acknowledges us. We are at bottom in the same boat as Oedipus, even if we don't know it. As far as the father that Oedipus knew is concerned, he only becomes the father, as Freud's myth indicates, once he is dead.

It is thus there, as I've said a hundred times, that one finds the paternal function. In our theory the sole function of the father is to be a myth, to be always only the Name-of-the-Father, or in other words nothing more than the dead father, as Freud explains in *Totem and Taboo*. But for this to be developed fully, of course, the human adventure has to be carried through to its end, if only in outline; that zone Oedipus enters after having scratched out his eyes has to be explored.

It is always through some beneficial crossing of the limit that man experiences his desire. Others have expressed the idea before me. The whole meaning Jones discovers in connection with aphanisis is related to this; it is linked to the important risk, which is quite simply the loss of desire. Oedipus's desire is the desire to know the last word on desire.

When I tell you that the desire of man is the desire of the Other, I am reminded of something in a poem by Paul Eluard that says "the difficult desire to endure" *(le dur désir de durer)*. That is nothing more than the desire to desire.

For the ordinary man, given that Oedipus's mourning is at the origin of the superego, the double limit – from the real death risked to the preferred or the assumed death, to the being-for-death – only appears as veiled. It is a veil that Jones calls hate. You can grasp in this the reason why any alert author locates the final term of the psychic reality we deal with in the ambivalence between love and hate.

The external limit that keeps man in the service of the good is the *primum vivere*. It is fear, we are told, but you can see how superficial its influence is.

Between the two for the ordinary man lies the exercise of his guilt, which is a reflection of his hatred for the creator, whoever he may be – for man is creationist – who made him such a weak and inadequate creature.

All this nonsense is meaningless for the hero, for the one who has entered that zone, for Oedipus who goes as far as the $\mu\dot{\eta}\varphi\hat{\nu}\nu\alpha\iota$ of true being-for-death, goes as far as a malediction he acquiesces in or an engagement with annihilation that is taken to be the realization of his wish. There is nothing else here except the true and indivisible disappearance that is his. Entry into that zone for him is constituted of a renunciation of goods and of power that is supposed to be a punishment, but is not, in fact, one. If he tears himself free from the world through the act of blinding himself, it is because only he who escapes from appearances can achieve truth. This was known in antiquity; the great Homer was blind and so was Tiresias.

For Oedipus the absolute reign of his desire is played out between the two, something that is sufficiently brought out by the fact that he is shown to be unyielding right to the end, demanding everything, giving up nothing, absolutely unreconciled.

I showed you the reverse and derisory side of this topology, which is the topology of tragedy, in connection with poor Lear, who doesn't understand a thing and who makes the ocean and the earth echo because he tried to enter the same region in a salutary way with everyone agreeing. He appears in the end as still not having understood a thing and holding dead in his arms the object of his love, who is, of course, misrecognized by him.

Thus defined, that region enables us to posit the limits that illuminate a certain number of problems that are raised by our theory and our experience. We have never stopped repeating that the interiorization of the Law has nothing to do with the Law. Although we still need to know why. It is possible that the superego serves as a support for the moral conscience, but everyone knows that it has nothing to do with the moral conscience as far as its most obligatory demands are concerned. What the superego demands has nothing to do with that which we would be right in making the universal rule of our actions; such is the ABC of psychoanalytic truth. But it is not enough to affirm the fact; it must be justified.

I believe that the schema I have proposed to you is capable of doing that, and that if you stick with it you will find a way of not getting lost in that labyrinth.

Next time, I will start out on the path that all this has been leading to – a more precise grasp of catharsis and of the consequences of man's relationship to desire.

June 29, 1960

XXIV

The paradoxes of ethics
or
Have you acted in conformity with your desire?

THE COMIC DIMENSION
THE FABLE OF THE CASH REGISTER
DESIRE AND GUILT
GIVING GROUND RELATIVE TO ONE'S DESIRE
RELIGION, SCIENCE AND DESIRE

We come now to our final talk.

By way of conclusion I propose to make a certain number of comments, some of which are conclusive and others experiential or suggestive. You will not be surprised, for we haven't brought our discussion to a close, and it's not easy to find a medium when one has to conclude on a subject that is by its very nature excentric. Let's say that today I am proposing "a mixed grill."[1]

1

Since one should always start up again with a definition, let's say that an ethics essentially consists in a judgment of our action, with the proviso that it is only significant if the action implied by it also contains within it, or is supposed to contain, a judgment, even if it is only implicit. The presence of judgment on both sides is essential to the structure.

If there is an ethics of psychoanalysis — the question is an open one — it is to the extent that analysis in some way or other, no matter how minimally, offers something that is presented as a measure of our action — or it at least claims to. At first sight the idea may occur to someone that it offers a return to our instincts as the measure of our action. Such seems to belong to a time long past, but there are perhaps those here and there whom that prospect frightens. I have even had someone raising objections of that kind to me in a

---

[1] In English in the original.

philosophical society, objections that I thought had disappeared over forty years ago. But it is true to say that by now everyone has been sufficiently reassured on that topic; nobody seems to fear a moral cleansing of that kind as the result of an analysis.

I have often shown you that in, so to speak, constructing the instincts, in making them the natural law of the realization of harmony, psychoanalysis takes on the guise of a rather disturbing alibi, of a moralizing hustle or a bluff, whose dangers cannot be exaggerated. That's a commonplace as far as you are concerned, and I won't pursue it.

To limit ourselves to something that can be said right off, that everyone has known for a long time now, and that is one of the most modest features of our practice, let us say that analysis progresses by means of a return to the meaning of an action. That alone justifies the fact that we are interested in the moral dimension. Freud's hypothesis relative to the unconscious presupposes that, whether it be healthy or sick, normal or morbid, human action has a hidden meaning that one can have access to. In such a context the notion of a catharsis that is a purification, a decantation or isolation of levels, is immediately conceivable.

That hardly seems to me to qualify as a discovery; rather, it is the minimal position that is fortunately not too obscured in the common notion of psychoanalysis: in what goes on at the level of lived experience there is a deeper meaning that guides that experience, and one can have access to it. Moreover, things cannot be the same when the two layers are separated.

That doesn't take us very far. It is the embryonic form of a very old γνῶθι σεαυτόν, though it obviously has its own particular emphasis, which is related to an excessively general form of all that goes under the name of inner progess. But it is already enough to situate the sharp difference I have emphasized this year that is introduced, if not by analytical experience, then at least by Freudian thought.

What does this difference consist of? It may be measured in the response given to the question that ordinary people ask themselves, a question that we answer more or less directly. The question is, once it is over, once the return to the meaning of an action has been accomplished, once the deep meaning has been liberated – that is to say, separated out through a catharsis in the sense of decantation – will everything work out all right by itself? Or, to be precise, will there be nothing but goodness?

That takes us back to a very old question. A certain Mencius, as he was called by the Jesuits, tells us that it can be judged in the following way. In the beginning, goodness was natural to man; it was like a mountain covered with trees. Only the inhabitants of the surrounding area started to cut the trees down. The blessing of the night was that it gave rise to a fresh growth of suckers, but in the morning the herds returned to eat them and in the end the mountain was denuded, so that nothing grew on it.

You see that the problem is not a new one, then. The goodness in question is so far from being confirmed in our experience that we start out from what is modestly called the negative therapeutic reaction, something that at the more remarkable level of literary generality I last time called a malediction assumed or agreed to in the μή φύναι of Oedipus. Not that the problem doesn't remain whole; that is decided beyond the return to sense.

I asked you this year to enter into a mental experiment, an *experimentum mentis* as Galileo called it – contrary to what you may think he was much better acquainted with mental experiments than with those of the laboratory, and without it in any case he would certainly not have taken the decisive step. The *experimentum mentis* that I have been proposing to you throughout the year is directly connected to something that our experience points to whenever we try to articulate it in its own topology, in its own structure, instead of reducing it to a common denominator or common standard, instead of making it fit into preexisting pigeon-holes. The experiment consisted in adopting what I called the point of view of the Last Judgment. And I mean by that choosing as the standard of that reconsideration of ethics to which psychoanalysis leads us, the relationship between action and the desire that inhabits it.

To make you understand this relationship, I had recourse to tragedy, that is to a reference one cannot avoid, as is proved by the fact that Freud was obliged to make use of it from the beginning. The ethics of psychoanalysis has nothing to do with speculation about prescriptions for, or the regulation of, what I have called the service of goods. Properly speaking, that ethics implies the dimension that is expressed in what we call the tragic sense of life.

Actions are inscribed in the space of tragedy, and it is with relation to this space, too, that we are led to take our bearings in the sphere of values. Moreover, this is also true of the space of comedy, and when I started to talk to you about the formations of the unconscious, it was, as you know, the comic that I had in mind.

Let us say by way of a preliminary sounding that the relationship between action and the desire which inhabits it in the space of tragedy functions in the direction of a triumph of death. And I taught you to rectify the notion as a triumph of being-for-death that is formulated in Oedipus's μή φύναι, a phrase in which one finds that μή, the negation that is identical to the entrance of the subject supported by the signifier. There lies the fundamental character of all tragic action.

A preliminary sounding of the space of comedy shows it is less a question of a triumph than of a futile or derisory play of vision. However little time I have thus far devoted to the comic here, you have been able to see that there, too, it is a question of the relationship between action and desire, and of the former's fundamental failure to catch up with the latter.

The sphere of comedy is created by the presence at its center of a hidden signifier, but that in the Old Comedy is there in person, namely, the phallus. Who cares if it is subsequently whisked away? One must simply remember that the element in comedy that satisfies us, the element that makes us laugh, that makes us appreciate it in its full human dimension, not excluding the unconscious, is not so much the triumph of life as its flight, the fact that life slips away, runs off, escapes all those barriers that oppose it, including precisely those that are the most essential, those that are constituted by the agency of the signifier.

The phallus is nothing more than a signifier, the signifier of this flight. Life goes by, life triumphs, whatever happens. If the comic hero trips up and lands in the soup, the little fellow nevertheless survives.

The pathetic side of this dimension is, you see, exactly the opposite, the counterpart of tragedy. They are not incompatible, since tragi-comedy exists. That is where the experience of human action resides. And it is because we know better than those who went before how to recognize the nature of desire, which is at the heart of this experience, that a reconsideration of ethics is possible, that a form of ethical judgment is possible, of a kind that gives this question the force of a Last Judgment: Have you acted in conformity with the desire that is in you?

This is not an easy question to sustain. I, in fact, claim that it has never been posed with that purity elsewhere, and that it can only be posed in the analytical context.

Opposed to this pole of desire is traditional ethics – not completely, of course, for nothing is new, or everything is new, in human thought. That's something I wanted to make you feel by choosing the example of the antithesis of the tragic hero in a tragedy, an antithesis who nevertheless embodies a certain heroic quality, and that is Creon. With reference to this example, I spoke to you of the service of goods that is the position of traditional ethics. The cleaning up of desire, modesty, temperateness, that is to say, the middle path we see articulated so remarkably in Aristotle; we need to know what it takes the measure of and whether its measure is founded on something.

An attentive examination shows that its measure is always marked with a deep ambiguity. In the end the order of things on which it claims to be founded is the order of power, of a human – far too human – power. We are not the ones to say so, but it is obvious that it can hardly take two steps in expressing itself without sketching in the ramparts that surround the place where, as far as we are concerned, the signifiers are unleashed or where, for Aristotle, the arbitrary rule of the gods holds sway – insofar as at this level gods and beasts join together to signify the world of the unthinkable.

The gods? We don't mean by that the prime mover, but mythological gods. We, of course, know how to contain the unleashing of the signifiers, but it is not because we have staked almost everything on the No/Name-of-the-Father that the question is simplified. If you go and take a close look at it – and it's worth the trouble – you will see that Aristotle's morality is wholly founded on an order that is no doubt a tidied-up, ideal order. But it is nevertheless one that corresponds to the politics of his time, to the organization of the city. His morality is the morality of the master, created for the virtues of the master and linked to the order of powers. One shouldn't be contemptuous of the order of powers – these are not the comments of an anarchist – one simply needs to know their limit with relation to our field of inquiry.

As far as that which is of interest to us, namely, that which has to do with desire, to its array and disarray, so to speak, the position of power of any kind in all circumstances and in every case, whether historical or not, has always been the same.

What is Alexander's proclamation when he arrived in Persepolis or Hitler's when he arrived in Paris? The preamble isn't important: "I have come to liberate you from this or that." The essential point is "Carry on working. Work must go on." Which, of course, means: "Let it be clear to everyone that this is on no account the moment to express the least surge of desire."

The morality of power, of the service of goods, is as follows: "As far as desires are concerned, come back later. Make them wait."

2

It is worth recalling here the line of demarcation with reference to which the question of ethics is raised for us. It is also a line that marks an essential end in the development of philosophy.

Kant is the person I have in mind because he renders us the greatest service by introducing the topological milestone that distinguishes the moral phenomenon. And by that I mean the field that is of interest to moral judgment as such. It is a limited categorical opposition no doubt, purely ideal, but it was essential that someone someday articulate it by purifying it – catharsis – of all interest, which does not mean of the interests linked to mental pathology, to the *pathologisches,* but simply to sensible, vital human interests. For it to be valorized as the properly ethical field, none of our interests must be in any way involved.

A decisive step is taken there. Traditional morality concerned itself with what one was supposed to do "insofar as it is possible," as we say, and as we are forced to say. What needs to be unmasked here is the point on which that morality turns. And that is nothing less than the impossibility in which we recognize the topology of our desire. The breakthrough is achieved by Kant when he posits that the moral imperative is not concerned with what may or may not be done. To the extent that it imposes the necessity of a practical reason, obligation affirms an unconditional "Thou shalt." The importance of this field derives from the void that the strict application of the Kantian definition leaves there.

Now we analysts are able to recognize that place as the place occupied by desire. Our experience gives rise to a reversal that locates in the center an incommensurable measure, an infinite measure, that is called desire. I showed you how one can easily substitute for Kant's "Thou shalt" the Sadean fantasm of *jouissance* elevated to the level of an imperative – it is, of course, a pure and almost derisory fantasm, but it doesn't exclude the possibility of its being elevated to a universal law.

Let us stop here and look at the prospects on the horizon. If Kant had only designated this crucial point for us, everything would be fine, but one also sees that which the horizon of practical reason opens onto: to the respect and the admiration that the starry heavens above and the moral law within inspires in him. One may wonder why. Respect and admiration suggest a personal relationship. That is where everything subsists in Kant, though in a demystified form. And that is where my comments on the basis furnished by analytical experience relative to the dimension of the subject in the signifier are essential. Let me illustrate this briefly.

Kant claims to find a new proof of the immortality of the soul in the fact that nothing on earth satisfies the demands of moral action. It is because the soul remains hungry for something more that it needs an afterlife, so that the unrealized harmony may be achieved somewhere or other.

What does that mean? That respect and that admiration for the starry skies had already grown fragile at that moment in history. Did they still exist in Kant's time? As far as we are concerned, when we look at the vast universe, doesn't it seem to us that we are in the middle of a huge construction site surrounded by various nebulae with one funny little corner, the one we live in, that has always been compared to a watch that someone forgot? Apart from that, it is easy to see if there is no one there, if, that is, we give a meaning to what might be construed as a presence. And there is no other articulatable meaning to give this divine presence except that which functions for us as a criterion of the subject, namely, the dimension of the signifier.

The philosophers can speculate all they want on the Being in whom act and knowledge are one, the religious tradition is not misled: only that which can be articulated by means of a revelation has the right to be recognized as one or more divine persons. As for us, only one thing could convince us that the heavens are inhabited by a transcendent person and that is a signal. What signal? Not the one that defines the theory of communication, which spends its time telling us that one can interpret the warning rays that traverse space in terms of signs. Distance creates mirages. Because these things come from far off, people believe that they are messages we are receiving from stars three hundred light-years away. But they are no more messages than when we look in a bottle. It would only be a message if some explosion of a star at these immense distances corresponded to something that was written down somewhere in the Great Book – in other words, something that would make a reality of what was happening.

Some of you recently saw a film that didn't exactly excite me, but since then I have revised my impression, for there are some interesting details. It's Jules Dassin's film, *Never on Sunday*. The character who is presented to us as marvelously at one with the immediacy of his supposedly primitive feelings, in a small bar in Piraeus, starts to beat up those who are sitting around because they haven't been speaking properly, that is to say in conformity with moral norms. On other occasions, in order to express his immense excitement and his happiness, he picks up a glass and shatters it on the ground. And every time a glass is shattered, we see the cash register vibrate frenetically. I see that as a beautiful touch, a stroke of genius. That cash register defines very clearly the structure that concerns us.

The reason why there is human desire, that the field can exist, depends on the assumption that everything real that happens may be accounted for somewhere. Kant managed to reduce the essence of the moral field to something pure; nevertheless, there remains at its center the need for a space where accounts are kept. It is this that is signified by the horizon represented by his immortality of the soul. As if we hadn't been plagued enough by desire on earth, part of eternity is to be given over to keeping accounts. In these fantasms one finds projected nothing but the structural relationship that I attempted to indicate on the graph with the line of the signifier. It is insofar as the subject is situated and is constituted with relation to the signifier that the break, splitting or ambivalence is produced in him at the point where the tension of desire is located.

The film I just referred to, in which I learned afterwards the director, Dassin, plays the role of the American, presents us with a nice and curious model of something that can be expressed as follows from a structural point of view. The character who plays the satirical role, the role that is offered for our derision, namely, Dassin as the American, finds himself to be as the producer and creator of the film in a position that is more American than those whom he makes fun of, that is, the Americans.

Don't misunderstand me. He is there in order to undertake the reeducation of a good-hearted whore. And the irony of the screenwriter is to be found in the fact that in carrying out this pious mission he is in the pay of the one whom we might call the Grand Master of the brothel. The deeper meaning is signaled to us by the placing before our eyes of an enormous pair of black glasses – he is someone whose face is for good reason never shown. Naturally, when the whore learns that it is the character who is her sworn enemy who is paying the piper, she eviscerates the beautiful soul of the American in question, and he who has conceived such great hopes is made to look very foolish.

If there is a dimension of social criticism in this symbolism – that it to say that what one finds hidden behind the brothel are the forces of order, so to speak – it is somewhat naive to make us hope at the end of the screenplay that all that is needed to solve the problem of the relations between virtue and desire is to close down the brothel. There runs constantly throughout the film that old *fin de siècle* ambiguity, which involves identifying classical antiquity with the sphere of liberated desire. It is not to have gone beyond Pierre Louÿs to believe that it is somewhere outside her own situation that the good Athenian prostitute can focus all the light of the mirages she is at the center of. In a word, Dassin didn't have to confuse what flows from the sight of this attractive figure with a return to Aristotelian morality, which he fortunately doesn't spell out in detail.

Let's get back on track. This shows us that on the far edge of guilt, insofar as it occupies the field of desire, there are the bonds of a permanent bookkeeping, and this is so independently of any particular articulation that may be given of it.

Part of the world has resolutely turned in the direction of the service of goods, thereby rejecting everything that has to do with the relationship of man to desire – it is what is known as the postrevolutionary perspective. The only thing to be said is that people don't seem to have realized that, by formulating things in this way, one is simply perpetuating the eternal tradition of power, namely, "Let's keep on working, and as far as desire is concerned, come back later." But what does it matter? In this tradition the communist future is only different from Creon's, from that of the city, in assuming – and it's not negligible – that the sphere of goods to which we must all devote ourselves may at some point embrace the whole universe.

In other words, this operation is only justified insofar as the universal State is on the horizon. Yet nothing indicates that even at that limit the problem will disappear, since it will persist in the consciousness of those who live with that view of things. Either they imply that the properly statest values of the State will disappear, that is organization and policing, or they introduce a term such as the universal concrete State, which means no more than supposing things will change on a molecular level, at the level of the relationship that constitutes the position of man in the face of various goods, to the extent that up till now his desire was not there.

Whatever happens to that point of view, nothing is structurally changed. The sign of this is, first, that, although the divine presence of an orthodox kind is absent, the keeping of accounts certainly is not and, second, that for the inexhaustible dimension that necessitates the immortality of the soul for Kant, there is substituted the notion of objective guilt, which is precisely articulated as such. From a structural point of view in any case, nothing is resolved.

I think I have now sufficiently outlined the opposition between the desiring center and the service of goods. We can now come to the heart of the matter.

3

It is in an experimental form that I advance the following propositions here. Let's formulate them as paradoxes. Let's see what they sound like to analysts' ears.

I propose then that, from an analytical point of view, the only thing of which one can be guilty is of having given ground relative to one's desire.

Whether it is admissible or not in a given ethics, that proposition expresses quite well something that we observe in our experience. In the last analysis, what a subject really feels guilty about when he manifests guilt at bottom always has to do with – whether or not it is admissible for a director of conscience – the extent to which he has given ground relative to his desire.

Let's take this further. He has often given ground relative to his desire for a good motive or even for the best of motives. And this shouldn't astonish us. For guilt has existed for a very long time, and it was noticed long ago that the question of a good motive, of a good intention, although it constitutes certain zones of historical experience and was at the forefront of discussions of moral theology in, say, the time of Abelard, hasn't enlightened people very much. The question that keeps reappearing in the distance is always the same. And that is why Christians in their most routine observances are never at peace. For if one has to do things for the good, in practice one is always faced with the question: for the good of whom? From that point on, things are no longer obvious.

Doing things in the name of the good, and even more in the name of the good of the other, is something that is far from protecting us not only from guilt but also from all kinds of inner catastrophes. To be precise, it doesn't protect us from neurosis and its consequences. If analysis has a meaning, desire is nothing other than that which supports an unconscious theme, the very articulation of that which roots us in a particular destiny, and that destiny demands insistently that the debt be paid, and desire keeps coming back, keeps returning, and situates us once again in a given track, the track of something that is specifically our business.

Last time I opposed the hero to the ordinary man, and someone was upset by that. I do not distinguish between them as if they were two different human species. In each of us the path of the hero is traced, and it is precisely as an ordinary man that one follows it to the end.

The fields that I sketched out last time – the inner circle to which I gave the name being-for-death, in the midst of desires, renouncing entry into the external circle – are not in opposition to the triple field of hatred, guilt and fear as the ordinary man is in opposition to the hero. That's not the point at all. That general form is definitely traced by the structure in and for the ordinary man. And it is precisely to the extent that the hero guides himself correctly there that he experiences all the passions in which the ordinary man is entangled, except that in his case they are pure and he succeeds in supporting himself there fully.

Someone among you has baptized the topology that I have sketched out for you this year with the apt and somewhat humorous phrase, the zone between-two-deaths. Your vacation will give you the time to consider whether its rigor seems to you to be especially effective. I ask you to think it over.

In Sophocles you will encounter again the dance between Creon and Antigone. It is obvious that to the extent that his presence in the zone indicates that something is defined and liberated, the hero bears his partner into that zone along with him. At the end of *Antigone* Creon henceforth speaks loudly and clearly of himself as someone who is dead among the living, and this is because he has literally lost all other goods as a result of the affair. As a consequence of the tragic act, the hero frees his adversary too.

There is no reason to limit the exploration of this field simply to Antigone. Take the example of *Philoctetes*, where you will learn other aspects of the question, that is to say, that a hero doesn't have to be heroic to be a hero. Philoctetes isn't much of a man. He went off all excited and full of enthusiasm to die for his country on the shores of Troy, and he wasn't even wanted for that. He was dumped on an island because he smelled so bad. He spent ten years there consumed with hatred. The first fellow who comes looking for him, a nice young man called Neoptelemes, cons him like a baby, and in the end he nevertheless goes off to the shores of Troy because Hercules appears as a *deux ex machina* to offer a solution to all his sufferings. This *deus ex machina* isn't nothing, but everybody has known for a long time that he simply serves as a frame and limit to tragedy, that we don't have to take any more account of it than we do of the supports that define the area of the stage.

What makes Philoctetes a hero? Nothing more than the fact that he remains fiercely committed to his hate right to the end, when the *deus ex machina* appears like the curtain falling. This reveals to us not only that he has been betrayed and he is aware that he has been betrayed, but also that he has been betrayed with impunity. This is emphasized in the play by the fact that Neoptelemes, who is full of remorse because he betrayed the hero and thereby demonstrates his noble soul, comes to make proper amends and gives him back the bow that plays such an essential role in the tragic space of the play

– because it operates there like a subject that is spoken about and addressed. It is the space of the hero and for good reason.

What I call "giving ground relative to one's desire" is always accompanied in the destiny of the subject by some betrayal – you will observe it in every case and should note its importance. Either the subject betrays his own way, betrays himself, and the result is significant for him, or, more simply, he tolerates the fact that someone with whom he has more or less vowed to do something betrays his hope and doesn't do for him what their pact entailed – whatever that pact may be, fated or ill-fated, risky, shortsighted, or indeed a matter of rebellion or flight, it doesn't matter.

Something is played out in betrayal if one tolerates it, if driven by the idea of the good – and by that I mean the good of the one who has just committed the act of betrayal – one gives ground to the point of giving up one's own claims and says to oneself, "Well, if that's how things are, we should abandon our position; neither of us is worth that much, and especially me, so we should just return to the common path." You can be sure that what you find there is the structure of giving ground relative to one's desire.

Once one has crossed that boundary where I combined in a single term contempt for the other and for oneself, there is no way back. It might be possible to do some repair work, but not to undo it. Isn't that a fact of experience that demonstrates how psychoanalysis is capable of supplying a useful compass in the field of ethical guidance?

I have, therefore, articulated three propositions.

First, the only thing one can be guilty of is giving ground relative to one's desire.

Second, the definition of a hero: someone who may be betrayed with impunity.

Third, this is something that not everyone can achieve; it constitutes the difference between an ordinary man and a hero, and it is, therefore, more mysterious than one might think. For the ordinary man the betrayal that almost always occurs sends him back to the service of goods, but with the proviso that he will never again find that factor which restores a sense of direction to that service.

We come finally to the field of the service of goods; it exists, of course, and there is no question of denying that. But turning things around, I propose the following, and this is my fourth proposition: There is no other good than that which may serve to pay the price for access to desire – given that desire is understood here, as we have defined it elsewhere, as the metonymy of our being. The channel in which desire is located is not simply that of the modulation of the signifying chain, but that which flows beneath it as well; that is, properly speaking, what we are as well as what we are not, our being and our non-being – that which is signified in an act passes from one signifier of the chain to another beneath all the significations.

I explained this last time with the metonymy of "eating the book" that no doubt just came to me, but if you examine it a little more closely, you will see that it is the most extreme of metonymies – something that shouldn't surprise us on the part of Saint John, the man who placed the Word at the beginning. It really is a writer's idea, and he was an incomparable one. But eating the book is, after all, something that confronts what Freud imprudently told us is not susceptible to substitution and displacement, namely, hunger, with something that isn't really made to be eaten, a book. In eating the book we come into contact with what Freud means when he speaks of sublimation as a change of aim and not of object. That's not immediately clear.

The hunger in question, sublimated hunger, falls in the space between the two, because it isn't the book that fills our stomach. When I ate the book, I didn't thereby become book any more than the book became flesh. The book became *me* so to speak. But in order for this operation to take place – and it takes place everyday – I definitely have to pay a price. Freud weighs this difference in a corner of *Civilization and Its Discontents*. Sublimate as much as you like; you have to pay for it with something. And this something is called *jouissance*. I have to pay for that mystical operation with a pound of flesh.

That's the object, the good, that one pays for the satisfaction of one's desire. And that's the point I wanted to lead you up to, so as to shed a little light on something that is essential and that isn't seen enough.

It is, in effect, there that the religious operation lies, something that is always interesting for us to consider. That good which is sacrificed for desire – and you will note that that means the same thing as that desire which is lost for the good – that pound of flesh is precisely the thing that religion undertakes to recuperate. That's the single trait which is common to all religions; it is coextensive with all religion, with the whole meaning of religion.

I can't develop this further, but I will give you two applications that are as expressive as they are brief. In a religious service the flesh that is offered to God on the altar, the animal sacrifice or whatever, is consumed by the people of the religious community and usually simply by the priest; they are the ones who stuff themselves with it. The form is an exemplary one; but it is just as true of the saint, whose goal is, in effect, access to sublime desire and not at all his own desire, for the saint lives and pays for others. The essential element in saintliness resides in the fact that the saint consumes the price paid in the form of suffering at two extreme points: the classic point of the worst ironies relative to religious mystification, such as the priests' little feast behind the altar, and the point of the last frontier of religious heroism as well. There, too, we find the same phenomenon of recuperation.

It is in this respect that great religious work is distinguished from what goes on in an ethical form of catharsis, which may bring together things as apparently foreign to each other as psychoanalysis and the tragic spectacles of the Greeks. If we found our measure there, it is not without reason. Catharsis has the sense of purification of desire. Purification cannot be accomplished, as is clear if one simply reads Aristotle's sentence, unless one has at least established the crossing of its limits that we call fear and pity.

It is because the tragic *epos* doesn't leave the spectator in ignorance as to where the pole of desire is and shows that the access to desire necessitates crossing not only all fear but all pity, because the voice of the hero trembles before nothing, and especially not before the good of the other, because all this is experienced in the temporal unfolding of the story, that the subject learns a little more about the deepest level of himself than he knew before.

For anyone who goes to the *Théâtre-Français* or the Theater of Athens, it will last as long as it lasts. But if, in the end, Aristotle's formulations mean anything, it is that. One knows what it costs to go forward in a given direction, and if one doesn't go that way, one knows why. One can even sense that if, in one's accounts with one's desire, one isn't exactly in the clear, it is because one couldn't do any better, for that's not a path one can take without paying a price.

The spectator has his eyes opened to the fact that even for him who goes to the end of his desire, all is not a bed of roses. But he also has his eyes opened – and this is essential – to the value of prudence which stands in opposition to that, to the wholly relative value of beneficial reasons, attachments or pathological interests, as Mr. Kant says, that might keep him on that risky path.

I have given you there an almost prosaic interpretation of tragedy and its effects, and however vital its peaks may be, I am not happy to have reduced it to a level that might lead you to believe that what I take to be essential in catharsis is pacificatory. It may not be pacificatory for everybody. But it was the most direct way of reconciling what some have taken to be the moralizing face of tragedy with the fact that the lesson of tragedy in its essence is not at all moral in the ordinary sense of the word.

Of course, not every catharsis can be reduced to something as external as a topological demonstration. When it is a matter of the practices of those whom the Greeks called $\mu\alpha\iota\nu\acute{o}\mu\epsilon\nu\text{o}\iota$, those who go crazy through a trance, through religious experience, through passion or through anything else, the value of the catharsis presupposes that, in a way that is either more-or-less directed or wild, the subject enters into the zone described here, and that his return involves some gain that will be called possession or whatever – Plato doesn't hesitate to point this out in the cathartic procedures. There is a whole range there, a spectrum of possibilities, that it would take a whole year to catalogue.

The important thing is to know where all that is to be located in the field whose limits I have outlined for you this year.

4

And now a word in conclusion.

The field that is ours by reason of the fact that we are exploring it is going to be in one way or another the object of a science. And, you are going to ask me, will this science of desire belong to the field of the human sciences?

Before leaving you this year, I would like to make my position on the subject very clear. I do not think, given the way that field is being laid out, and I assure you it is being done carefully, that it will amount to anything else but a systematic and fundamental misunderstanding of everything that has to do with the whole affair that I have been discussing here. The fields of inquiry that are being outlined as necessarily belonging to the human sciences have in my eyes no other function than to form a branch of the service of goods, which is no doubt advantageous though of limited value. Those fields are in other words a branch of the service of those powers that are more than a little precarious. In any case, implied here is a no less systematic misunderstanding of all the violent phenomena that reveal that the path of the triumph of goods in our world is not likely to be a smooth one.

In other words, in the phrase of one of the exceptional politicians who has functioned as a leader of France, Mazarin, politics is politics, but love always remains love.

As for the kind of science that might be situated in that place I have designated the place of desire, what can it be? Well, you don't have to look very far. As far as science is concerned, the kind that is presently occupying the place of desire is quite simply what we commonly call science, the kind that you see cantering gaily along and accomplishing all kinds of so-called physical conquests.

I think that throughout this historical period the desire of man, which has been felt, anesthetized, put to sleep by moralists, domesticated by educators, betrayed by the academies, has quite simply taken refuge or been repressed in that most subtle and blindest of passions, as the story of Oedipus shows, the passion for knowledge. That's the passion that is currently going great guns and is far from having said its last word.

One of the most amusing features of the history of science is to be found in the propaganda scientists and alchemists have addressed to the powers that be at a time when they were beginning to run out of steam. It went as follows: "Give us money; you don't realize that if you gave us a little money, we would be able to put all kinds of machines, gadgets and contraptions at your service." How could the powers let themselves be taken in? The answer to the question is to be found in a certain breakdown of wisdom. It's a fact that they did let themselves be taken in, that science got its money, as a consequence of which we are left with this vengeance. It's a fascinating thing, but as far as those who are at the forefront of science are concerned, they are not without a keen consciousness of the fact that they have their backs against a wall of hate. They are themselves capsized by the turbulent swell of a heavy sense of guilt. But that isn't very important because it's not in truth an adventure that Mr. Oppenheimer's remorse can put an end to overnight. It is moreover there where the problem of desire will lie in the future.

The universal order has to deal with the problem of what it should do with that science in which something is going on whose nature escapes it. Science, which occupies the place of desire, can only be a science of desire in the form of an enormous question mark; and this is doubtless not without a structural cause. In other words, science is animated by some mysterious desire, but it doesn't know, any more than anything in the unconscious itself, what that desire means. The future will reveal it to us, and perhaps among those who by the grace of God have most recently eaten the book – I mean those who have written with their labors, indeed with their blood, the book of Western science. It, too, is an edible book.

I spoke about Mencius earlier. After having made the statements that you would be wrong to consider optimistic about the goodness of man, he explains very well that what we are most ignorant about is the laws that come to us from heaven, the same laws as Antigone's. His proof is absolutely rigorous, but it is too late for me to repeat it here. The laws of heaven in question are the laws of desire.

Of him who ate the book and the mystery within it, one can, in effect, ask the question: "Is he good, is he bad?" That question now seems unimportant. The important thing is not knowing whether man is good or bad in the beginning; the important thing is what will transpire once the book has been eaten.

July 6, 1960

ACKNOWLEDGMENTS

When Jacques Lacan died on September 9, 1981, in Paris, he had planned that the publication of a complete edition of his *Seminar* would continue according to the principles outlined in the notice and postscript of the first volume that appeared, *The Four Fundamental Concepts* (Paris: Le Seuil, 1973; New York: Norton, 1981), principles I referred to in a pamphlet, *Entretien sur le Séminaire avec François Ansermet* (Paris: Navarin, 1985).

This edition of Book VII has benefitted from the work of Mrs. Judith Miller on the Greek references, especially the Sophoclean references. Mr. Franz Kaltenbeck verified the German quotations, notably the Freudian ones. Professors Quackelbeen of the University of Ghent and Rey-Flaud of the University of Montpellier obtainaed for me T. H. Van de Velde's *Ideal Marriage* and the text of Arnaud Daniel, respectively. Mr. François Wahl of the Editions de Seuil reread the manuscript. Doctor Danièle Silvestre, Doctor Patrick Valas, Ms. Elisabeth Doisneau and Ms. Annie Staricky helped with the correction of the proofs. I thank them all as I thank in advance any reader who would like to collaborate in the revision of a text that is the object of continuing work. Comments should be forwarded c/o my publisher.

J.-A. Miller

BIBLIOGRAPHY

The following are works referred to in the body of the Seminar in English language editions where they exist.

Anouilh, Jean (1946). *Antigone*. Paris: La Table Ronde.
Aristotle (1968). *The Nicomachean Ethics* (Bilingual with an English trans. by H. Rackham). Cambridge: Harvard University Press, Loeb Classical Library.
Bataille, Georges (1986). *Erotism: Death and Sensuality* (Mary Dalwood, Trans.). San Francisco, CA: City Lights.
Bentham, Jeremy (1932). *The Theory of Fictions*. London: K. Paul, Trench, Tribner.
Bergler, Jacques (1960). *Le matin des magiciens*. Paris: Gallimard.
Bernfeld, Siegfried (1921). *Bemerkungen über Sublimierung* [Observations on Sublimation]. *Imago*, VIII.
Blanchot, Maurice (1963). *Lautréamont et Sade*. Paris: Minuit.
Breton, André (1937). *L'Amour fou*. Paris: Gallimard.
—— (1932). *Les Vases Communicants*. Paris: Cahiers Libres.
Breuer, Joseph, & Freud, Sigmund (1893–95). Studies on Hysteria. In J. Strachey (Ed. and Trans.), *The Standard Edition of the Complete Psychological Works of Sigmund Freud* (Vol. 2). New York: Norton.
Capellanus, Andreas (1990). *Art of Courtly Love* (J.J. Parry, Trans.). New York: Columbia University Press.
Claudel, Paul (1935). *Introduction à la peinture hollandaise*. Paris: Gallimard.
Colette (1987). *Enfant et les Sortilèges*. Videorecording with music by Maurice Ravel. National Video Corporation: Mass.
Corbin, Henry (1969). *The Creative Imagination in the Sufism of Ibn Arabi* (R. Manheim, Trans.). Princeton, NJ: Princeton University Press.
Daniel, Arnaut (1981). *The Poetry of Arnaut Daniel* (James J. Wilhelm, Trans.). New York: Garland Publishing.
Deutsch, Helen (1944–1945). *The Psychology of Women: A Psychoanalytic Interpretation*. New York: Grune and Stratton.
—— (1965) *Neuroses and Character Types: Clinical Psychoanalytical Studies* (John D. Sutherland and M. Masud R. Kahn, Eds.). London: Hogarth Press.
Diderot, Denis (1956). *Rameau's Nephew and Other Works* (J. Barzun & R. Bowen, Trans.). Garden City, NY: Doubleday.

—— (1964). *Supplement au Voyage de Bougainville*. In *Oeuvres Philosophiques* (Paul Vernière, Ed.). Paris: Garnier.

Ellis, Havelock (1936). *Studies in the Psychology of Sex*. New York: Random House.

Eluard, Paul (1968). Capitale de la Douleur. In *Oeuvres Complètes* I. Paris: Gallimard, Bibliothèque de la Pléiade.

Engels, Friedrich, & Marx, Karl (1959). *Basic Writings on Politics and Philosophy*. Garden City, NY: Doubleday.

Erasmus, Desiderius, & Luther, Martin (1961). *Discourse on Free Will* (E.F. Winter, Trans.). New York: Unger.

Febvre, Lucien (1982). *The Problem of Unbelief in the Sixteenth Century* (B. Gottlieb, Trans.). Cambridge, MA: Harvard University Press.

Fourier, Charles (1901). *Selections from the Works of Fourier*. London: Sommenschein.

Freud, Sigmund (1900–1901). The Interpretation of Dreams. In J. Strachey (Ed. and Trans.), *The Standard Edition of the Complete Psychological Works of Sigmund Freud* (Vols. 4 & 5). New York: Norton.

—— (1905). Three Essays on the Theory of Sexuality. In *The Standard Edition* (Vol. 7, pp. 125–245). New York: Norton.

—— (1910[1909]). Five Lectures on Psycho-Analysis. In *The Standard Edition* (Vol. 11, pp. 1–56). New York: Norton.

—— (1913[1912–13]). Totem and Taboo. In *The Standard Edition* (Vol. 13, pp. 1–162). New York: Norton.

—— (1914). On Narcissism: An Introduction. In *The Standard Edition* (Vol. 14, pp. 67–107). New York: Norton.

—— (1915–1917). Introductory Lectures on Psycho-Analysis. In *The Standard Edition* (Vols. 15 & 16). New York: Norton.

—— (1917[1918]). Mourning and Melancholia. In *The Standard Edition* (Vol. 14, pp. 238–260). New York: Norton.

—— (1919). Introduction to *Psycho-Analysis and the War Neuroses*. In *The Standard Edition* (Vol. 17, pp. 205–215). New York: Norton.

—— (1920). Beyond the Pleasure Principle. In *The Standard Edition* (Vol. 18, pp. 1–64). New York: Norton.

—— (1930[1929]). Civilization and Its Discontents. In *The Standard Edition* (Vol. 21, pp. 57–145). New York: Norton.

—— (1937). Analysis Terminable and Interminable. In *The Standard Edition* (Vol. 23, pp. 209–253). New York: Norton.

—— (1939[1934–38]). Moses and Monotheism. In *The Standard Edition* (Vol. 23, pp. 1–137). New York: Norton.

—— (1950[1895]). Project for a New Scientific Psychology. In *The Standard Edition* (Vol. 1, pp. 281–397). New York: Norton.

Freud, Sigmund, & Fliess, Wilhelm (1985). *The Complete Letters of Sigmund Freud and Wilhelm Fliess, 1887–1904* (Jeffrey Mousaieff Masson, Trans. and Ed.). Cambridge: Harvard University Press.

Fromm, Erich (1959). *Sigmund Freud's Mission*. New York: Harper & Bros.

Glover, Edward (1931). Sublimation, Substitution and Social Anxiety. *The International Journal of Psychoanalysis*.

Hegel (1967). *The Phenomenology of Mind* (J. B. Baillie, Trans.). London: Allen & Unwin.

Heidegger, Martin (1969). *Identity and Difference* (J. Stambaugh, Trans.). New York: Harper & Row.
—— (1968). *What Is a Thing?* (W.B. Barton & V. Deutsch, Trans.). Chicago: Henry Regnery & Co.
Jones, Ernest (1948). Hatred, Culpability and Fear. In *Papers on Psychoanalysis* (5th ed.). London: Bailliere, Tindall & Cox.
Kant, Immanuel (1987). *The Critique of Judgment* (W. S. Pluhar, Trans.). Indianapolis, IN: Hackett.
—— (1956). *The Critique of Practical Reason* (L.W. Beck, Trans.). New York: Liberal Arts Press.
—— (1966). *The Critique of Pure Reason* (F.M. Muller, Trans.). Garden City, NY: Doubleday.
Klein, Melanie (1948). *Contributions to Psychoanalysis: 1921–1945*. London: Hogarth Press.
—— (1975). *The Writings of Melanie Klein* (Roger Money-Kyrle, Ed.). London: Hogarth Press & the Institute of Psychoanalysis.
Krafft-Ebing, R. (1991). *Psychopathia Sexualis: Or the Antipathic Sexual Instinct*. American Institute of Psychiatry.
Lacan, Jacques (1955 / 56). The Freudian Thing. In Jacques Lacan (1977), *Ecrits: A Selection* (A. Sheridan, Trans.) (pp. 114–145). New York: Norton.
—— (1958). The direction of the treatment and the principles of its power. In *Ecrits: A Selection* (pp. 226–80). New York: Norton.
Lambin, Denys (1820). *Aristotelis Ethicorum Nicomacheorum*. Heidelberg.
Lautréamont, Comte de (1987). *Maldoror* (A. Lyliard, Trans.). New York: Schocken.
Lévi-Srauss, Claude (1967). *Structural Anthropology* (Claire Jacobson & Brooke Grundfest Schoepf, Trans.). New York: Basic Books.
—— (1969). *The Elementary Structures of Kinship* (H. Bell, J.R. von Sturmer & R. Needham, Trans.). London: Eyre and Spottiswoode.
Luther, Martin (1983). *Sermons* (J. N. Lenker, Ed.). Grand Rapids, MI: Baker Books.
—— (1952). *Table Talk*. New York: World Pub. Co.
Mandeville, Bernard de (1989). *The Fables of the Bees*. New York: Viking Penguin.
Marx, Karl (1964). Contribution to the Critique of Hegel and The Jewish Question. In *Early Writings* (T.B. Bottomore, Trans.). New York: McGraw-Hill.
Miller, Henry (1965). *Nexus*. New York: Grove.
—— (1963). *Plexus*. London: Weidenfeld & Nicholson.
—— (1950). *Sexus*. Paris: The Obelisk Press.
Mirabeau, Gabriel-Honoré de Riqueti, comte de (1984). *L'Oeuvre Libertine du Comte de Mirabeau*. Sainte-Maxime: D'Aujourd'hui.
Navarre, Marguerite de (1984). *The Heptameron* (P.A. Chilton. Trans.). Harmondsworth, England: Penguin.
Nelli, René (1929). *Oeuvre romanesque complète*. Paris: A. Michel.
—— (1953). *Spiritualité de l'Hérésie: Le Catharisme*. AMS.
Pascal, Blaise (1963). *Oeuvres Complètes*. Paris: Seuil.
Piéron, Henry (1952). *The Sensations: Their Functions, Processes, and Mechanisms*. London: F. Miller.
Rauh, Fritz (1969). *Das Sittliche Leen des Menschen im Licht des gleichenden Verhaltensforschung*. Kevelaer, Rheinland: Butzen und Bercker.

Réage, Pauline (1972). *Histoire d'Eau.* Paris: Jean-Jacques Pauvert.
Régis, E., & Hesnard, A. (1914). *La Psychoanalyse des Nevroses et des Psychoses.* Paris.
Reinhardt, Karl (1979). *Sophocles.* Oxford: Blackwell.
Rohde, Erwin (1972). *Psyche: The Cult of Souls and Belief in Immortality Among the Ancient Greeks.* Freeport, NY: Books for Libraries.
Rougement, Denis de (1956). *Love and the Western World.* New York: Pantheon.
Sacher-Masoch, Leopold von (1989). *Venus in Furs.* New York: Blast Books.
Sade, Marquis de (1965). *Philosophy in the Boudoir and Other Writings.* New York: Grove.
—— (1968). *The Story of Juliette.* New York: Grove.
—— (1970). *Idées sur le Roman.* Bordeaux: Ducros.
Saint Augustine (1961). *Confessions* (R.S. Pine-Coffin, Trans.). New York: Viking Penguin.
Saint Paul (1967). Epistle to the Romans. In the *Holy Bible.* New York: Oxford University Press.
Sartre, Jean Paul (1976). *Critique of Dialectical Reason.* London: Humanities Press.
Sharpe, Ella (1950). *Collected Papers on Psycho-Analysis.* London: Hogarth Press.
Sophocles (1956–1961). Antigone. In *Sophocles* (Bilingual with an English trans. by F. Storr). Cambridge: Harvard University Press, Loeb Classical Library.
Sperber, Hans (1914). Ueber den Einfluss Sexueller Momente auf Entstehung und Entwicklung de Sprache [On the Influence of Sexual Factors on the Origin and Development of Language]. *Imago, I.*
Stendhal (1947). *On Love.* New York: Liveright.
Sterba, Richard (1930). Problematik der Sublimierungslehre. *Internationale Zeitschrift für Psychoanalyse, XVI.*
Terence (1967). The Self-Tormenter. In *The Comedies of Terence* (Frank O. Copley, Trans.). Indianapolis: Bobbs-Merrill.
Vailland, Roger (1960). *La Fête.* Paris: Gallimard.
Valéry, Paul (1956). Monsieur Teste. In J. Mathews (Ed.), *The Collected Works of Paul Valéry* (vol. 6). New York: Pantheon.

INDEX

Abfuhr, 49
abreaction, 244
adultery, 78
Aeschylus, 271, 273
affects, psychology of, 102–3
aggressions, primal and inverted, 106, 115
agricultural work, as symbolic copulation, 164
Ajax (Sophocles), 271
Akhenaton, 173, 180
Allacoque, Marie, 188
Allais, Alphonse, 13–14
allgemeine, 76–77
altruism, 187, 195
Ambassadors, The (Holbein), 135, 140
amor intellectualis Dei, 180
Amour fou, L' (Breton), 154
Analysis Studies, 159
"Analysis Terminable and Interminable" (Freud), 299
anamorphosis:
  in *Antigone,* 272–73, 282
  in architecture, 135, 140
  in art, 135–36, 140–41, 272–73
  courtly love as, 139–54
Andersen, see Other
anger, 103
animal realm:
  anger and, 103
  symbols and, 45
animal totem, 177
Anthology of Sublime Love, The (Perret), 148
Antigone (Sophocles), 240, 241–87, 306, 320, 325
  anamorphosis in, 272–73, 282
  Antigone as hero of, 258, 262–66, 270, 276–83
  Antigone's beauty in, 247–48
  Antigone's entombment and hanging in, 248, 268–69, 280, 286, 299
  Antigone's self-justification in, 254–56
  Atè in, 262–64, 267, 270, 277, 281, 283, 286, 300
  desire in, 247
  importance of, 243, 257, 273, 284
  translations of, 254, 270

anti-morality, 78
antiquity, love in, 98–99
anxiety, 103
Apocalypse, 294
aporia, 274–75
appetitive process, 33
architecture, 175
  anamorphosis in, 135, 140
  emptiness and, 135–36
Aristophanes, 297
Aristotle, 60, 121, 124, 216, 221, 252, 255, 273, 277, 292, 314–15, 318, 323
  on catharsis, 244, 245, 246, 257–58, 287
  ethics and, 5, 10–11, 12, 13, 22–23, 27, 29, 36, 186
Ars Amandi (Ovid), 153
art:
  anamorphosis in, 135–36, 140–41, 272–73
  in caves, 139–40
  Ding and, 131, 141
  emptiness and, 130, 136, 140
  history and, 141–42
  imitation vs. non-imitation in, 141
  real and, 141
  rewards and, 144–45
  see also creativity, sublimation and
ascetic experience, 7
Atè, 262–64, 267, 270, 277, 281, 283, 286, 300
atherapy, 107
atomism, 32–33, 102
Aufbau, 40, 51
Aufhebung, 193
Augustine, Saint, 97, 220, 233–34
authenticity, as psychoanalytic ideal, 9–10
avoidance, 63–64

Bahnungen (facilitation), 31, 222
  of language, 45
  of memory, 58
  of pleasure principle, 36, 39, 41, 63, 137
Bataille, Georges, 201

331

beautiful, beauty, 257, 261, 269, 286–87, 295, 296, 297, 301
  desire and, 237–39, 248–49
  function of, 298
  good vs., 217
Befriedigungserlebnis, 39, 53, 93
Begriff, 259
behaviorism, 47
being, Being vs., 214, 248
belief (faith), 54, 62–63, 130–31, 170–71
"Bemerkungen über Sublimierung" ("Observations on Sublimation") (Bernfeld), 144, 155, 159
Bentham, Jeremy, 12, 187, 228
Bernays, Jakob, 246–47
Bernays, Michael, 246
Bernfeld, Siegfried, 111, 144, 145, 203–4, 211, 212
  critique of, 155–60
Besetzung, 49–50, 137
bestiality, 5
Bewegung, 48
Bewusstsein, see conscious
beyond-of-the-signified, 54
Beyond the Pleasure Principle (Freud), 21, 185, 213, 222
Bible, 68, 122
  see also ten commandments; *specific books*
Blanchot, Maurice, 200–201
blindness, truth and, 310
Boehme, Jakob, 215
Bornibus, 120–21
Breton, André, 154
Breuer, Joseph, 244
Brücke, Ernst Wilhelm von, 29
Buddhism, 175, 176
burning bush, as *Ding*, 174, 180

calumny, 78
Camus, Albert, 201*n*
"ça parle, Le," 206*n*
Capellanus, Andreas, 146
castration, 299, 307, 308
Cathars, 123–24, 153, 215, 245
catharsis, 244–46, 257–58, 287, 310, 312, 315
Cathar Writings (Book of Two Principles) (Nelli, ed.), 124
Catholic church, 123–24
causality, 72
causa noumenon, 73
causa pathomenon, 97
cave art, 139–40
censor, 3
"Certain Aspects of Sublimation and Delirium" (Sharpe), 107
César (Pagnol), 69*n*
character, ethics and, 10
child in man, 24, 25
Chinese language, 167
Chrétien de Troyes, 151, 153
Christ, 96, 97, 174
Christianity:
  atheistic message in, 178
  crucifixion image in, 262
  and death of God, 193
  doing good and, 319
Civilization and Its Discontents (Freud), 6–7, 13, 27, 34, 37, 89, 90, 96, 98, 143, 179, 184–86, 199, 207, 302, 322
Claudel, Paul, 298
Clement of Alexandria, Saint, 299
clothes, symbolism of, 226–28
Cohen, Gustave, 112
Colette, 115
collecting, psychology of, 113–14, 117
Combat, 155
comedy, function of, 90, 313–14
Communicating Vases, 91
complicationes, 40
component drive, 5, 194–95
Concerning the Heptameron (Febvre), 131
Confessions (Augustine), 220
conscience, consciousness vs., 122*n*
conscious, 44
  endopsychic perception and, 49
  perception and, 49–51, 61, 74
  preconscious and unconscious and, 37, 61–62
  reality principle and, 48
consciousness, 122*n*, 213–14, 223–24
consolamentum, 215
contiguity and continuity, 33
Contributions to Psychoanalysis (Klein), 115
"Contribution to the Critique of Hegel's Philosophy of Law, The" (Marx), 208
Corbin, Henry, 148, 149
counteraggression, 115
countertransference, 291
courtly love *(Minne)*, 99, 109, 235
  as anamorphosis, 139–54
  Eastern religions and, 149, 153
  heresy and, 125
  Lady and, 126, 146, 148, 149, 150–51, 162–63
  Liebe vs., 125
  poetry and poets of, 145–52, 161–63, 214–15
  as sublimation, 128, 131, 136, 142, 160, 161–63, 215
  unconscious traces of, 112, 131–32
covetousness, 82–83
creation:
  ex nihilo, 121–22, 212–14, 225, 260–61, 262
  of signifiers, 119
creationism, 124, 126, 212, 261
Creative Imagination, The (Corbin), 148
creativity, sublimation and, 106–7, 115–17, 238
crime, as transgression, 260
Critique of Dialectical Reason (Sartre), 226
Critique of Judgment, The (Kant), 249, 261, 287
Critique of Practical Reason, The (Kant), 72, 76, 78, 80, 97
Critique of Pure Reason, The (Kant), 77, 78, 108
crucifixion image, 262
culture:
  nature vs., 67–68, 77–78, 274
  sublimation and, 107
  see also society
Cyril, Saint, 68

Index

Da, Fort vs., 65, 169
danger, etymology of, 84
Daniel, Arnaud, 161–63, 215
Dante Alighieri, 149, 163
Dassin, Jules, 317–18
David, King of Israel, 81
De Arte Amandi (Capellanus), 146
death drive, 2, 6, 236, 239, 295
   in *Antigone*, 281, 282, 286
   Bernfeld on, 203–4
   nature of, 211–13
defense systems:
   organic, 73
   sublimation and, 95
De Libero Arbitrio (Erasmus), 97
"Denegration" ("Die Verneinung") (Freud), 37, 46, 52, 58
De Officiis (Cicero), 160
dependence, prophylaxis of, 10
Descartes, René, 103, 206
desire, 134, 216, 237, 300
   action and, 310–25
   of analyst, 300–301
   in *Antigone*, 247, 248–49
   beauty and, 237–39, 248–49
   compromise and, 105
   definition of, 321
   desire of, 14
   function of, 209, 246, 257, 265
   genitalization of, 8
   guilt, 319, 321
   law and, 82–84
   Law and, 170
   man's relationship to, 306, 310, 318
   morality and, 3, 5
   naturalist liberation of, 3–4
   natural vs. perverse, 232
   need vs., 207, 225
   normalization of, 181
   object and, 113
   of Oedipus, 309
   pain and, 80
   pleasure of, 152
   power and, 315
   repression of, 6
   science of, 324
   and transgression of pleasure principle's limits, 109–10
destrudo, 194
Deuteronomy, 80–81
Deutsch, Helene, 9
Diabolus, 92
diachrony, synchrony vs., 285
Diderot, Denis, 4, 177
Ding, 43–70, 253
   burning bush as, 174, 180
   centrality of, 97, 105
   distance between subject and, 69, 73, 105
   drives and, 111
   as emptiness, 129–30
   ethics and, 103, 104, 105
   evil and, 124

   as extimacy, 139
   as *Fremde*, 52
   genital act and, 300
   inaccessibility of, 159, 203
   incest and, 68, 70
   Law and, 83–84, 186
   mythic body of the mother and, 106
   Nebenmensch and, 51
   object and, 101–14, 126
   as Other of subject, 52, 71
   reality principle and, 45, 66
   repetition demanded by, 75
   Sache vs., 43–45, 62–63
   sublimation and, 95, 99, 115, 117, 126, 129, 131, 134, 158
   vacuole and, 150
   veiled nature of, 118
   Vorstellung and, 57–62, 63
Dionysionism, 198
discharge, 53, 244
doctor-love, 8
Dolce Vita, La, 253
Domnei, 149, 150
don de merci, le, 152
Don Quixote (Cervantes), 153
dreams, 62, 133
drives, 87–100, 144
   aim of, 110, 111
   component, 5, 194–95
   Ding and, 111
   ego assisted by, 159
   as English translation, 110, 249*n*
   as fundamental ontological notion, 127
   jouissance as satisfaction of, 209
   pleasure principle as realm of, 96
   satisfaction of, 111
   source of, 93
   sublimation and, 110, 238
   see also instincts
Dumont, Etienne, 12
duty, 7–8

Eckhart, Johannes (Master Eckhart), 63
ego, 37, 51, 137
   drives' assistance to, 159
   libido vs., 157
   organic defense by, 73
   Spaltung of, 171
   as unconscious, 49
Einführung des Ichs (Freud), 49, 95, 97
Einführung des Narzissmus (Freud), 111
Eleanor of Aquitaine, 126, 146
Electra (Sophocles), 271
Ellis, Havelock, 195
Eluard, Paul, 154, 309
Emma (patient), 73–74
émoi pulsionnel, 249
emptiness:
   architecture and, 135–36
   art and, 130, 136, 140
   Ding as, 129–30
   female sexual organ and, 169, 215

emptiness (*continued*)
  of God, 196
  sublimated forms of, 130
"Empty Space" (Mikailis), 116
endogamy, 67
endopsychic perception, 49
energy/matter equivalence, 122
Enfant et les Sortilèges, L' (Colette), 115
Entwurf (Project for a Scientific Psychology) (Freud), 35–42, 57, 73, 130, 222
  Ding and, 45–47, 54, 101
  importance of, 30, 35
  original German vs. translations of, 37, 39, 40, 74
  pleasure/reality opposition in, 27, 31, 32, 35, 36–42
  as theory of neuronic apparatus, 47
Epimenides, 82
Epistles, 83
epopteia, 259–60
Erasmus, 97
Erlebnis, 54
Eros, 93, 99, 142, 231
eroticism, erotics, 4, 9, 14, 84, 100, 142, 145, 152, 188
Erscheinung, 60, 114
Es, 137, 206n
Essay on Negative Greatness (Kant), 189
Essays and Lectures (Heidegger), 120
étant, l', 214, 248
ethics:
  Antigone's importance to, 243
  Aristotelian, 5, 10–11, 12, 13, 22–23, 27, 29, 36, 186
  central problem of, 121
  definition of, 311
  Ding and, 103, 104, 105
  faults vs. misfortunes and, 89
  Hegelian, 105
  historical evolution of, 11–14
  ideology and, 182
  importance of, 3
  innovation and, 14–15
  Kantian, 72–73, 76–78, 79, 80, 108–9, 188–89, 259
  Lacan's choice of term, 2
  as mediator, 95
  paradoxes of, 311–25
  pleasure/reality opposition and, 35
  and pleasure vs. good, 36
  question formulation of, 19
  rites and, 258
  Sadian, 78–80, 188, 191, 197, 199–203, 209, 210–11, 212
  as science of character, 10
  sublimation and, 107–8
  see also morality; moral law
être, l', 214, 248
Euripides, 263, 264–65, 273
evil, 73, 97, 197
  beauty and, 217
  Freud and, 104, 106

jouissance as, 179, 184–90
  search for source of, 123–24
  Supreme-Being-in, 215
evolutionism, 126, 213–14
excluded interior, 101
exhibitionism, reciprocal, 158
existentialism, 122
ex nihilo creation, 121–22, 212–14, 225, 260–61, 262
experience, process of, 33
experimentum mentis, 313
extimacy, 139

Fable of the Bees, The (Mandeville), 69
facilitation, *see Bahnungen*
faith (belief), 54, 62–63, 130–31, 170–71
Fanny (Pagnol), 69n
fantasms, 115, 144, 239, 298, 316, 317
  of phallus, 299, 301
  in Sade, 261
  speech and, 80
  symbolization of, 99
father:
  castration by, 307
  Father as, 181
  as he who acknowledges, 309
  as idiot or thief, 308
  and image of God, 308
  incest by, 67
  murder of, 2, 5, 143, 176–77, 180, 304
  as myth, 309
Father, 228
  death of, 126–27
  as father, 181
  Freud and, 96–97, 100, 126, 170–78
  human nature of, 181
  see also God
fear and pity:
  catharsis of, 244, 245, 247–48, 257–58
  as lacking in martyrs, 267, 273
Febvre, Lucien, 131
Fechner, Gustav Theodor, 40
Fellini, Federico, 253
female sexual organ, metaphor and, 168–69, 227
feminine sexuality, 298–99
  psychoanalytical avoidance of, 9
fictitious, definition of, 12
figurative, concrete vs., 120
Five Lectures on Psychoanalysis (Freud), 90
Fixierarbeit, 88
Fléchier, Esprit, 199
Fliess, Wilhelm, 27, 28, 35, 50, 53, 59
Folignio, Angela de, 188
fool, foolery, 182–83, 195
foreplay, 152
"Formulierungen über die Zwei Prinzipen des Psychischen Geschehens" (Freud), 27
Fort, Da vs. 65, 169
Fourier, Charles, 225
François de Sales, Saint, 97
Franju, Georges, 70n

Index

Freud, Anna, 113
Freud, Sigmund:
  auto-analysis of, 26, 30
  belief as obsession of, 130
  Bernays family and, 246–47
  as collector, 113
  and evolution of ethics, 11, 12–14
  as father, 181–82
  gnomic formulas of, 129
  impotency of, 26
  intellectual decline of, 172
  as non-progressive humanitarian, 183–84, 207–8
  as not to be measured, 206
  psychoanalysis handed to women by, 182
  relationship between father and, 308–9
  schism of disciples of, 92
  Sovereign Good denied by, 70, 95, 300
  "What does woman want?" question of, 9
  see also specific works
Freudian aesthetics, 159
"Freudian Thing, The" (Lacan), 132
Fromm, Erich, 26
"fuck" metaphor, 168

genital act, 300
genital love, 8
genital objecthood, 293
Gesammelte Werke (Freud), 91, 95, 156
Geviert, 65–66
Giraudoux, Jean, 263
Gleichbesetzung, 49, 51
Gleichzeitigkeit, 65
Glover, Edward, 111, 115
Gnade, 146
gnomic formulas, 129
God, 121, 122, 124, 294
  death of, 126–27, 143, 177–78, 179–81, 184, 193
  emptiness of, 196
  as guarantor of Law, 194
  hatred for, 308
  as "I am that I am," 81, 173
  libertine challenge to, 34
  radical elimination of, 213–14
  see also Father
Goethe, Johann Wolfgang von, 248, 250, 254, 255, 258, 268, 278
good, 259, 292
  beauty vs., 217
  Ding and, 72
  Freud's denial of, 96
  function of, 218–30, 233–34
  Law and, 220–21
  pain and, 240
  pleasure principle and, 33–34, 36, 216, 221–22, 224–25
Gospels, 96
grace, 171, 261
grenouille, 227n
guilt, 57, 318
  calming of, 4

  desire and, 319, 321
  omnipresence of, 3
gute Wille (good will), 77

habits, 222
  acquisition of, 22
  dimension of, 10
Haftbarkeit, 88
hallucination, 33, 52–53, 137, 138
Hamlet (Shakespeare), 251
happiness:
  demand for, 291–301
  etymology of, 13
hate, 306, 309
"Hatred, Culpability and Fear" (Jones), 306
hedonism, 185
Hegel, G. W. F., 133, 178, 198, 206, 208, 258
  on *Antigone*, 235–36, 240, 243, 248, 249, 254
  ethics and, 105
  in history of philosophy, 234
  Lacan as influenced by, 134, 249
  and position of the master, 11–12, 23
Heidegger, Martin, 65–66, 120, 276, 297
Heine, Heinrich, 122, 147
Helmholtz, Hermann Ludwig Ferdinand von, 29
Heptameron, The (Navarre), 131
Heraclites, 299
Herbart, Johann Friedrich, 30
hero, ordinary man vs., 319–21
Herodotus, 255
He Who Punishes Himself (The Self-Tormentor) (Terence), 89
Hilflosigkeit, 303–4
Hinduism, 149, 153
Hippocrates, 245
Holbein, Hans, the Younger, 135, 140
Hölderlin, Freidrich, 65, 66
homeostasis, 46, 59, 118, 119
homo faber, 214
humanization of the planet, 233
hysteria, 53, 54, 73, 129, 138, 205–6

"I," 56
"I am that I am," 81
Ich, see ego
Ichgerechte, 156
Ich-ideal, Ideal-ich vs., 98, 234
Ichlibido/Objektlibido, 95, 98
Ichziele, 144, 156, 157, 158
idealism, 30
idealization, of object, 100, 111, 160
Ideals on the Novel (Sade), 199
Iliad (Homer), 172, 281–82
imaginary, 11, 20
Imago, 155, 164
immobility, 49
incest, 78, 304
  Ding and, 68, 70
  as fundamental desire, 67, 76
  in ten commandments, 69
individuation, 198

"Infant Analysis" (Klein), 115
"Infantile Anxiety Situations Reflected in a Work of Art and in the Creative Impulse" (Klein), 115–17
Inquisition, 124
instincts, 106, 109, 204, 209, 301
   artistic reward and, 145
   masochism in economy of, 14, 15
   as measure of action, 311–12
   plasticity of, 91
   satisfaction of, 293
   search for, 99
   see also drives
instinctual excitement, 249
intellectual comfort, 192
intellectuals, left vs. right wing, 182–83, 195, 207
intemperance, 23, 29
Interpretation of Dreams, The (Traumdeutung) (Freud), 14, 27, 31, 37
"intersaid," 65
Introduction to Psychoanalysis (Freud), 14
Introductory Lectures on Psychoanalysis (Freud), 7, 90, 91
"It speaks," 206

Jakobson, Roman, 12
jealousy, 237
Jederman, 194
"Jewish Question, The" (Marx), 208
Jews, history of, 174
John, Saint, 322
Jones, Ernest, 9, 25, 159, 163–64, 182, 226–27, 246, 306, 308, 309
jouissance, 229, 298, 316
   as accessible to other, 237
   as evil, 179, 184–90
   murder of father and, 176
   as satisfaction of drive, 209
   sublimation and, 322
   taming of, 4–5
   of transgression, 177, 191–204
   Vorstellung and, 61
Joy of Love, The (Perdu), 148
Jung, Carl, 92
juvenile mentality, 25

Kant, Immanuel, 55, 70, 84, 97, 206, 207, 249, 257, 261, 269, 286–87, 295, 301, 315–16, 317, 323
   ethical fable of, 108–9, 188–89
   ethics and, 72–73, 76–78, 79, 80, 259
Kaufmann, Pierre, 155–56, 158, 159, 161, 203–4, 211, 295
Kierkegaard, Søren, 198
King Lear (Shakespeare), 305
Kjar, Ruth, 116–17
Klein, Melanie, 106, 115–17, 307
Kleinian theory, 73, 106–7, 111, 115–17
knave, knavery, 182n, 183–84, 195, 199
knowledge, theory of, 60–61, 171

known, unknown vs., 33
Krafft-Ebing, Richard von, 195

La Fontaine, Jean de, 55
Lambin, Denis, 245
language:
   artifice and, 136
   dominance of, 45
   inquiry through, 43
   of love, 65
   schizophrenia and, 44
   sexual roots in, 167–68
   unconscious and, 32, 44–45
langue d'oc, 146, 162
Laocoon (Lessing), 297
Laplanche, Jean, 38, 65, 66, 95, 133, 137
Last Judgment, 313, 314
Lautréamont (Isidore Lucien Ducasse), 201
law:
   desire and, 82–84
   philosophy of, 105
Law, 188, 192–93
   desire and, 170
   Ding and, 83–84, 186
   function of, 177
   God as guarantor of, 194
   good and, 220–21
   interiorization of, 310
Lebensneid, 237
Lee, M., 106
Lefebvre, Henri, 155
Lefèvre-Pontalis, Jean-Bertrand, 38, 44, 46, 50
Lessing, Gotthold Ephraim, 297
Lévi-Strauss, Claude, 67, 68, 75, 143, 274, 282, 285, 287
libertine thought, 4, 79, 131, 215
libido, 298
   archaic forms of, 93–94
   demand by, 91–92
   desexualization of, 102, 111
   ego vs., 157
   object and, 94, 109, 144, 158
Libidoziel, 157
lies:
   paradox of, 73
   prohibition against, 81–82
logos, 6, 179
love:
   as analytical ideal, 8–9
   in antiquity, 98–99
   hate and, 309
   language of, 65
   of neighbor, 177–78, 179–90, 193–94, 196
   philanthropy vs., 186
   sublime, 259
   as sublimation of feminine object, 109, 112
   see also courtly love
Love and the Myths of the Heart (Nelli), 148
Luke, Gospel of, 96
Lust-Ich, 101, 103
Lustprinzip, see pleasure principle

Lust/Unlust polarity, 58, 59, 72
Lustziele, 157
Luther, Martin, 92–93, 97, 122

Macaulay, Thomas Babington, 25
Mandeville, Bernard de, 69
Manicheism, 215
Map of Love (*Carte du Tendre*), 146
Marius (Pagnol), 69n
Mark, Gospel of, 96
Martin, Saint, 186, 226, 228
Marx, Harpo, 55
Marx, Karl, 206, 208–9, 225–26, 227
masochism:
  in economy of instincts, 14, 15
  moral, 20
  nature of, 239–40
master, function of, 11–12, 23, 292, 315
master-fools, 182–83
masturbation, collective, 158
match box fable, 113–14
Matthew, Saint, 96, 133
"Me!," 56
mechanism, 29
méchant, 89
mediation, 133–34
melancholia, 89, 116
même, 198
Memoirs on the Great Days in Auvergne (Fléchier), 199
memory, 209, 223
  of forgotten things, 231
  Niederschriften and, 50–51
  unconscious discourse of, 236
  Vorstellung and, 58
Mencius, 312, 325
metamorphosis, 264–65
metaphor and metonymy, laws of, 61, 168
metipsemus, 198, 203
Mikailis, Karin, 116
Miller, Henry, 200, 233
Minne, see courtly love
Mirabeau, Honoré-Gabriel Riquetti, comte de, 4, 79
mirror function, 151
mise en scène, 252–53
Mittel, action as, 53
mobility, 49
Molière, 244
monogamy, 8, 105
monotheism, 172, 174
monotonous qualities, 42, 49
moods, causes of, 48, 59
moral action:
  definition of, 76
  as experience of satisfaction, 56
moral conscience:
  paradox of, 89
  sublimation as, 87
  superego as support for, 310
moral imperative, 20, 21
moralisches Entgegenkommen, 306

morality:
  anti-, 78
  desire and, 3, 5
  genealogy of, 35–36
  origin of, 5, 143
  of power, 315
  see also ethics
moral law, 71–84
  real and, 20, 76
  rejection of, 175, 176–77
  Sade's reversal of, 78–79
  ten commandments and, 80–83
  see also ethics
morbidity, transgression and, 2
Morin, André, 126
Moses, 142, 171, 173–74, 180
Moses and Monotheism (Freud), 90, 130, 142, 145, 171–72, 175, 181
mother, 143, 307
  incest with, 67–70
  mythic body of, 106, 111, 115, 117
Motorische Neuronen, 41, 59
"Mourning and Melancholia" (Freud), 307
murder:
  of Christ, 174
  of father, 2, 5, 143, 176–77, 180, 304
  prohibition against, 81
music, catharsis and, 245–46
mysticism, 149, 187
myth, function of, 143

narcissism, 37, 95, 98, 112, 151
nature, culture vs., 67–68, 77–78, 274
Navarre, Marguerite de, 131
ne, 64, 305–6
Nebenmensch, 39, 51, 76, 151
need, desire vs., 207, 225
negative therapeutic reaction, 313
Nelli, René, 124, 148
Netz der Triebe, 91, 92
neuronenwahl, 54
neuronic apparatus, 46–47, 57, 58
neurosis, 35
"Neutralisation and Sublimation" (Bernfeld), 159
Never on Sunday, 317–18
New Justine, The (Sade), 200
Newtonian physics, 76
Nicolas of Cuse, 75
Nicomachean Ethics, The (Aristotle), 5, 10, 23, 27, 36
Niederschriften, memory and, 50–51
Nietzsche, Friedrich, 35, 198
"No and Yes," 132–33
Nobel Prize, 201–2
No/Name, paternal (Nom-*de*-père), 65
No/Name of the Father (Nom-*du*-père), 65, 142, 181, 314
non-dependence, as psychoanalytic ideal, 10
Non-Thing, 136
Nostre-Dame, Michel de (Nostradamus), 145–46
Not des Lebens, 46, 48, 58

nudity, function of, 227
Numbers, 81
numen, 172

object, 53
  bad, 73
  change of, 293
  in collecting vs. psychoanalysis, 113
  cultural loss of, 99
  Ding and, 101–14, 126
  elaborations on, 99
  good, 73
  idealization of, 100, 111
  libido and, 94, 109, 144, 158
  narcissistic foundations of, 112
  overevaluation of, 109
  part, 202
  pathological, 76
  pleasure principle and, 58
  refound, 118
  sublimation of, 109–14
objectalité genitale, l', 293
objectification, 33
objective chance, 154
object relations, 98
obligation, sense of, 3, 315
obsessional neurosis, 54, 203
Oedipus at Colonus (Sophocles), 250, 257, 271, 272, 284–85
Oedipus complex, 244, 304, 307
Oedipus myth, 142, 181, 304–7, 313, 324
Oedipus Rex (Sophocles), 243, 271–72
On Love (Stendhal), 146
"On the Influence of Sexual Factors on the Origin and Development of Language" (Sperber), 163
operational thought, 104–5
organic defense, 73
orthopedics, 10
Other, 53, 152, 192–93, 202
  assault on image of, 195
  Atè and, 277
  Ding as, 52, 71
  jouissance as accessible to, 237
  man deprived of good by, 234
  pain of, 80
  self-discovery as Other of, 66
Ovid, 146, 153, 265

Pagnol, Marcel, 69n
pain:
  desire and, 80
  ethics and, 108
  limit of, 59–60
  pleasure and/or, 189
  see also masochism
Palladio, Andrea, 136
Pan, 163, 178, 198
paranoia, 54, 129, 130
part object, 202
pastoral, domain of, 88–89

pathologisches Objekt, 76
patients, 1, 2
Paul, Saint, 83, 95, 97, 170, 177, 189
peccant humors, 244
Péguy, Charles, 103
Peirce, C. S., 91
penis:
  comparisons of size of, 158
  see also castration
perception, 41, 65
  consciousness and, 49–51, 61, 74
  hallucination and, 52–53
  thought vs., 33
Perdu, Pierre, 148
Perret, Benjamin, 148
perspective, in art, 136, 140
perverse drive, 5
perversion, 109–10, 194–95, 232
Phaedrus (Plato), 257, 259, 268
phallus, fantasm of, 299, 301
Phenomenology of Mind, The (Hegel), 235
philanthropy, 196
  love vs., 186
Philoctetes (Sophocles), 271, 272, 320
Philosophical Works (Marx), 208
Philosophy in the Boudoir (Sade), 78
Philosophy of Law (Hegel), 208
Phoenissae (Euripides), 264
physics:
  nature's integration and, 236
  Newtonian, 76
Picasso, Pablo, 118
Piéron, Henry, 47
Pignarre, Robert, 254
pity, *see* fear and pity
Plato, 105, 141, 182, 216, 221, 257, 259, 260, 323
pleasure function, 11, 12, 13
pleasure principle (primary process), 52, 53, 239
  Bahnung and, 36, 39, 41, 63, 137
  beyond, 184, 188
  as dominance of signifier, 134
  field of, 104
  function of, 27, 72, 119
  good and, 33–34, 36, 216, 221–22, 224–25
  pain and/or, 189
  reality principle vs., 20–21, 25–26, 30–34, 35, 36–42, 43, 48, 74, 137, 225
  as realm of drives, 96
  regulation of, 55
  satisfaction vs., 41
  search for object governed by, 58
  signifier and, 137–38
  tragedy and, 246
  transgression of, 109
  unconscious and, 48, 63
  Vorlust and, 152
  Vorstellung governed by, 57, 61, 63
  will and, 125
Poetics (Aristotle), 244, 245
poetry:
  as childhood ego goal, 144–45, 157

of courtly love, 145–52, 161–63
  metamorphosis in, 264–65
  romantic vs. metaphysical, 24–25
Poitiers, Guillaume de, 148, 151–52
Politics (Aristotle), 245
pot fable, 120–21
potlatch, 235
preconscious:
  conscious, unconscious and, 37, 61–62
  language and, 45
  reality principle and, 48
Prévert, Jacques, 114, 275
Primal Cavity, The (Spitz), 133
primary process, *see* pleasure principle
primum vivere, 306, 309
Problem of Unbelief in the Sixteenth Century, The (Febvre), 131
Project for a Scientific Psychology (Freud), *see* Entwurf
Proudhon, Pierre Joseph, 82
Psychanalyse, La, 276
Psyche (Rohde), 250, 285
psychic reality, 21, 33, 43, 130
psychoanalysis:
  "American way" of, 219
  demand for happiness and, 291–301
  as ethical order, 88
  goal of, 4
  good and, 218–19
  as handed to women, 182
  ideals of, 8–10
  Kleinian school of, 73, 106–7, 111, 115–17
  moral action and, 21–22
  moral goals of, 302–10
  as moralizing hustle, 312
  and psychology of affects, 103
  sublimation foregrounded by, 128
  termination of, 300, 303–4
psychoanalysts:
  desire of, 300–301
  transference and, 291
psychology:
  of affects, 102–3
  atomism and, 102
  of collecting, 113–14, 117
  dreams and, 62
  moral agency promoted by, 57
Psychology for the Use of Neurologists (Freud), 26–27
Psychopathia Sexualis (Krafft-Ebing), 195
puberty, 156

Q quantity, 46
Qη quantity, 46–47
Qualitätszeichen, 47, 50, 52

Raised Curtain, The (Mirabeau), 79
Rauh, Fritz, 3
Ravel, Maurice, 115
Reaktionsbildung (reaction formation), 94–95, 156–57

real, 118, 223
  art and, 141
  definition of, 70
  hole in, 121
  man and, 11, 129
  moral law and, 20, 76
  of psychic organization, 101
  as rational, 180
  structuralization of, 75
  unitarianism of, 173
Real-Ich, 101, 102
reality, weight of, 108
reality principle (secondary process):
  Aufbau and, 40
  Ding and, 45, 66
  good and, 222, 224
  paradox of, 46
  pleasure principle vs., 20–21, 25–26, 30–34, 35, 36–42, 43, 48, 74, 137, 225
  precariousness of, 30
  rectification and, 28
  subject isolated from reality by, 46
reason, weight of, 108
rectification, 28
reification, 132, 134
religion:
  Ding displaced in, 131, 134
  emptiness and, 130
Religionsschwärmereien, 84
repetition, principle of, 41
repetition compulsion, 222–23
represent, representation vs., 71–72
repression, 54, 293
  paradox of, 64–5
  signifier and, 44
  sublimation and, 156
  ten commandments as, 69
"Repression" ("Die Verdränung") (Freud), 44
Rhetoric (Aristotle), 255, 287
rites, 224, 258
Rohde, Erwin, 250, 251, 285
romanticism, 24–25
Rougemont, Denis de, 123, 149

sabbath, 81
Sache:
  definition of, 45
  Ding vs., 43–45, 62–63
Sacher-Masoch, Leopold von, 239
Sacy, Silvestre de, 68
Sade, Marquis de, 4, 70, 185, 207, 219, 220–21, 231, 233, 248, 260, 295, 316
  ethics of, 78–80, 188, 191, 197, 199–203, 210–11, 212
Saint-Just, Louis Antoine Léon de, 292
saintliness, 322
Samuel, second Book of, 81
Sartre, Jean-Paul, 226
satisfaction:
  moral action as experience of, 56
  pleasure principle vs., 41

schizophrenia, language and, 44
Schlüsselneuronen, 41
Schopenhauer, Arthur, 104, 212
science, 77, 129
　biblical roots of, 122
　Ding repudiated by, 131, 134
　as structuralization of realty, 75
　Unglauben and, 130
secondary process, *see* reality principle
second death, 211, 248, 254, 260, 294–95
secretorisch, 59
self:
　etymology of, 198
　integration of, 209
Self-Tormentor, The (Terence), 89n
Senhal, 151
Sensations, The (Piéron), 47
sensory organs, as sieve, 47
sentiment, 79
Sermons (Luther), 92
service of goods, 303, 304, 305, 313–15, 318–19, 321, 324
se tailler, 168
sexuality, feminine, *see* feminine sexuality
Shakespeare, William, 251, 265, 305
shame, 298
Sharpe, Ella, 106, 107, 139
Sicherung, 73, 83
Sigmund Freud's Mission (Fromm), 26
signifiers, 43, 301
　Adam and Eve and, 227
　as at beginning, 213–14
　creation of, 119
　first system of, 65
　Freudian aesthetics and, 159
　function of, 153, 168, 295
　hysteria and, 205
　man as between real and, 129, 134, 236
　omnipotence identified with, 234
　pleasure principle and, 137–38
　power of, 236
　refound object and, 118–19
　repression and, 44
　tools vs., 120, 123
　unleashing of, 314
signs:
　definition of, 91
　man as, 75
　repetition of, 72–73
"Similar and Divergent Unconscious Determinants, which Subtend the Sublimations of Pure Art and Pure Science" (Sharpe), 107
sin, 84, 170, 177, 189
society:
　individual vs., 105, 110
　see also culture
Socrates, 22
Songs of Maldoror (Lautréamont), 201
Sophocles, 257, 258, 269, 271–72, 273, 284, 285, 304, 320
soul, 105, 316, 318

Sovereign Good, 97
　Aristotle and, 11, 22
　Freud's refutation of, 70, 95, 300
　Kant's detachment from, 77
Spaltung, 102, 171, 209
speech:
　as distance between subject and *Ding*, 69
　fantasms and, 80
　and law and desire, 82
Sperber, Hans, 163–64, 167, 168
spezifische Aktion, 41, 53
Spinalneuronen, 40
state, 318
　function of, 105
Stendhal, 146, 183
Sterba, Richard, 111, 157
Stimmungen, 26
Story of Juliette, The (Sade), 197, 200, 202, 210, 220
Story of O, The (Réage), 202
subject, 204, 224
　and access to relationship to death, 295
　Ding as Other of, 52, 71
　distance between *Ding* and, 69, 73, 105
　first apprehension of reality by, 51
　and isolation from reality, 46
　signifier and, 44
　Spaltung and, 102
sublimation, 85–164
　artistic reward and, 144–45
　collective, 99
　courtly love as, 128, 131, 136, 142, 160, 161–63, 215
　creativity and, 106–7, 115–17, 238
　death drive as, 212
　definition of, 144, 293
　Ding and, 95, 99, 115, 117, 126, 129, 131, 134, 158
　drives and, 110, 238
　emptiness in, 130
　ethics and, 107–8
　of feminine object, 109, 112
　function of Father and, 181
　importance of, 128
　jouissance and, 322
　in Kleinian doctrine, 117
　limits of, 91–92, 94
　of object, 109–14
　as prohibition, 87
　projection of, 203
　reaction formation and, 156–57
　repression and, 156
　satisfaction of instinct and, 293
"Sublimation, Substitution and Social Anxiety" (Glover), 111
subsidence, 265–66
summum bonum, 160
superego, 6, 7, 37, 66, 143, 176, 194, 302, 307, 308, 310
Supreme-Being-in-evil, 215
Surrogate, 94

symbolic, 11, 12, 20
  animals and, 45
  diabolic and, 92–93
  Ding and, 57
symbolism, of clothes, 226–28
synchrony, 66
  diachrony vs., 285

Table Talk (Luther), 92
Taoism, 123
Technical Writings (Freud), 234
temple, destruction of, 175
Temps Modernes, Les, 134
ten commandments, 66, 79–83, 173–74
  as moral law, 80–83
  as prohibitions, 68–69
Tête contre les Murs, La, 70n
"Theory Concerning Creation in the Free Arts, A" (Lee), 106
Theory of Fictions, The (Bentham), 228
Thing, see *Ding*
Thomas Aquinas, Saint, 221, 238, 249
thought, 213–14
  individual and collectivity and, 94
  operational, 104–5
  perception vs., 33
  as unconscious, 48
  Vorstellung and, 61
Three Essays on the Theory of Sexuality (Freud), 88, 90, 94, 152, 156
Totem and Taboo (Freud), 5, 171, 180, 181, 309
Trachiniae, The (Sophocles), 271, 272
tragedy:
  action in, 250–52, 313
  author-subject conflict in, 250–51
  centrality of, 243–44
  Chorus in, 252
  heroic isolation in, 271, 272
  mise en scène in, 252–53
  nature of, 244, 246, 247, 257–58
  subsidence in, 265–66
transcendental aesthetics, 77
transference, 291
transgression, 207
  attraction of, 2
  crime as, 260
  jouissance of, 177, 191–204
  morbidity and, 2
  origin of, 6
  of pleasure principle, 109
  translator's choice of term, 1n
Traumdeutung (The Interpretation of Dreams) (Freud), 14, 27, 31, 37
Trieb, see drives
Triebregung, 249
troubadours, trouvères, 145, 148, 149, 161–63
truth:
  blindness and, 310
  truth about, 184

Uberich, see superego
Uberschätzung, 109
Unbewusst, see unconscious
Übung, 51
unconscious:
  centrality of, 224
  conscious, preconscious and, 37, 61–62
  ego as, 49
  as field of non-knowledge, 236–37
  as function of the symbolic, 12
  incest and, 68
  language as structure of, 32, 44–45
  and laws of metaphor and metonymy, 61
  lies in, 73
  memorizing discourse of, 236
  as memory of forgotten things, 231
  negation in, 137
  pleasure principle and, 48, 63
  representation in, 71–72
  Wahrnehmungsbewusstsein and, 51
"Unconscious, The" (Freud), 44
Unglauben, 130–31
unknown, known vs., 33
unmasking, psychoanalysis as, 9, 10
utilitarian conversion, 11, 36
utilitarianism, 160, 187, 216, 228

vacuole, 150, 152
Vailland, Roger, 73
Valéry, Paul, 296n
values, theory of, 14, 87
vase fable, 119–21, 122, 129, 168
Ventadour, Bernard de, 149
Verdrängung, 156
"Verdrängung, Die" ("Repression") (Freud), 44
vermeidet, 63–64
Verneinung, 64–65, 144
"Verneinung, Die" ("Denegation") (Freud), 37, 46, 52, 58
Versagen des Glaubens, 54
Verschiebbarkeit, 91, 92
Verwerfung, 65, 131
virtue:
  function of, 292
  science of, 10
vital needs, 46
Vorbewusstsein, see preconscious
Vorlesungen (Introductory Lectures on Psychoanalysis) (Freud), 7, 90, 91
Vorrat, 49, 51
Vorratskammer, 51
Vorstellung, 57–62, 63, 74, 91, 93, 137–38
Vorstellungsrepräsentanzen, 61, 71, 102, 103, 118, 137

Wahrnehmungsbewusstsein, 49–51, 61, 74
  definition of, 49–50
Walter, Robert, 144
Whitman, Walt, 93
Wieder zu finden, 58

will, 212, 259
  general, 195
  good and bad, 104, 125
Wille, 104, 212
Wirklichkeit, 26, 29
Wohl, 72, 76
women:
  in feudal society, 147
  "grenouille" term for, 227*n*
  psychoanalysis handed to, 182
  see also courtly love; feminine sexuality
"word," in French vs. German, 55
Wordsworth, William, 24

Wortvorstellung, 44, 45, 49
Wunsch, 24, 31, 72

yin and *yang*, 223
"You," *Ding* and, 56

Zielablenkung, 144
Zur Einführung des Narzissmus ("On Narcissism: An Introduction") (Freud), 95
"Zur Problematik der Sublimierungslehre" ("On the Problematic of the Doctrine of Sublimation") (Sterba), 111

The Good Body —
Winkler + Cole.

Acetosin in integumy
 cultin.
 Yale.